STROKE PREVENTION

STROKE PREVENTION

Edited by

John W. Norris, M.D.
and
Vladimir Hachinski, M.D.

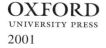

OXFORD
UNIVERSITY PRESS
2001

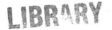
Athens   Auckland   Bangkok   Bogotá   Buenos Aires   Calcutta
Cape Town   Chennai   Dar es Salaam   Delhi   Florence   Hong Kong   Istanbul
Karachi   Kuala Lumpur   Madrid   Melbourne   Mexico City   Mumbai
Nairobi   Paris   São Paulo   Shanghai   Singapore   Taipei   Tokyo   Toronto   Warsaw

and associated companies in
Berlin   Ibadan

Copyright © 2001 by Oxford University Press, Inc.

Publishes by Oxford University Press, Inc.,
198 Madison Avenue, New York, New York, 10016
http://www.oup-usa.org

Oxford is a registered trademark of Oxford University Press.

Library of Congress Cataloging-in-Publication Data
Stroke prevention / edited by John W. Norris, Vladimir Hachinski.
p. cm.   ISBN 0-19-513382-X
1. Cerebrovascular disease—Prevention.
I. Norris, John W.   II. Hachinski, Vladimir.
RC388.5 .S8529 2001   616.8'1—dc21   00-041673

9 8 7 6 5 4 3 2 1

Printed in the United States of America
on acid-free paper

PREFACE

In 1991 we published our first book on the prevention of stroke. So many discoveries and advances have been made in the last decade that we felt obliged to revisit the same subject, but with a completely different organization, content, and authorship. Because of changing concepts of stroke prevention, we organized this new volume into three distinct parts: primary prevention, secondary prevention, and the effort to translate policy into practice.

The section on primary prevention presents fresh information on established risk factors, such as atrial fibrillation, smoking, and hypertension, as well as newly discovered risk factors, such as homocysteinemia and the paradoxical role of alcohol. In addition, we include much new data on the protective effects of lifestyle changes and indicate that diet, exercise, and estrogen are beginning to enter into prevention strategies. Despite several large, multicenter studies on both sides of the Atlantic, the roles of carotid endarterectomy, angioplasty, and stenting for asymptomatic carotid stenosis remain controversial.

The section on secondary prevention addresses the importance of cardiac anomalies, such as patent foramen ovale and atrial septal aneurysm, which are increasingly revealed by high-definition cardiac imaging. It also revisits the controversies surrounding the oldest antiplatelet agent, aspirin, and evaluates several new antiplatelet drugs now on the market. Carotid endarterectomy has been clearly defined as the single most effective strategy in secondary prevention, while a large scale multicenter trial comparing carotid surgery to stenting has just been initiated.

The transfer of findings from clinical trials to actual clinical practice is coming under intensified scrutiny, and we feel that it warrants a section in itself. Showing that an intervention such as carotid endarterectomy works is not enough; we need to know whether it is applied appropriately. Patients in clinical trials are highly selected, closely monitored, and provided with the highest standard of care. The restricted conditions of clinical trials are seldom reproduced in the larger world, and a benefit clearly demonstrated in a clinical trial may be quickly cancelled by applying the intervention to inappropriate patients or by applying it appropriately but with a higher complication rate. Costs increasingly dictate clinical practice. Interventions that may be effective when costs are not a consideration rapidly run into the realities of affordability and the competing demands of an aging population. An evidence-based approach is helpful in the unending balancing act between the ideal and the affordable, yet only a fraction of what is learned in clinical trials is ever applied. The benefits of treating hypertension for the prevention of stroke are substantial and uncontestable, yet it is estimated that only one-fifth of American hypertensives have their blood pressures controlled. The unacceptable gap between clinical trials and clinical practice must be breached. This book focuses on stroke prevention as it is practiced in North America, Europe, and Australia, but stroke is a worldwide problem, and we include a chapter on the global perspective.

We set a high standard for authorship by enlisting international experts who know not only their subject but also how to convey it clearly. Moreover, we asked that whenever possible they write the chapters themselves and avoid the common practice of having a junior associate do most of the work, with editing by the senior author. The fact that so many prominent authors accepted our invitation speaks to the importance of stroke prevention and their commitment to it. The result is a broad-based, lucidly written book that is founded on evidence and that provides logical bridges to daily practice where the evidence falls short.

Stroke is the leading cause of serious disability in adults. Thus, it behooves neurologists, geriatricians, internists, neurosurgeons, vascular surgeons, family physicians, health planners, and all those involved in lightening this burden to learn the latest strategies of stroke prevention.

We would like to acknowledge the invaluable help of our personal assistant Ms. Donna Huber, who not only spent many hours painstakingly editing the text of most chapters, but gave help and suggestions in reorganizing some of the text. Mr. Jeff House, Senior Editor of Oxford University Press was a major factor in ensuring that the prose and grammar were direct, correct and clear, and ruthlessly corrected ambiguous passages.

North York, Ontario, Canada   J.W.N
London, Ontario, Canada   V.H.

CONTENTS

CONTRIBUTORS

HAROLD P. ADAMS, JR., M.D.
Professor and Director
Division of Cerebrovascular Diseases
Department of Neurology
University of Iowa College of Medicine
Iowa City, Iowa

H.J.M. BARNETT, O.C. M.D.,
  FRCP(C)
John P. Robarts Research Institute
London, Ontario
Canada

J. BOGOUSSLAVSKY, M.D.
Professor and Chairman
Department of Neurology
Lausanne, Switzerland

RUTH BONITA, M.D., M.P.H.,
  PH.D.
Director
NCD Surveillance
World Health Organization
Geneva, Switzerland

NATHAN M. BORNSTEIN, M.D.
Professor of Neurology
Stroke Unit
Department of Neurology
Tel Aviv Sourasky Medical Center
Sackler Faculty of Medicine
Tel Aviv, Israel

MARTIN M. BROWN, M.D., F.R.C.P.
Professor of Stroke Medicine
University College London
Institute of Neurology
The National Hospital for Neurology &
  Neurosurgery
Queen Square
London, United Kingdom

G. DEVUYST, M.D.
Department of Neurology
Lausanne, Switzerland

GEOFFREY A. DONNAN, M.D.,
F.R.A.C.P.
Professor of Neurology
National Stroke Research Institute
Melbourne University
Austin and Repatriation Medical Centre
Heidelberg, Victoria
Australia

J. DONALD EASTON, M.D.
Professor and Chairman
Department of Clinical Neurosciences
Brown University School of Medicine
and
Rhode Island Hospital
Providence, Rhode Island

THOMAS E. FEASBY, M.D.
Professor and Head
Department of Clinical Neurosciences
University of Calgary
Calgary, Alberta
Canada

PHILIP B. GORELICK, M.D.,
M.P.H., F.A.C.P.
Professor and Director
Center for Stroke Research
Department of Neurological Sciences
Rush Medical Center
Chicago, Illinois

VLADIMIR HACHINSKI, M.D., D.Sc.
Professor
Department of Clinical Neurological
    Sciences
London Health Sciences Centre
The University of Western Ontario
London, Ontario
Canada

GRAEME J. HANKEY, M.D., F.R.C.P.,
F.R.C.P. EDIN., F.R.A.C.P.
Clinical Associate Professor
Department of Neurology
Royal Perth Hospital
University of Western Australia
Perth, Western Australia
Australia

HEATHER E. MELDRUM, B.A.
John P. Robarts Research Institute
London, Ontario
Canada

E. JOHN NASRALLAH, M.D.
Division of Cerebrovascular Diseases
Department of Neurology
University of Iowa College of Medicine
Iowa City, Iowa

JOHN W. NORRIS, M.D., F.R.C.P.
Professor of Neurology
University of Toronto
Canada

JEAN-MARC ORGOGOZO, M.D.
Professor and Head
Department of Neurology
CHU Pellegrin
University of Bordeaux and INSERM
    Epidemiology Unit U-330
Bordeaux, France

DIANA B. PETITTI, M.D., M.P.H.
Director of Research
Kaiser Permanente Medical Care
    Program
Southern California Region
Pasadena, California

SERGE RENAUD, M.D.
Unité INSERM U330
Université de Bordeaux II
Bordeaux, France

RALPH L. SACCO, M.S., M.D.
Associate Chair of Neurology for Clinical
    Research and Training
Associate Professor of Neurology and
    Public Health (Epidemiology)
Associate Director of the Stroke Division
Neurological Institute
College of Physicians and Surgeons
Columbia University
New York, New York

DAVID SHERMAN, M.D.
Ross J. Sibert Distinguished Chair
Division of Neurology
Department of Medicine
University of Texas Health Science Center
San Antonio, Texas

PHILIP A. WOLF, M.D.
Professor of Neurology
Boston University School of Medicine
Boston, Massachusetts

STROKE PREVENTION

The aim of medicine is to prevent disease and prolong life, the ideal of medicine is to eliminate the need of a physician.

William Mayo (1861–1939)

1

PREVENTION OF STROKE: A PERSPECTIVE

John W. Norris and Vladimir Hachinski

Humans have never been healthier. The greatest benefit to humans from the explosion of scientific advances in the twentieth century has been the conquest of disease and advancement of health and well-being.[1] This applies to both the "developed" and "developing" worlds. The anguish of childhood death and crippling disability and the plagues that decimated the world not so long ago have been greatly reduced, but as people live longer and better, degenerative diseases of the brain and blood vessels exact their toll.

Fifty years ago, cardiovascular disease was almost unknown in the developing world, but with economic growth comes increased life expectancy, so that the traditional risk factors of infection, parasitic disease, and malnutrition are being replaced by obesity, hypertension, and coronary artery disease. People can afford to smoke more, exercise less, and switch from largely vegetarian diets to those rich in animal fats. A global epidemic of cardiovascular disease (and stroke) is predicted to encompass a large part of the world's population that lives in China, India, Indonesia, and the former Soviet Union (Fig. 1.1).[2] Conversely, as these diseases increase in the developing world, health education is bringing healthier lifestyles to the Western world, where cardiovascular diseases and stroke are diminishing in incidence.

The incidence and mortality of stroke have declined substantially in the United States (the best-documented country) since the 1920s, reaching an annual rate of

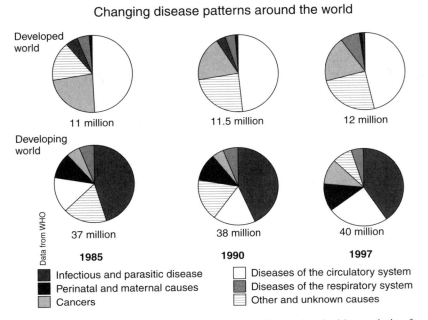

FIGURE 1.1. Changing disease patterns around the world. Reprinted with permission from Ref. 2.

decline of 5% by the 1970s.[3] This decline has slowed in recent decades because of both successful treatment and successful prevention, while computerized tomography (CT) brain scanning is revealing many minor cases of stroke that were previously attributed to other lesions.[4]

CT scanning partly explains the apparent fall in stroke severity, but a true shift to less severe strokes was documented in the Framingham study. This was not due to any change in the proportions of ischemic or hemorrhagic stroke but represented a real increase in patients with minor neurological deficits compared with patients admitted in unconscious states with more devastating lesions.[5]

According to epidemiologists, the explanations for these favorable changes can only be found by careful analysis of stroke incidence and fatality,[6] but epidemiologic studies often overlook the importance of verifying the presence and type of stroke using clinical and brain imaging methods. Data from family physician surveys and death certificates can be of dubious value or frankly misleading.

PRIMARY PREVENTION OF STROKE

Five factors must be considered in the primary prevention of stroke. These include nonmodifiable risk factors, modifiable risk factors, medical prevention, surgical prevention, and public health strategies.

Nonmodifiable Risk Factors

Nothing at present can be changed regarding age, sex, or family history, although genetic engineering is likely to play an increasingly major role in all forms of disorders. Males have always suffered the lion's share of vascular disease in the heart, brain, and peripheral blood vessels, and the prevalence rises steeply with age. In developing countries, the number of old people (over 60 years) is predicted to increase from 171 million in 1998 to 1.594 billion by 2050.[7]

The contributions of nurture and nature in stroke incidence remain uncertain, but clear epidemiological evidence indicates that nurture plays the major role. The high prevalence of all forms of stroke in Japan (one of the world's stroke "hot spots") declines with westward emigration. The decrease in stroke frequency from Japan through Hawaii to the United States indicates that whatever prognosis the genetic basis provides, it is strongly influenced by lifestyle.[3]

Modifiable Risk Factors

Details of lifestyle modification and treatable risk factors are presented in later chapters. Major changes in the way people live, exercise, smoke, drink, and eat have had profound effects on the incidence, mortality, and severity of all forms of vascular disease.

The lay public tends to believe that stroke and heart attack are due to stress. In ancient times, "apoplexy" was attributed to "emotion, sloth, drunkenness, and gluttony."[8] Although there is convincing evidence from many sources that sudden cardiac death can be precipitated by acute emotional events, such as the threat of death, no such relationship has ever been demonstrated in stroke. In ischemic stroke this is hardly surprising, since the commonest cause is thrombo embolism from the extracranial arteries or heart.

Attempts to relate the "type A" personality to stroke remain strikingly unsuccessful. The idea that sudden, precipitous rises in blood pressure can produce hemorrhagic stroke is more plausible. It was claimed that this occurred in Israel during the Persian Gulf crisis.[9]

Fruit and vegetables have been promoted for many years as health foods, in part because of the supposedly protective effects of their high potassium content. Epidemiologic studies demonstrated a reduction of both vascular disease and cancer in people with large vegetarian moieties in their diet. The explanation offered was that antioxidant vitamins (beta carotene and vitamins B and C) interfere with oxidative damage to DNA and lipoproteins. [10] At present insufficient evidence exists to recommend vitamin supplements, pending the results of ongoing randomized trials, but it is becoming clear that factors previously considered irrelevant, such as diet and cholesterol, are as important in cerobrovascular as in cardiovascular disease.[11]

The role of the contraceptive pill as a stroke risk factor has become increasingly controversial in recent years. Early studies using high-dose estrogen (>100 micrograms) and primitive methodology were performed before CT scanning was widely used. Studies in recent years using low-dose pills (<50 micrograms) and carefully performed cohort and case control studies indicate either infinitesimal or no risk increase of either ischemic or hemorrhagic stroke.[12] Moreover, mounting evidence suggests that estrogen replacement therapy protects against ischemic cardiac and cerebral disease.[13]

Although hypertension is the major preventable risk factor for all forms of vascular disease, surpassed only by malnutrition and smoking as a cause of death worldwide,[14] its control only partly explains the decline in mortality from stroke noted in previous decades and probably accounts for only 15%.[15] Nevertheless, observational studies indicate that small reductions in diastolic blood pressure have enormous impact at a population level. It is estimated that 2 mm. average blood pressure reduction would result in a 17% decrease in the prevalence of hypertension, a 6% reduction in coronary heart disease, and a 15% reduction in stroke.[16]

Cholesterol has emerged only in recent years as a risk factor for stroke.[17] An in-depth analysis of randomized trials published in 1998 concluded that in hyperlipidemic patients without previous stroke the use of 3-hydroxy-3-methyl glutaryl co-enzyme A (HMG CoA) reductase inhibitors (which lower blood lipid levels) reduce the subsequent incidence of stroke in these patients.[18]

In patients with previous coronary heart disease, the picture is much clearer. In the Long-Term Intervention with Pravastatin in Ischemic Disease (LIPID) study, where pravastatin was given to patients with prior coronary artery disease, stroke risk was significantly reduced over the seven years of follow-up ($p < 0.048$).[19]

One problem in determining the role of cholesterol as a stroke risk factor is its compounding effect with hypertension. Where hypertension is sufficiently controlled to reduce hypertensive strokes, dyslipidemia is unmasked as a stroke risk factor.[20]

In a pooled study of nearly 125,000 persons in China and Japan, hypertension and cholesterol had no synergistic effect. Lower cholesterol levels were associated with a lower ischemic stroke rate but a higher rate of hemorrhagic stroke. The author's conclusion was that population-wide changes in eastern Asia, such as lower salt intake, higher potassium intake (fruit), more exercise, less obesity, and wider availability of effective antihypertensive drugs would have a major impact on health.[21]

New risk factors have emerged in recent years but have not yet assumed an established role, such as the metabolic disturbance of hyperhomocysteinemia. Increases in this amino acid in turn raise levels of free radical activation, damaging vascular endothelium. The antidote is to increase levels of folic acid as well as vitamins B-12 and B-6, and therapeutic trials are in progress.[22]

The gram negative bacterium chlamydia pneumoniae affects most of the population in childhood, but elevated titers of the antibody are found in patients with coronary artery disease and, more recently, cerebrovascular disease.[23] It is postulated that chronic vascular infection initiates or accelerates atherosclerosis and plaque formation. Evidence so far is inconclusive.

Medical Prevention

For some years, the media, taking an oversimplified and overdramatic stance, have promoted the daily use of aspirin (usually one 325 mg. tablet) to ward off heart attacks and strokes. More than half the patients attending cardiology and stroke prevention clinics have been taking aspirin, often for years before the event. Although two well-documented trials (one in the United States and one in the United Kingdom) of chronic ingestion of 350–500 mg/day of aspirin in asymptomatic male physicians demonstrated a decrease in ischemic cardiac events, no such effect was seen on stroke.[3] Added to these negative results is the chance of gastrointestinal bleeding related to the dose of aspirin, which may prove fatal, especially with increasing age. There is simply no justification for asymptomatic persons to take aspirin daily to prevent stroke. Unfortunately, data are scanty for patients with asymptomatic carotid stenosis, but the only published randomized trial showed no stroke prophylactic effect with long-term aspirin ingestion.[24]

The broadly aggressive approach of treating all types of vascular disease (including that of the heart, brain, and limbs), as in some recent antiplatelet trials,[25] has proven effective in preventing events in other vascular territories in patients without symptoms. Cardiologists lagged behind neurologists for years in endorsing the relationship between atrial fibrillation and embolic stroke, but anticoagulant trials in recent years have demonstrated beyond doubt that warfarin considerably reduces the risk of cardioembolic stroke in both symptomatic and asymptomatic patients.[26] Unfortunately, many physicians regard anticoagulant therapy as too dangerous in the very old (over 80 years), even though evidence from trials suggests the opposite. Consequently, only a minority of patients (probably less than 25%) receive anticoagulant therapy, though five separate trials have demonstrated a 68% reduction in stroke outcome.[26] A search is underway for alternative anticoagulants that do not require the inconvenience and expense of blood monitoring,[27] and devices to monitor coagulation parameters in the home are being tested.[28]

Surgical Prevention

The studies that have probably had greatest effect are the carotid endarterectomy trials for symptomatic patients, because they have fundamentally established guidelines for surgical practice.[29] The value of carotid surgery in asymptomatic patients and in those undergoing cardiac surgery is more questionnable. A national survey of Canadian neurologists specializing in stroke concluded that there was insufficient evidence to recommend carotid endarterectomy in asymptomatic carotid stenosis, and, further, the authors did not endorse screening even for asymptomatic patients with risk factors for vascular disease.[30]

The role of carotid surgery for asymptomatic carotid stenosis remains unsettled, and strong lobbies exist both for and against surgical intervention. The definitive trial, the Asymptomatic Carotid Atherosclerosis Study (ACAS),[31] which enrolled 1662 patients with >60% stenosis and followed them over 2.7 years, showed an absolute risk reduction for stroke of only 1% annually. Women had scarcely any benefit at all.

To show benefit, carotid endarterectomy trials must demonstrate a minimal combined risk from angiography and surgery. In ACAS, this was 2.3% for stroke and death, with more risk from angiography (1.2%) than from surgery (1.1%). Since all data from trials are gathered from state-of-the-art procedures, higher risks may mean the benefit will become negligible in practice, where guidelines are blurred or ignored. For instance, in a survey of Toronto teaching hospitals from 1994 to 1996, the stroke and death rate for asymptomatic carotid surgery was 3.8%,[32] raising concerns that the relatively low complication rates achieved by ACAS surgeons could not be matched, even in centers with extensive experience outside trial conditions.

There is no obvious solution to this problem. A search for a subgroup of high-risk patients who will benefit from surgical intervention so far has not been fruitful. Attempts to identify these special risk patients have targeted those with rapidly progressing stenoses using ultrasound[33] and those with falling cerebral blood flow values.[34] To compound this issue, those at highest risk of stroke may also have the highest risk of ischemic heart disease,[33] so that the very patients most needing carotid surgery are the ones that are most at risk on the operating table.

Angioplasty and stenting have not yet found a clear place in surgical intervention for symptomatic or asymptomatic disease. Preliminary data suggest that these procedures are too hazardous in asymptomatic patients and are only just acceptable in certain high-risk, symptomatic patients.[35] The results of current international trials may shed more light.

Public Health Strategies

Risk factor profiles of potential stroke patients are now well enough established to exert pressure on public health policies aimed at changing lifestyles and screening patients at high risk. To do this, extensive and expensive national campaigns are required to educate not just the public but also physicians. The apparently huge expenditure should be offset by equivalent cost savings from stroke prevention, to say nothing of the reduced toll of suffering.

Screening is ideal in principle, but often poor in practice. In a survey of elderly people (>65 years old) for atrial fibrillation in the United Kingdom, 4.7% of 4843 people had atrial fibrillation. Using standard criteria based on published trials, 61% would have benefited from anticoagulation therapy, but in practice only 23% received treatment. The authors concluded that anticoagulants were "underused and misdirected." Physicians need to be educated not only concerning anticoagulants but also in the use of hypertensive drugs.

Despite the proven efficacy of drugs to control high blood pressure, compliance is poor, and patients lose enthusiasm, so that even in developed countries many hypertensives remain untreated.[36]

Public health strategies, including screening for surgical prevention of stroke, are even more complex and uncertain. The spectacular success of carotid endarterectomy in stroke prevention in symptomatic patients, following the publication of surgical trials,[29] encouraged attempts at repeating these successes in asymptomatic patients. Whether the asymptomatic patient with a 70% carotid stenosis has carotid surgery depends on the individual surgeon, the method of assessing the target artery, the patient's preference, the hospital, and even the country of residence. The ease and safety of noninvasive vascular imaging has encouraged the use of this procedure on a massive scale. Screening people in supermarkets or other public areas yields a 5%–6% rate of detectable carotid stenoses, of which at most 1%–2% will be eligible for surgery.[37] Some unscrupulous physicians even advertise to the public "free" carotid doppler examinations on the assumption that a small number will request surgery once a carotid lesion is found. Because 67 people with carotid stenoses need to be treated to prevent one stroke, the major costs of screening, neurovascular imaging, and surgery, with it's attendant complications, make this strategy impractical.

SECONDARY PREVENTION OF STROKE

Prevention of further strokes in patients who have already experienced transient ischemic attacks (TIAs) or stroke (secondary prevention) is less effective compared to primary prevention, although patients are more likely to follow advice after something happens to them. In a minority of patients, this means a transient ischemic attack, but the vast majority suffer a stroke. The patients at highest risk of having a stroke are those who already have had one. The mainstay of secondary prevention comprises control of risk factors, enhancement of protective factors, drug treatment, and other interventions.

Control of Risk Factors

Hypertension remains the most important treatable risk factor for stroke in secondary prevention, as it is in primary prevention. This is true for women and men, for systolic and diastolic blood pressure, and for ischemic and hemorrhagic stroke[38] (see Chapter 5). Growing evidence supports a role also for hypertension in cognitive decline; new data suggest that treatment of hypertension may mitigate or prevent this decline.[39] In addition, it appears that treatment with the angiotension-converting enzyme inhibitor ramipril in patients who have already had a stroke reduces the risk of stroke by one-third.[40]

Smoking represents a risk factor for all types of arterial disease (peripheral, coronary, and cerebrovascular) in both primary and secondary stroke prevention[41] (see Chapter 2). About one-third of individuals still smoke in developed countries and a growing number in the developing world. The WHO has made an antismoking campaign its top priority.

Lipids have long been known as risk factors for coronary disease, but no relationship was established with stroke until recently. Now it is clear that statins decrease the risk of coronary disease, and the evidence suggests a similar fact for stroke prevention. The mechanism remains unclear; it may be lipid lowering, endothelium protection, or both[42] (see Chapter 4).

Atrial fibrillation is a serious complication of valvular heart disease. It is an escalating problem in the elderly everywhere, as the prevalence of atrial fibrillation doubles every decade. Fortunately warfarin and, to a lesser extent, aspirin are effective in both primary and secondary prevention[43] (see Chapter 6).

Homocystinemia is clearly associated with carotid atherosclerosis. What remains to be demonstrated is whether treatment with vitamins will slow, arrest, or reverse the process.[41]

Many other risk factors have been described. Some are common, such as diabetes, strict treatment of which makes little difference to large vessel disease but prevents small vessel diseases that lead to retinopathy, nephropathy, and neuropathy. Others are rare, such as lupus anticoagulant, and still others are uncertain, such as migraine, which may be a marker of increased risk rather than a risk factor itself.

Protective Factors

Good exercise, diet, and drink are powerful protective factors against stroke, along with estrogen replacement for postmenopausal women. Exercise in moderation seems to be good for everything from maintaining health to preventing and treating virtually all ailments. A diet rich in fruit and vegetables, hence high in potassium, seems to protect not only the heart, but the brain.[44] A drink or two a day may keep the stroke doctor away, although much needs to be clarified regarding the precise role of the ethanol molecule and its various vehicles[45] (see Chapter 3). Despite controversy, estrogen replacement therapy for postmenopausal women seems to protect against cardiovascular disease[46] (see Chapter 8).

Interventions

The value of carotid endarterectomy in symptomatic patients with carotid stenosis >70% has been established beyond a reasonable doubt, providing that it can be done within well defined limits of perioperative complications[47] (see Chapter 12). Angioplasty and stenting are gaining ground as promising techniques, with overall complication rates approaching those of carotid endarterectomy[48] (see Chapter 13). However, the role of carotid endarterectomy in secondary prevention is both clear and durable, whereas experience with angioplasty and stenting is brief and controversial. The time has come for a direct comparison. Otherwise, the procedures will fall into a quandary similar to that that clouds the role of angioplasty in peripheral vascular disease almost three decades after it was first attempted.

Drug Therapy

Antiplatelet agents have proven to be effective in decreasing the risk of further stroke after a transient ischemic attack or minor stroke. Aspirin remains the drug of choice, although the right dose continues to be debated[49] (see Chapter 10). Ticlopidine, clopidogrel, and dipyridamole may offer better alternatives[50] (see Chapter 11).

The only clear role of anticoagulants in secondary prevention is in reducing the risk of recurrent cardiac embolism[43,51] (see Chapters 6 and 9). Aspirin decreases the risk of a recurrent stroke, but whether it prevents cardiac embolism or reduces the risk of other strokes to which the patient is prone remains uncertain.

PREVENTION: POLICY AND PRACTICE

Stroke poses such a ubiquitous threat of death and disability that an urgent plan of stroke prevention is needed worldwide. Eighty percent of stroke deaths occur in the poor countries of the world, and the number will rise as some of the most populous countries witness a doubling in the number of their elderly. A hierarchy of values of various interventions for stroke must be clarified[52] (see Chapter 14).

The challenges are formidable. Even in developed countries, where costs are not insuperable, highly effective measures are seldom implemented to their fullest[53] (see Chapter 7). Only a fraction of the people who should receive anticoagulant treatment are getting it, and only one in five American hypertensives has his or her blood pressure controlled.[54]

An intervention can be overused or misused as well as underused. This is exemplified by carotid endarterectomy, the best documented surgical procedure for stroke prevention[55] (see Chapter 16).

Translating the results of clinical trials into clinical practice has major limitations[56] (see Chapter 15). Patients in clinical trials are selected, receive extraordinary care, and are seldom representative of the general population. Although we have made evidence-based medicine an ideal, there will never be enough evidence from clinical trials to address all pressing health problems. While the results of clinical trials provide the best odds that a particular treatment will benefit patients, they do not directly address whether a particular patient will respond to a specific intervention. More research is needed into the basis of individualizing therapy and the best strategies for acquiring and applying knowledge.

As usual, the ideal clashes with the affordable[57] (see Chapter 17). Not all measures have equal value, and no method is acceptable to all. Eventually, some common measure of value for invested money may emerge, such as disability adjusted life years (DALY) lost, to judge what each society or individual can or wants to afford. This may vary widely, given the great diversity in wealth, priorities, and cultures. Even so, different cultures can make decisions better in reference to a common currency.

CONCLUSIONS

Any discussion of the feasibility and costs of primary stroke prevention must factor in cost savings. Lifetime costs (as compared to acute care costs) are at least twice as high as most quoted figures. A study in the United States in 1997 estimated costs, depending on the type of stroke, at between $90 and $230 thousand per patient, based on 1990 data.[58] In one Canadian study, costs plummeted from Can$27,500 in 1993 to Can$10,000 in 1997, reflecting more than medical factors, such as earlier hospital discharge and a shift of burden to family and social services.[59,60]

A meaningful attack on significant risk factors can occur only after accurate evaluation of epidemiologic data. People at high risk of stroke due to high blood pressure need treatment, but treatment at lower levels of hypertension has progressively less influence on disease trends. Nevertheless, resources must be mobilized worldwide to combat the rising epidemic of vascular disease. One should also bear in mind a note of caution concerning the ethical dimension of "health promotion" sounded by the Irish epidemiologist McCormick: "Health promotion . . . falls far short of meeting the ethical imperatives for screening procedures. General practitioners would do better to encourage people to live lives of modified hedonism, so that they may enjoy to the full, the only life they are likely to have".[61]

It is known that most risk factors are not thresholds, but gradients. This applies to hypertension as well as lipid and homocysteine levels. This implies that there are different cost benefit ratios at different ends of the spectrum and calls for more sophisticated analyses about the effects of treatment.

Protective factors are emerging as important contributors of individual resistance to disease and its recurrence. Although much has been learned, much more needs to be discovered. If all known risk factors for stroke were abolished today, only about half of all strokes would be prevented[53] (see Chapter 7). Much more research is needed into the interaction of the environment and genetics, not only in disease development, but in disease protection and individual response to treatment.

REFERENCES

1. Porter R. The *Greatest Benefit to Mankind*. London: Harper Collins, 1997.
2. Husten L. Global epidemic of cardiovascular disease predicted. *Lancet* 1998;352: 1530.
3. Bronner LL, Kanter DS, Manson JE. Primary prevention of stroke. *N Engl J Med* 1995;333:1392–1400.
4. Broderick JP, Phillips SJ, Whisnant JP, et al. Incidence rates of stroke in the eighties. *Stroke* 1989;20:577–582
5. Wolf PA, D'Agostino RB, O'Neal MA, et al. Secular trends in stroke incidence and mortality. *Stroke* 1992;23:1551–1555.
6 Bonita R, Broad JB, Beaglehole R. Changes in stroke incidence and case-fatality in Auckland, New Zealand, 1981-91. *Lancet* 1993;342:1470–1473.
7. The hidden epidemic of cardiovascular disease. *Lancet* 1998;352:1795 (editorial).
8. Schneck MJ. Is psychological stress a risk factor for cerebrovascular disease? *Neuroepidemiology* 1997;16:174–179.
9. Kleinman Y, Korn-Lubetzki I, Eliashiv S, Abramsky O, Eliakim M. High frequency of hemorrhagic strokes in Jerusalem during the Persian Gulf War. *Neurology* 1992;42: 2225–2226.
10. Greenberg ER, Sporn MB. Antioxidant vitamins, cancer, and cardiovascular disease. *N Engl J Med* 1996;334:1189–1190.
11. Gorelick PB. Stroke Prevention: Windows of opportunity and failed expectations? *Neuroepidemiology* 1997;16:163–173.
12. Schwartz SM, Petitti DB, Siscovick DS, et al. Stroke and use of low-dose oral contraceptives in young women. *Stroke* 1998;29:2277–2284.
13. Gurwitz D. Oestrogen replacement therapy in postmenopausal women. *Lancet* 1999;353:674.
14. Murray CJLM, Lopez AD. Evidence-based health policy—lessons from the Global Burden of Disease Study. *Science* 1996;274:740–743.
15. Bonita R, Beaglehole R. Increased treatment of hypertension does not explain the decline in stroke mortality in the United States, 1970–1980. *Hypertension* 1989;13 (suppl 1):I-69–I-73.
16. Cook NR, Cohen J, Hebert PR, et al. Implications of small reductions in diastolic blood pressure for primary prevention. *Arch Intern Med* 1995;155: 701–709.
17. Gorelick PB, Schneck M, Bergland LF, Feinberg W, Goldstone J. Status of lipids as a risk factor for stroke. *Neuroepidemiology* 1997;16:107–115.
18. The long-term intervention with pravastatin in ischemic disease (LIPID) study group. *N Engl J Med* 1998;339:1349–1357.
19. Bucher HC, Griffith LE, Guyatt GH. Effective HMGcoA reductase inhibitors on stroke. *Ann Intern Med* 1998;128:89–95.
20. Spence JD. Statins for prevention of stroke. *Lancet* 1998;352:909.

21. Eastern Stroke and Coronary Heart Disease Collaboration Research Group. Blood pressure, cholesterol, and stroke in eastern Asia. *Lancet* 1998;352:1801–1807.
22. Welch GN, Loscalzo J. Homocysteine and atherothrombosis. *N Engl J Med* 1998;328: 1042–1050.
23. Fagerberg B, Gnarpe J, Gnarpe H, et al. Chlamydia pneumoniae but not cytomegalovirus antibodies are associated with future risk of stroke and cardiovascular disease. *Stroke* 1999;30:299–305.
24. Cote R, Battista RN, Abrahamowicz M, et al. Lack of effect of aspirin in asymptomatic patients with carotid bruits and substantial carotid narrowing. *Ann Intern Med.* 1995;123:649–655.
25. CAPRIE Steering Committee. A randomised, blinded trial of clopidogrel versus aspirin in patients at risk of ischaemic events (CAPRIE). *Lancet* 1996;348:1329–1339.
26. Albers GW. Atrial fibrillation and stroke—three new studies, three remaining questions. *Arch Intern Med* 1994;154:1443–1448.
27. Fihn SD. Aiming for safe anticoagulation. *N Engl J Med* 1995;333:54–55.
28. Hirsh J, Weitz JI. New antithrombotic agents. *Lancet* 1999;353:1431–1436.
29. Barnett HJM, Eliasziw M, Meldrum HE. Drugs and surgery in the prevention of ischemic stroke. *N Engl J Med* 1995;332:238–248.
30. Perry JR, Szalai JP, Norris JW. Consensus against both endarterectomy and routine screening for asymptomatic carotid artery stenosis. *Arch Neurol* 1997;54:25–28.
31. Executive committee for the asymptomatic carotid atherosclerosis study. *JAMA* 1995; 273:1421–1428.
32. Smurawska LT, Bowyer B, Rowed D, Maggisano R, Oh P, Norris JW. Changing practice and costs of carotid endarterectomy in Toronto, Canada. *Stroke* 1998; 29: 2014–2017.
33. Chambers BR, Norris JW. Outcome in patients with asymptomatic neck bruits. *N Engl J Med* 1986; 315:860–865.
34. Frey JL. Asymptomatic carotid stenosis: Surgery's the answer, but that's not the question. *Ann Neur* 1996; 39:3:405–406.
35. Norris JW, Nadareishvili ZG, Rowed DW, Bowyer B, Magigisano R. Are the hazards of carotid stenting unacceptably high? *Neurology* 1999;52(suppl):A269.
36. Caro JJ, Salas M, Speckman JL, Raggio G, Jackson JD. Persistence with treatment for hypertension in actual practice. *CMAJ* 1999;160(1):31–37.
37. O'Leary DH, Polak JF, Krournal RA, et al. Distribution and correlates of sonographically detected carotid artery disease in the Cardiovascular Health Study. *Stroke* 1991;23:1752–1760.
38. Taylor TN, David PH, Torner JC, Holmes J, Meyer JW, Jacobson MF. Lifetime cost of stroke in the United States. *Stroke* 1996;27:1459–1466.
39. Forette F, Stewx M-L, Staessen JA, et al. Prevention of dementia in randomized, doubleblind, placebo controlled Systolic Hypertension in Europe (Syst-Eur) trial. *Lancet* 1998;352:1347–1351.
40. The Heart Outcomes Prevention Evaluations Study Investigators. Effects of an angiotensin-converting-enzyme inhibitor, ramipril, on cardiovascular events in high-risk patients. *N Engl J of Med* 2000;342:145–153.
41. Sacco, chapter 2, this volume.
42. Adams, chapter 4, this volume.
43. Sherman, chapter 6, this volume.
44. Joshipura, KJ, Ascherio A, Manson JE, Stampfer MJ, Rimm EB, Speizer FE, Hennekens CH, et al. Fruit and vegetable intake in relation to risk of ischemic stroke. *JAMA* 1999;282(13):1233–1239.

45. Orgogozo, chapter 3, this volume.
46. Petitti, chapter 8, this volume.
47. Barnett, chapter 12, this volume.
48. Brown, chapter 13, this volume.
49. Bornstein, chapter 10, this volume.
50. Easton, chapter 11, this volume.
51. Bogousslavsky, chapter 9, this volume.
52. Bonita, chapter 14, this volume.
53. Gorelick, chapter 7, this volume.
54. Wolf PA. Prevention of stroke. *Stroke* 1998;352(suppl):15–18.
55. Feasby, chapter 16, this volume.
56. Donnan, chapter 15, this volume.
57. Hankey, chapter 17, this volume.
58. Taylor TN, David PH, Tomer JC, et al. Lifetime costs of stroke in the United States. *Stroke* 1996;27:1459–1466.
59. Smurawska LT, Alexandrov AV, Bladin CF, Norris JW. Cost of acute stroke care in Toronto, Canada. *Stroke* 1994;25:1628–1631.
60. Tran C, Nadareishvili Z, Smurawska L, Oh PIT, Norris JW. Decreasing costs of stroke hospitalization in Toronto. *Stroke* 1999;30:185–186.
61. McCormick J. Health promotion: the ethical dimension. *Lancet* 1994;344:390–391.

I

PRIMARY PREVENTION

2

STROKE RISK FACTORS: AN OVERVIEW

Ralph L. Sacco

Ranked as the second leading cause of death worldwide, stroke is far more often disabling than fatal and results in enormous costs measured in both health care dollars and lost productivity. Approximately 730,000 people have a new or recurrent stroke each year, and there are over 4 million stroke survivors in the United States. The estimated cost of stroke-related health care is a staggering $20 to $40 billion measured in both health care dollars and lost productivity.[1]

Over the next three decades, the public health impact of stroke is likely to increase. The proportion of the population over age 65 is expected to rapidly grow. The aging of the population and the changing race/ethnic composition of certain nations could lead to an increased absolute number of strokes per year, resulting in greater incidence, mortality, morbidity, and cost.

In recent years great strides have been made in understanding the pathophysiology of ischemic stroke and in testing and applying treatments for acute stroke aimed at reducing morbidity and mortality after stroke. However, the most effective way to reduce the burden of stroke is through prevention. Stroke risk factors have been elucidated, and clinical trials have indicated the benefits of treatments for persons with hypertension, atrial fibrillation, hypercholesterolemia, and asymptomatic carotid disease. Stroke prevention strategies can occur at multiple stages: in the healthy, stroke-free population (primary prevention): among those who have developed recognizable risk factors and may have subclinical disease (late primary or early secondary prevention); and after the development of neurological symptoms of stroke or transient ischemic attack, or TIA (late secondary or tertiary prevention). The process requires changes in national health policy directed at public health practices to promote healthy lifestyles, recognition of who is at increased risk of stroke, and modification of this risk whenever possible to prevent stroke.

CLASSIFICATION AND DETERMINATION OF STROKE RISK FACTORS

Every stroke prevention strategy begins with an understanding of stroke risk factors. A risk factor is any exposure that leads to an increase in the probability of stroke among those with the factor relative to those without the factor. Some factors are not modifiable and may be better characterized as risk markers, while others are amenable to behavioral, medical, or surgical modification. Risk markers may include age, gender, race–ethnicity and heredity. Modifiable risk factors may include environmental or even genetic exposures that when modified, lead to reductions in the risk of stroke. Conditions such as hypertension and hyperlipidemia are good examples of factors that may have both environmental and genetic determinants, but where control of the condition can lead to a reduction in stroke risk.

Epidemiologic studies such as case control and cohort studies have identified stroke risk factors. In case control studies the odds of exposure to a specific condition are assessed in cases with stroke compared to controls without stroke. The potency of the risk factor is measured by the odds ratio. Problems can be encountered because the exposure is usually measured after the onset of disease, and selection biases lead to a collection of cases who do not adequately reflect all individuals with stroke and controls who are not representative of the general population. These problems can be improved by using population-based study designs in which all the cases of stroke within a specific area are included and controls are randomly derived from the same community. Methods to measure exposures that reflect the pre-disease status can help reduce the problems of the retrospective design. Despite these limitations, case control studies can provide cost-effective insights into risk factors that are less prevalent.

In cohort studies, the risk or incidence of disease is determined among those with and without the factor of interest to calculate the relative risk or rate. Moreover, the attributable risk, or etiologic fraction, can be readily calculated as is a measure of the proportion of cases explained or attributed to the exposure. Prospective cohorts usually require systematic, lengthy follow-up after a baseline assessment. Retrospective cohort studies circumvent this problem by identifying individuals who had some baseline measurements made years before the study was conceived and then determine who subsequently developed stroke. The clear advantage to cohort studies is the measurement of the exposure pre-stroke and the ability to determine the prevalence of the exposure in the general population. However these studies are time consuming, expensive, and require large numbers of subjects.

Experimental epidemiologic studies, such as the randomized, controlled clinical trial, are the mainstay of demonstrating that modification of a risk factor can lead to a reduction in stroke risk. The population at risk usually has already been selected, with the risk factor based on inclusion and exclusion criteria. Subjects are randomly assigned to an intervention or not and then followed for the occurrence of a specific outcome, such as stroke. Randomization is used to help ensure that the groups are balanced for known and unknown factors that could increase the risk of stroke and serve as confounders. While these studies can also be expensive and require large numbers of patients, they are essential to the development of evidence-based guidelines for stroke prevention.

NONMODIFIABLE RISK MARKERS

Four nonmodifiable factors are generally considered to increase a person's risk of stroke. They include age, sex, race/ethnicity, and heredity.

Age and Sex

Age is one of the strongest determinants of stroke (Table 2.1). Stroke incidence rises with age, nearly doubling every decade after age 55, and the majority of strokes occur in persons older than 65.[1] Most of the future predicted increase in the number of strokes occurring each year is largely due to the aging of populations.

Stroke incidence is greater for men than women, with rates about 25% to 30% greater for men.[2] In Sweden, Italy, and Taiwan, stroke incidence was 66%, 35%, and 16% greater in men than women, respectively.[3-5] Women, however, have a greater life expectancy; hence, the prevalence of stroke in a population is usually greater among women. Differential incidence rates by sex vary by stroke

TABLE 2.1. Nonmodifiable Risk Markers for Incident Ischemic Stroke

FACTOR	EFFECT ON STROKE INCIDENCE	REFERENCE(S)
Age	Doubles per decade after age 55	2
Sex	24%–30% greater for men	2–5
Race/ethnicity	2.4-fold increase for African Americans 2.0-fold increase for Hispanics Increased among Chinese	7,16,17
Heredity	1.9-fold increase among first-degree relatives	21

subtype, with rates among men greater for cerebral infarction, rates for men and women similar for intracerebral hemorrhage, and rates among women greater for subarachnoid hemorrhage.[2,6] Some issues in stroke prevention are specific to women, such as oral contraceptives and postmenopausal estrogen use.

Race/Ethnicity

Despite a decline in stroke mortality in all race and sex groups, the relative difference between races in stroke mortality has remained fairly uniform, with nearly a two-fold increased stroke mortality in blacks compared to whites.[7] Few studies, however, have had enough of a race/ethnic mixture to compare stroke incidence in multiethnic groups in the same region. Various studies have found that blacks had a greater incidence and prevalence of stroke than whites of comparable age, sex, and residence.[8–14] In the National Health and Nutrition Survey, the relative risk of stroke for blacks was higher than for whites, even after adjustment for age, hypertension, and diabetes.[15] In northern Manhattan, the overall age-adjusted one-year stroke incidence rate for blacks was 2.4 times that of whites in a population-based stroke incidence study among white, black, and Hispanic residents.[16]

By contrast with blacks, Hispanics have rarely been identified separately in epidemiologic studies of stroke. In northern Manhattan, Hispanics, predominately from the Dominican Republic, had an overall age-adjusted one-year stroke incidence rate 2 times that of whites.[16] Finally, in other studies, Asians, particularly Chinese and Japanese, have exceedingly high stroke incidence rates that seem to be decreased among those who have migrated to Hawaii and California.[17]

The explanation for the increased mortality from stroke in African Americans, Hispanics, and Asians continues to be investigated. One explanation is that increased mortality is directly related to increased incidence. However, others have shown that different groups have a unique burden of stroke risk factors after controlling for differences in socioeconomic status and other demographic variables.[18] One way to look at differential burdens in stroke risk is to calculate the attributable risk of the risk factor. The ability to identify differences in risk factor profiles across racial/ethnic groups will allow more targeted and better justified therapeutic or preventative interventions.

Heredity

The hereditability, or genetic risk, of cerebrovascular disease has been under-emphasized. Stroke is predominantly a complex disease, influenced by both genetic and environmental factors. Although there are more than 50 monogenic disorders associated with stroke, most are rare and account for a small percentage of stroke cases. Stroke is likely caused by several different genes whose individual effects are determined by certain environmental triggers in a complex gene–environmental interaction causal model. Studies in different populations have demonstrated familial aggregation of stroke. Twin studies have found a significantly greater concordance of stroke in monozygotic than in dizygotic twins.[19] Cohort studies in different populations have demonstrated an association between parental stroke death and an increased risk of stroke in offspring.[20] Variations in the incidence of ischemic stroke in racial groups support the notion of a genetic component.[21] Relatives of people with ischemic stroke often share the same risk factors, making it difficult to separate genetic factors from shared environment.

The familial effect is thought to represent indirect genetic influences that likely operate through well-documented risk factors such as hypertension, diabetes mellitus, cardiac diseases, and abnormal lipid states. Each of these risk factors is itself under genetic influence that may or may not interact with environmental factors, and this observation argues against the notion that any single gene is a sufficient or necessary cause of stroke. Knowledge about these possible indirect genetic causes of stroke is incomplete. Potential genetic stroke risk factors include apolipoprotein E and lipoprotein α, as well as genetic markers of thrombosis, such as factor V Leiden, and fibrinogen.[22]

The identification of genetic determinants for stroke would allow early identification of persons with increased risk of stroke through genetic screening. At present, genetic screening is not available for atherosclerosis or stroke. In the future it may be possible to alter genes with molecular biological techniques and modify the risk of stroke. Prior to these advances, the detection of a genetic factor could also lead to more intensive environmental risk factor modification.

MODIFIABLE RISK FACTORS

Major reductions in stroke morbidity and mortality are more likely to arise from identification and control of modifiable factors in the stroke-prone individual. Modifiable stroke risk factors include hypertension, cardiac disease (particularly atrial fibrillation), diabetes, dyslipidemia, cigarette use, alcohol abuse, physical inactivity, diet, asymptomatic carotid stenosis, and transient ischemic attacks (Table 2.2).

Hypertension

After age, hypertension is the most powerful stroke risk factor. It is prevalent in both men and women and is of even greater significance in African Americans. The risk of stroke rises proportionately with increasing blood pressure. Isolated systolic hypertension is increasingly prevalent with age and increases the risk of stroke by 2 to 4 times, even after controlling for age and diastolic blood pressure.[2]

TABLE 2.2. Estimated Relative Risk, Prevalence, and Identification of Important Modifiable Risk Factors for Ischemic Stroke. The Prevalence of the Risk Factor in the General Population Varies by Age, Sex, Race/Ethnicity, and Definition of the High Risk Factor

STROKE RISK FACTOR	ESTIMATED RELATIVE RISK	ESTIMATED PREVALENCE (%)	DEFINITIONS
Hypertension	3.0–5.0	25–40	SBP ≥ 140mmHg DBP ≥ 90 mmHg
Atrial fibrillation	5.0–18.0	1–2	Irregular pulse Confirmation–Holter/EKG
Diabetes mellitus	1.5–3.0	4–20	FBS > 126 mg/dl
Dyslipidemia	1.0–2.0	6–40	TC ≥ 200; LDL ≥ 100 mg/dl HDL <35 mg/dl TG > 200 mg/dl
Cigarette smoking	1.5–2.5	20–40	Current smoking (within 5 years)
Heavy alcohol use	1.0–3.0	5–30	Heavy drinking (≥5 drinks per day)
Physical inactivity	2.7	20–40	< 30–60 min per day of exercise 3–4 times per week

Reduction of both systolic and diastolic blood pressure in hypertensives substantially reduces stroke risk. A large multicenter hypertension detection and follow-up program trial, comparing standardized stepped care with routine care, showed a 35% reduction in total strokes and a 44% reduction in fatal strokes over a five-year period.[23] Reduction of isolated systolic hypertension to < 140 mm Hg in elderly individuals is clearly beneficial.[24,25,26] The Syst-Eur trial demonstrated that treatment of older patients with isolated systolic hypertension led to a 42% reduction in stroke risk with no significant decline in overall mortality.[27] Meta-analyses of prospective randomized controlled trials indicated that a decrease in diastolic blood pressure of 5 to 6 mm Hg reduced the risk for stroke by 42%, with similar magnitudes of risk reduction for men, women, and subjects of all ages.[28,29]

Current guidelines for treatment of hypertension have been published by the Joint National Committee on Prevention, Detection, Evaluation, and Treatment of High Blood Pressure.[30] Definitions of hypertension have been broadened to include individuals who were once considered "borderline hypertensive." Because the attributable stroke risk for hypertension (proportion of strokes explained by hypertension) ranges from 35% to 50% depending on age, even a slight improvement in the control of hypertension could translate into a substantial reduction in stroke frequency.[31] The National Stroke Association recommends that to help decrease the risk for a first stroke, the three following things should be done: (1) blood pressure should be controlled in patients with hypertension who are most likely to develop stroke, (2) physicians should check the blood pressure of all their patients at every visit, and (3) patients with hypertension should monitor their blood pressure at home.[32]

Cardiac Diseases

Various cardiac conditions have been clearly associated with an increase in the risk of ischemic stroke (Table 2.3). Because certain stroke risk factors, like hypertension, may also be determinants of cardiac disease, some cardiac conditions may be viewed as intervening events in the causal chain for stroke. Cardiac factors that have been documented independently to increase the risk of stroke include atrial fibrillation, valvular heart disease, myocardial infarction, coronary artery disease, congestive heart failure, and electrocardiographic evidence of left ventricular hypertrophy. Improved cardiac imaging has led to the increased detection of potential stroke risk factors, such as mitral annular calcification, patent foramen ovale (PFO), aortic arch atherosclerotic disease, atrial septal aneurysms, spontaneous echo contrast (a smoke-like appearance in the left cardiac chambers visualized on transesophageal echocardiography), and valvular strands.

Nonvalvular atrial fibrillation (AF) is a potent predictor of stroke, causing a nearly fivefold increase in the relative risk of stroke.[33] It has been estimated that AF affects more than 2 million Americans and becomes more frequent with age, ranking as the leading cardiac arrhythmia in the elderly. For each advancing

TABLE 2.3. Cardiac Risk Factors for Incident Ischemic Stroke

DEFINITE	POSSIBLE
Atrial fibrillation	
Myocardial Disease	
Coronary artery disease	Patent foramen ovale
Cardiac failure	Atrial septal aneurysm
Left ventricular hypertrophy	Spontaneous echo contrast
Intracardiac thrombus	
Cardiac Valve Abnormalities	
Mitral stenosis	
Mitral annular calcification	Valve strands
Prosthetic valves	
Endocarditis	
Aortic arch plaque	

decade of age, the incidence of AF nearly doubles. The overall prevalence of AF is approximately 1%, but the prevalence among those older than 65 years is close to 6%. Therefore, the attributable risk of stroke from AF increases significantly with age, approaching that of hypertension among those 80 to 89 years old.

Clinical trials have demonstrated conclusive evidence of the efficacy of oral anticoagulants for stroke prevention among individuals with nonvalvular atrial fibrillation.[34] Aspirin may also have some efficacy among lower-risk groups or those who have relative contraindications to anticoagulants. Stroke prevention in atrial fibrillation (SPAF III) demonstrated that warfarin with an international normalized ratio (INR) of 2–3 was far superior to aspirin and mini-dose warfarin with an INR < 1.5 in the prevention of stroke among high-risk patients with nonvalvular atrial fibrillation.[35] The recommendation from the fifth American College of Chest Physicians Consensus Conference on Antithrombotic Therapy was that long-term oral warfarin therapy (INR 2.0–3.0, target 2.5) be used in patients with atrial fibrillation who are eligible for anticoagulants, except in patients less than 60 years of age who have no associated cardiovascular disease.[36] It has been estimated that for every 1000 patients with nonvalvular atrial fibrillation treated with warfarin for one year, 35 thromboembolic events can be prevented at a cost of one major bleed.

Stroke risk nearly doubles in those with antecedent coronary artery disease, triples with left ventricular hypertrophy, and nearly quadruples in subjects with cardiac failure.[33] Acute myocardial infarction has been associated with stroke. Even uncomplicated angina, non–Q wave infarction, and silent myocardial infarction were found to be stroke risk factors in the Framingham Study cohort. The attributable risk of stroke for coronary heart disease was approximately 12% and ranged from 2.3% to 6.0% for cardiac failure, depending on age.

Mitral stenosis, endocarditis, and prosthetic heart valves are some of the valvular diseases that can also increase the risk of stroke. After adjusting for other risk factors in the Framingham cohort, the presence of mitral annular calcification (MAC) was associated with a relative risk of stroke of 2.1.[37] Mitral valve prolapse (MVP) has a high prevalence in the general population and has been reported to be more frequent in young patients with unexplained stroke compared to controls. However, more recent studies with more stringent diagnostic criteria for MVP have failed to demonstrate a convincing independent increase in stroke risk.[38,39]

Diabetes Mellitus

Diabetes is a determinant of atherosclerosis and microangiopathy of the coronary, peripheral, and cerebral arteries. Death from cerebrovascular disease is greatly increased among subjects with elevated blood glucose values.[40] Cohort studies have demonstrated an independent effect of diabetes on stroke risk after controlling for other risk factors, with relative risks ranging from 1.5 to 3.0.[2,41,42,43] Some studies have shown conflicting data regarding the relative risk of stroke in diabetic women as compared with men. A Swedish study showed a 6-fold rise in the risk of stroke in diabetic males compared to a 13-fold rise in females.[44] In Rochester, Minn., diabetes was a significant risk factor for stroke among men, but not women.[45] Both studies found that the impact of diabetes on stroke risk was greater in older women. Among Hawaiian men of Japanese descent in the Honolulu Heart Program, those with diabetes had twice the risk of thromboembolic stroke compared with those without diabetes, independent of other risk factors.[46] In the Framingham study, at all ages of both men and women, the incidence of atherothrombotic infarction among diabetics was almost twice that of nondiabetics.[47]

In western Europe, insulin-dependent, or type 1, diabetes accounts for perhaps 10%–20% of all diabetic patients. Worldwide, there seems to be an extraordinary increase in type 2 diabetes, from an estimated 124 million at present to a predicted 221 million by the year 2010, with only 3% of all patients with type 1 diabetes.[48] Based on preliminary data from the Northern Manhattan Stroke Study, the prevalence of diabetes may be as high as 22% and 20% among elderly blacks and Hispanics, respectively, and the corresponding attributable risks of stroke were 13% and 20%.[49]

Intensive treatment of both type 1 and type 2 diabetes, aimed at maintaining near normal levels of blood glucose, can substantially reduce the risk of microvascular complications such as retinopathy, nephropathy, and neuropathy, but it has not been conclusively shown to reduce macrovascular complications, including stroke.[50,51,52] However, the UK Prospective Diabetes Study group reported that aggressive treatment of blood pressure (< 150/85 mm Hg) among type 2 diabetics helped significantly to reduce the risk of stroke by 44%.[53] Recent guidelines for management of diabetes have been published by the American Diabetes Association and have lowered the target fasting blood glucose level to 126 mg/dl.[54] The National Stroke Association (NSA) recommends rigorous comprehensive control of blood sugar levels for adherent patients with type 1 and type 2 diabetes mellitus to prevent microvascular complications.[32]

Dyslipidemias

Abnormalities of serum lipids (triglyceride, cholesterol, low-density lipoprotein [LDL], and high-density lipoprotein [HDL]) are clear risk factors for atherosclerotic disease, particularly coronary disease. Recent studies have helped clarify the relationship between lipids and stroke risk. Studies using ultrasound technology have established that total cholesterol or LDL cholesterol is directly associated and HDL cholesterol is inversely associated with extracranial carotid atherosclerosis and intima-media plaque thickness.[55–59] Case control studies have found the concentration of HDL to be lower in stroke cases, even after controlling for other stroke risk factors, and ischemic stroke mortality has been found to be related to lower HDL levels.[60-63] Most prospective studies have found no association between serum cholesterol and cerebral infarction, while some have demonstrated a relationship.[41,64] In the Multiple Risk Factor Intervention Trial, mortality from ischemic stroke was greater among men with high cholesterol.[65] In the Honolulu Heart Program, there was a continuous and progressive increase in both coronary heart disease CHD and thromboembolic stroke rates with increasing levels of cholesterol, with a relative risk of 1.4 comparing the highest and lowest quartiles.[64]

Meta-analyses among prospective studies have found either no or only a minimally increased relative risk of stroke due to elevated total cholesterol.[66,67] The absence of a consistent significant relationship between cholesterol and stroke may be partially explained by the recognition that there are multiple stroke subtypes that are not all attributed to atherosclerosis. Additionally, most prospective studies were done among younger populations and focused on cardiac outcomes, and lipoprotein fractions were not always evaluated separately from total cholesterol.

Clinical trials analyzing the efficacy of lipid-lowering strategies with statins have demonstrated impressive reductions in stroke risk in various high-risk populations with cardiac disease. In these studies, stroke was either a secondary endpoint or a nonspecified endpoint, determined based on post-hoc analyses.[68] Meta-analyses of some of these trials have found significant reductions in stroke risk, with a 29% reduced risk of stroke and a 22% reduction in overall mortality.[69,70] Secondary prevention trials showed a 32% stroke risk reduction, and primary trials demonstrated a 20% reduction. Two large trials in which stroke was prespecified as a secondary endpoint have also shown significant reductions using pravastatin among subjects with coronary artery disease and normal to only modest elevations of cholesterol.[71,72]

Using serial carotid ultrasound measurements, some clinical trials have also demonstrated carotid plaque regression with statins.[73-77] Thus, recent observational and clinical trial data provide mounting support for the role of lipoproteins as precursors of carotid atherosclerosis and ischemic stroke and the benefits of cholesterol lowering in stroke reduction. Individuals with cholesterol levels above 200 mg/dl and with cardiovascular risk factors should have a complete lipid analysis (total cholesterol, LDL, HDL, triglycerides) and most likely would benefit from cholesterol lowering regimens, including statins.[78]

Cigarette Smoking

Despite the clear evidence that cigarette smoking is an independent determinant of stroke and other diseases, it remains a major modifiable public health threat in every nation.[79] A wealth of data support the role of smoking as an important and prevalent stroke risk factor. In case control studies, the effect of cigarette smoking remained significant after adjustment for other factors, and a dose-response relationship was apparent.[80] Prospective studies have confirmed these findings in both men and women.[81,82] The Honolulu Heart Study demonstrated that smoking was an independent predictor of ischemic stroke, with adjusted relative risks of 2.5 for men and 3.1 for women. A meta-analysis of 32 studies found a summary relative risk of stroke for smokers of 1.5 (95% CI 1.4–1.6).[83] The risk decreased with age, and a slightly increased risk was noted for women compared to men. Stroke risk was increased twofold in heavy smokers (more than 40 cigarettes per day) compared to light smokers (less than 10 cigarettes per day). The stroke risk attributed to cigarette smoking was greatest for subarachnoid hemorrhage, intermediate for cerebral infarction, and lowest for cerebral hemorrhage. Even the effects of passive cigarette smoking exposure have been found to increase the risk of progression of atherosclerosis.[84]

Cigarette smoking is an independent determinant of carotid artery plaque thickness and the strongest predictor of severe extracranial carotid artery atherosclerosis.[85–88] Other biological mechanisms by which cigarettes may predispose to stroke include increased coagulability, blood viscosity, and fibrinogen levels; enhanced platelet aggregation; and elevated blood pressure.

No randomized clinical trial has been performed to measure the benefits of cigarette smoking cessation. However, ample evidence exists from observational epidemiologic studies that smoking cessation leads to a reduction in stroke risk. The Nurses' Health Study and the Framingham Study both demonstrated that the risk of ischemic stroke is reduced to that of nonsmokers after 2 years and 5 years, respectively.[89,90] It has been estimated that if cigarette smoking could be eliminated in the United States, the number of strokes occurring each year could be reduced by 61,500 with a saving of 3.08 billion stroke-related health-care dollars.[91] The NSA recommends the cessation of smoking as a stroke prevention measure, in accordance with guidelines by the Agency for Health Care Policy and Research that address various topics, including screening for tobacco use, advice to quit, interventions, smoking cessation pharmacotherapy, motivation to quit, and preventing relapses.[32,92]

Alcohol Use

The role of alcohol as a stroke risk factor is controversial and differs by dose as well as stroke subtype.[93,94] Almost all studies have shown an increased risk of hemorrhagic stroke associated with increasing alcohol consumption in a dose-dependent fashion.[95] Those studies that have investigated alcohol as a risk factor for ischemic stroke have found conflicting results. In a case control study among 205 predominantly black patients in Chicago, no significant effect of alcohol on stroke risk was found when controlled for confounders.[80] Other case control studies in New Haven,[96] Winnipeg, Canada,[97] London, U.K.,[98] and Milan, Italy,[99] similarly failed to find a significant association between alcohol and ischemic stroke. In northern Manhattan, a J-shaped relationship between alcohol and stroke was found, with an elevated stroke risk for heavy alcohol consumption and a protective effect in light to moderate drinkers (two or fewer drinks per day) when compared to nondrinkers (Figure 2.1).[100] The methodological problems in the case control approach to study alcohol and stroke have been summarized by Camargo and others.[94,98] For example, one investigation demonstrated that the odds ratio for stroke ranged from 0.73 (protective) to 1.93 (deleterious) depending upon whether controls were selected from a general hospital population, a population without potential alcohol-related diagnoses, or the community.[98]

Prospective cohort studies in predominantly white populations addressing the relationship of stroke to alcohol intake have found evidence of a protective effect of mild alcohol intake.[101–103] The large Nurses' Health Study, which examined different stroke subtypes, found a protective effect of mild alcohol consumption (up to 1.2 drinks per day in women) for ischemic stroke.[101] Other prospective cohort studies have failed to confirm this relationship.[104] Several studies of Japanese subjects that looked specifically at ischemic stroke failed to show any protective effect of alcohol, suggesting that alcohol's effect as a stroke risk factor may vary by race/ethnicity.[102,105]

The various mechanisms through which alcohol may increase the risk of stroke include hypertension, hypercoagulable states, cardiac arrhythmias, and cerebral

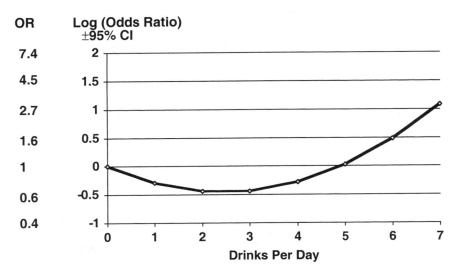

FIGURE 2.1. Quadratic, or J-shaped, relationship between alcohol exposure and ischemic stroke risk from the Northern Manhattan Stroke Study.

blood flow reductions. However, there is also evidence that light to moderate drinking can increase HDL-cholesterol, reduce the risk of coronary artery disease, and increase endogenous tissue plasminogen activator. The combination of deleterious and beneficial effects of alcohol is consistent with the observation of a dose-dependent relationship between alcohol and stroke. Elimination of heavy drinking can undoubtedly reduce the incidence of stroke. Since some ingestion of alcohol, perhaps up to two drinks per day, may actually help reduce the risk of stroke, drinking in moderation should not be discouraged for most of the public.[32]

Physical Activity

The cardiovascular benefits of physical activity have been emphasized by numerous organizations, including the Center for Disease Control, the National Institutes of Health, and the American Heart Assocation, based on accumulating data regarding the beneficial effects of physical activity in reducing the risk of heart disease and premature death.[106] Previous studies have evaluated the association between physical activity and the risk of stroke.[107–115] The beneficial effects have been predominately described among white populations, more apparent for men than women, and generally described for younger rather than older adults. The Honolulu Heart Program, which investigated older middle-aged men of Japanese ancestry, showed a protective effect of habitual physical activity from thromboembolic stroke only among the nonsmoking group.[108] The Framingham Study demonstrated the benefits of combined leisure and work physical activities for men, but not for women.[109] In the Oslo Study, among men aged 40 to 49, increased leisure physical activity was related to a reduced stroke incidence.[110] For women 40 to 65 years old, the Nurses' Health Study showed an inverse association between level of physical activity and the incidence of any stroke.[114] In the Northern Manhattan Stroke Study, the benefits of leisure-time physical activity were noted for all age, sex, and race/ethnic subgroups.[112] (Figure 2.2)

The optimal amount of exercise needed to prevent stroke is unclear, particularly for the elderly. Among subjects in a case control study in West Birmingham, United Kingdom, who were free of cardiovascular disease, recent vigorous exercise was no more protective than walking.[113] Among the older cohort of the Framingham Study, the strongest protection was detected in the medium tertile physical activity subgroup, with no benefit gained from additional activity.[109] The protective effect of physical activity may be partly mediated through its role in controlling various risk factors such as hypertension, diabetes, and obesity. Other than control of risk factors, biological mechanisms such as increased HDL and reduced homocysteine level also may be responsible for the effect of physical activity.[116,117]

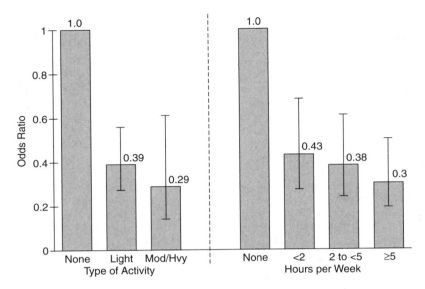

FIGURE 2.2. Dose response relationship by intensity and duration of physical activity (matched by age, sex, race/ethnicity, and adjusted for HTN, DM, PVD, smoking, cardiac disease, obesity, heavy alcohol use, activities limited for medical reasons, education, and season of enrollment).

Physical activity is a modifiable behavior that deserves greater emphasis in stroke prevention campaigns. The 1994 Behavioral Risk Factor Surveillance Survey found that 60% of adults did not achieve the recommended amount of physical activity, and people with the lowest incomes and less than 12th-grade education were more likely to be sedentary.[1] Moreover, 70% to 80% of older women report levels less than the recommended amount of physical activity.[118] Public health goals are to increase the percentage of people who engage in regular physical activity, and reduce the percentage of those who engage in no leisure-time physical activity, particularly among people aged 65 and older.[119] Leisure-time physical activity could translate into a cost-effective means of decreasing the public health burden of stroke and other cardiovascular diseases among the rapidly aging population.[32]

Dietary Factors

While data have suggested that diet may play an important role as a stroke risk factor, few studies have been able to clarify this relationship because of the complex issues associated with dietary intake and nutritional status (Table 2.4). Early, large ecological studies suggested that excess fat intake associated with migration may lead to increased risk of both coronary heart disease and stroke.[120] High daily dietary intake of fat is associated with obesity and may act as an inde-

TABLE 2.4. Dietary Factors Possibly Related to the
Risk of Stroke

Fats

Saturated fats
Cholesterol
Fish oil

Proteins

Homocysteinemia

Fruits and Vegetables

Antioxidants (Flavonoids)

Vitamins

Vitamin B6	Vitamin C
Folate	Vitamin E
Vitamin B12	Beta carotene

Minerals

Sodium	Calcium
Potassium	

pendent risk factor or may affect other stroke risk factors, such as hypertension, diabetes, hyperlipidemia, and cardiac disease. Results from the Framingham Study, however, suggested conflicting findings, with an inverse association between dietary fat and ischemic stroke.[121] Dietary sodium may also be associated with increased stroke risk. Specifically, increased sodium intake is involved with an increased risk of hypertension.[122]

Another important dietary component is homocysteine. Case control studies have demonstrated an association between moderately elevated homocysteine and vascular disease, including stroke.[123,124] Genetic and environmental causes of increased serum homocysteine have been implicated as a modifiable determinant of cardiovascular and cerebrovascular events.[125,126] The Framingham Study found that deficiencies in folate, B-12 levels, and pyridoxine accounted for the majority of elevated homocysteine levels in the study cohort.[127] Additionally, evidence from case control studies has suggested that increased dietary and supplemental intake of vitamin B-6 may decrease stroke risk.[128] Large studies, such as the Vitamin in Stroke Protection Trial (VISP), are currently investigating the protective effects of vitamin B-6, B-12, and folate for recurrent stroke.

Dietary intake of fruits and vegetables may reduce the risk of stroke. These foods may contribute to stroke protection through antioxidant mechanisms or through elevation of potassium levels.[129–132] Dietary antioxidants, including vitamin C, vitamin E, and beta-carotene, belong to a group of antioxidants called flavonoids that are found in fruits and vegetables. These scavengers of free radicals are thought to be associated with stroke risk reduction through the free-radical oxidation of LDL, which inhibits the formation of atherosclerotic plaques.[133] The large Western Electric cohort found a moderate decrease in stroke risk associated with a higher intake of both beta-carotene and vitamin C.[134] Other dietary factors associated with a reduced risk of stroke include milk and calcium[135] and fish oils.[136,137]

Extracranial Carotid Stenosis

Carotid stenosis has long been recognized as an important predictor of both TIA's and stroke. The occurrence of symptoms may be dependent on the severity and progression of the stenosis, the adequacy of collateral circulation, the character of the atherosclerotic plaque, and the propensity to form thrombus at the site of the stenosis. In the case of patients with symptomatic disease, the two-year risk of stroke is quite high, approaching 26% among medically treated patients with TIA or minor stroke and an ipsilateral carotid stenosis of >70%.[138] For those with asymptomatic carotid artery disease, the annual stroke risk is lower and reported to be 1.3% in those with stenosis of 75% or less, and 3.3% in those with stenosis of more than 75%, with an ipsilateral stroke risk of 2.5%.[139,140] The combined TIA and stroke risk was 10.5% per year in those with more than 75% carotid stenosis. The prevalence of asymptomatic carotid disease increases with age, occurring in 53.6% of subjects 65 to 94 years of age.[141]

The efficacy of carotid endarterectomy in asymptomatic carotid stenosis has been evaluated in a few clinical trials, including the Asymptomatic Carotid Artery Surgery Study (ACAS).[142] Patients eligible for ACAS were under age 80 with asymptomatic carotid stenosis greater than 60% and could not have any unstable cardiac disease. Overall, the 30-day ipsilateral stroke or death rate among the surgically treated patients was only 2.3%. The trial found a five-year ipsilateral stroke risk of 10.5% among the medical group and 4.8% in the surgical group. There was a 55% risk reduction of ipsilateral stroke associated with carotid endarterectomy. The benefit for men was greater than for women (risk reduction 69% vs. 16%). Given the right circumstances based on the degree of the stenosis, other co-morbid conditions, and the expertise of the surgeon, endarterectomy may be beneficial in certain asymptomatic persons.

Transient Ischemic Attacks

TIAs are a strong predictor of subsequent stroke, with annual stroke risks of 1% to 15%. The first year following a TIA is associated with the greatest stroke risk.

In hospital-referred patients, the average annual risk of stroke, myocardial infarction, or death was 7.5% after TIA.[143] Amaurosis fugax, or transient monocular blindness (TMB), had a better outcome than cerebral ischemic attacks, and stroke usually occurred in the same vascular territory as the initial TIA. Recommendations for the treatment of TIA include identification of the underlying etiology of the TIA, targeted risk factor prevention strategies, and the use of antithrombotic medications.[144–146]

OTHER POTENTIAL STROKE RISK FACTORS

Other potential stroke risk factors have been identified in some studies, but need confirmation and clarification through further epidemiologic investigations (Table 2.5).

New technology for the detection of polymorphisms has opened the field of genetic risk factors for stroke. Included among the potential genetic markers for lipids are α lipoprotein apo E. Hematologic testing has also suggested that various markers of hypercoagulable states may be independent stroke risk factors, such as antiphospholipid antibodies, lupus anticoagulant, factor V Leiden, free protein S and protein C deficiencies. Other risk factors, such as the use of oral

TABLE 2.5. Other Potential Stroke Risk Factors Under Further Epidemiologic Investigations

Genetic Markers

Lipoprotein fractions (Lp(a))
Apolipoprotein E
ACE polymorphism

Subclinical Markers

Intimal media carotid thickness
Endothelial reactivity
White matter hyperintensities
Aortic arch atheroma

Other Factors

Migraine

Hypercoagulable States

Antiphospholipid antibodies
Lupus anticoagulant
Protein C, free protein S deficiencies
Prothrombin fragment 1•2
Factor V Leiden

contraceptives and hormone replacement, are being investigated in large prospective studies. Finally, the interaction of these potential factors with known stroke risk factors needs to be investigated.

CONCLUSION

The Prevention of First Stroke Guidelines outlines evidence that can be used by clinicians for the prevention of first stroke.[32] These guidelines state that "preventing persons from having first stroke will require a comprehensive multidisciplinary strategy to identify and manage major risk factors and to promote adherence to preventive protocols." Based on the estimated prevalence of risk factors and their attributable risks for stroke in the United States, it is estimated that a significant percentage of strokes could be prevented through the control of these modifiable stroke risk factors.[147] Despite the wealth of data on the importance of stroke risk factors, control of these conditions remains inadequate due to poor patient compliance and adherence to behavior modifications as well as decreased detection and treatment by health care providers. Further reductions in the risk of stroke will require enhancements in our ability to detect, modify, and treat persons with risk factors.

REFERENCES

1. American Heart Association. *1999 Heart and Stroke Statistical Update*. Dallas: American Heart Association, 1998.
2. Sacco RL, Benjamin EJ, Broderick JP, Dyken M, Easton JD, Feinberg WM, Goldstein LB, Gorelick PB, Howard G, Kittner SJ, Manolio TA, Whisnant JP, Wolf PA. Risk Factors Panel—American Heart Association Prevention Conference IV. *Stroke* 1997;28:1507–1517.
3. Ricci S, Celani MG, La Rosa F, Vitali R, Duca E, Ferraguzzi R, Paolotti M, Seppoloni D, Caputo N, Chiurulla C, Scaroni R, Signorini E. SEPIVAC: A community-based study of stroke incidence in Umbria, Italy. *J Neurol Neurosurg Psych* 1991;54: 695–698.
4. Jerntorp P, Berglund G. Stroke registry in Malmo, Sweden. *Stroke* 1992;23:357–361.
5. Hu H-H, Sheng W-Y, Chu F-L, Lan C-F, Chiang BN. Incidence of stroke in Taiwan. *Stroke* 1992;23:1237–1241.
6. Sacco SE, Whisnant JP, Broderick JP, Phillips SJ, O'Fallon WM. Epidemiological characteristics of lacunar infarcts in a population. *Stroke* 1991;22:1236–1241.
7. Cooper R, Sempos C, Hsieh SC, Kovar MG. Slowdown in the decline of stroke mortality in the United States, 1978–1986. *Stroke* 1990;21:1274–1279.
8. Ostfeld AM, Shekelle RB, Klawans H, Tufo HM. Epidemiology of stroke in elderly welfare population. *Am J Publ Hlth* 1974;64:450–458.
9. Caplan LR, Gorelick PB, Hier DB. Race, sex and occlusive cerebrovascular disease: a review. *Stroke* 1986;17:648–655.
10. Gillum RF. Stroke in blacks. *Stroke* 1988;19:1–9.
11. Schoenberg BS, Anderson DW, Haerer AF. Racial differentials in the prevalence of stroke—Copiah County, Mississippi. *Arch Neurol* 1986;43:565–568.

12. Heyman A, Karp HR, Heyden S, Bartel A, Cassel JC, Tyroler HA, Cornoni J, Hames CG, Stuart W. Cerebrovascular disease in the bi-racial population of Evans County, Georgia. *Stroke* 1971;2:509–518.

13. Gross CR, Kase CS, Mohr JP, et al. Stroke in south Alabama: Incidence and diagnostic features—a population based study. *Stroke* 1984;15:249–255.

14. Friday G, Lai SM, Alter M, Sobel E, LaRue L, Gil-Peralta A, McCoy RL, Levitt LP, Isak T. Stroke in the Lehigh Valley: Racial/ethnic differences. *Neurology* 1989; 39:1165–1168.

15. Kittner SJ, White LR, Losonczy K, Wolf PA, Hebel JR. Black-white differences in stroke incidence in a national sample—the contribution of hypertension and diabetes mellitus. *JAMA* 1990;264:1267–1270.

16. Sacco RL, Boden-Albala B, Gan R, Kargman DE, Paik M, Shea S, Hauser WA, and the Northern Manhattan Stroke Study Collaborators. Stroke incidence among white, black and Hispanic residents of an urban community: the Northern Manhattan Stroke Study. *Am J Epidemiol* 1998;147:259–268.

17. Reed DM. The paradox of high risk of stroke in populations with low risk of coronary heart disease. *Am J Epidemiol* 1990;131:579–588.

18. Abel GA, Sacco RL, Lin IF, et al. Race-ethnic variability in etiologic fraction for stroke risk factors: The Northern Manhattan Stroke Study. *Stroke* 1998;29:277 (abstract).

19. Brass LM, Isaacsohn JL, Merikangas KR. A study of twins and stroke. *Stroke* 1991; 23(2)221–223.

20. Kiely DK, Wolf PA, Cupples LA, Beiser AS, Myers RH. Familial aggregation of stroke: The Framingham Study. *Stroke* 1993;24:1366–1371.

21. Halim A, Ottman R, Logroscino G, Gan R, McLaughlin C, Boden-Albala B, Hauser WA, Sacco RL. Familial aggregation of ischemic stroke in the Northern Manhattan Stroke Study. *Neurology* 1997;48:A161.

22. Alberts MJ (ed). *Genetics of Cerebrovascular Disease*. Armonk, NY: Futura Publications, 1999.

23. Hypertension Detection and Follow-Up Program Cooperative Group. Five-year findings of the Hypertension Detection and Follow-Up Program. III. Reduction in stroke incidence among persons with high blood pressure. *JAMA* 1982;247:633–638.

24. SHEP Cooperative Research Group. Prevention of stroke by antihypertensive drug treatment in older persons with isolated systolic hypertension: Final results of the Systolic Hypertension in the Elderly Program (SHEP). *JAMA* 1991;265:3255–3264.

25. Dohlof B, Lindholm LH, Hansson L, Scherst B, Ekbom T, Wester PO. Morbidity and mortality in the Swedish Trial in old patients with hypertension (STOP-Hypertension). *Lancet* 1991;338:1281–1285.

26. MRC Working Party. Medical Research Council trial of treatment of hypertension in older adults: Principle results. *BMJ* 1992;304:405–412.

27. Staessen JA, Fagard R, Thijs L, Celis H, Arabidze G, Birkenhager WH, Bulpitt C, Leeuw P, Dollery CT, Fletcher A, Forette F, Leonetti G, Nachev C, O'Brien E, Rosenfeld J, Rodicio JL, Tuomilehto J. Randomized double-blind comparison of placebo and active treatment for older patients with isolated systolic hypertension. *Lancet* 1997;350:757–764.

28. Hebert PR, Moser M, Mayer J, et al. Recent evidence on drug therapy of mild to moderate hypertension and decreased risk of coronary heart disease. *Arch Intern Med* 1993;153:578–581.

29. Collins R, Peto R, MacMahon S, et al. Blood pressure, stroke, and coronary heart

disease, part 2: Short-term reductions in blood pressure: Overview of randomized drug trials I their epidemiological context. *Lancet* 1990;335:827–737.

30. The Sixth Report of the Joint National Committee on Prevention, Detection, Evaluation, and Treatment of High Blood Pressure. *Arch Intern Med* 1997;157:2413–2446.

31. McMahon S, Rodgers A. The epidemiological association between blood pressure and stroke: Implications for primary and secondary prevention. *Hypertens Res* 1994; 17(suppl 1):S23–32.

32. Gorelick PB, Sacco RL, Smith DB, Alberts M, et al. Prevention of a first stroke: A review of guidelines and a multidisciplinary consensus statement from the National Stroke Association. *JAMA* 1999;281:1112–1120.

33. Wolf PA, Abbott RD, Kannel WB. Atrial fibrillation as an independent risk factor for stroke: The Framingham Study. *Stroke* 1991;22:983–988.

34. Stroke Prevention in Atrial Fibrillation Investigators. Stroke Prevention in Atrial Fibrillation Study—Final Results. *Circulation* 1991;84:527–539.

35. Stroke Prevention in Atrial Fibrillation Investigators. Adjusted-dose warfarin versus low-intensity, fixed-dose warfarin plus aspirin for high-risk patients with atrial fibrillation: Stroke prevention in atrial fibrillation III: Randomised clinical trial. *Lancet* 1996;348:633–638.

36. Laupacis A, Albers G, Dalen J, Dunn MI, Jacobson AK, Singer DE. Antithrombotic therapy in atrial fibrillation. *Chest* 1998;114(suppl):579S–589S.

37. Benjamin EJ, Plehn JF, D'Agostino RB, Belanger AJ, Comai K, Fuller DL, Wolf PA, Levy D. Mitral annular calcification and the risk of stroke in an elderly cohort. *N Engl J Med* 1992;327:374–379.

38. Gilon D, Buonanno FS, Joffe MM, et al. Lack of evidence of an association between mitral valve prolapse and stroke in young patients. *N Engl J Med* 1999;341:8–13.

39. Freed LA, Lev D, Levine RA, et al. Prevalence and clinical outcome of mitral-valve prolapse. *N Engl J Med* 1999;341:1–7.

40. Balkau B, Shipley M, Jarrett RJ, Pyorala K, Pyorala M, Forhan A, Eschwege E. High blood glucose concentration is a risk factor for mortality in middle-aged non-diabetic men. 20-year follow-up in the Whitehall Study, the Paris Prospective Study, and the Helsinki Policemen Study. *Diabetes Care* 1998;21(3):360–367.

41. Wolf PA, D'Agostino RB, Belanger AJ, Kannel WB. Probability of stroke: A risk profile from the Framingham Study. *Stroke* 1991;22:312–318.

42. Barrett-Connor E, Khaw K. Diabetes mellitus: An independent risk factor for stroke. *Am J Epidemiol* 1988;128:116–124.

43. Kuller LH, Dorman JS, Wolf PA. Cerebrovascular diseases and diabetes. In: National Diabetes Data Group, Department of Health and Human Services, National Institutes of Health, ed. *Diabetes in America: Diabetes Data Compiled for 1984.* Bethesda, MD: National Institutes of Health, 1985:1–18.

44. Lindegard B, Hillbom M. Associations between brain infarction, diabetes, and alcoholism: Observations from the Gothenberg population cohort study. *Acta Neurol Scand* 1987;75:195–200.

45. Davis PH, Dambrosia JM, Schoenberg BS, Schoenberg DG, Pritchard A, Lilienfeld AM, Whisnant JP. Risk factors for ischemic stroke: A prospective study in Rochester, Minnesota. *Ann Neurol* 1987;22:319–327.

46. Burchfiel CM, Curb JD, Rodriguez BL, Abbott RD, Chiu D, Yano K. Glucose intolerance and 22-year stroke incidence: The Honolulu Heart Program. *Stroke* 1994; 25:951–957.

47. Wolf PA, Cobb JL, D'Agostino RB. Epidemiology of Stroke. In: Barnett HJM, Mohr JP, Stein BM, Yatsu RM, eds: *Stroke: Pathophysiology, Diagnosis, and Management.* New York: Churchill Livingstone, 1992:3–27.

48. Watkins PJ, Thomas PK. Diabetes mellitus and the nervous system. *Journal of Neurology, Neurosurgery and Psychiatry* 1998;65(5):620–632.

49. Abel GA, Sacco RL, Lin IF, et al. Race-ethnic variability in etiologic fraction for stroke risk factors: The Northern Manhattan Stroke Study. *Stroke* 1998;29:277 (abstract).

50. Effect of intensive diabetes management on macrovascular events and risk factors in the Diabetes Control and Complications Trial. Am J Cardiol. 1995;75:894–903.

51. UK Prospective Diabetes Study Group. Intensive blood-glucose control with sulphonylureas or insulin compared with conventional treatment and risk of complications in patients with type 2 diabetes: UKPDS 33. *Lancet* 1998;352:837–853.

52. Diabetes Control and Complications Trial Research Group. The effect of intensive treatment of diabetes on the development and progression of long-term complications in insulin-dependent diabetes mellitus. *N Engl J Med* 1993;329(14):977–986.

53. UK Prospective Diabetes Study Group. Tight blood pressure control and risk of macrovascular and microvascular complications in type 2 diabetes: UK PDS38. *BMJ* 1998;317:703–713.

54. American Diabetes Association. Clinical practice recommendations 1998. *Diabetes Care* 1998;21(suppl 1):S1–S89.

55. Salonen R, Sappanen K, Rauramaa R, Salonen JT. Prevalence of carotid atherosclerosis and serum lipids in Eastern Finland. *Atheroslcerosis* 1988;8:788–791.

56. Dempsey RJ, Diana LA, Moore LD. Thickness of carotid artery atherosclerotic plaque and ischemic risk. *Neurosurgery* 1990;27:343–348.

57. Heiss G, Sharrett AR, Barnes R, Chambless LE, Szklo M, Alzola C, and the ARIC Investigators. Carotid atherosclerosis measured by B-mode ultrasound in populations: Associations with cardiovascular risk factors in the AIRC Study. *Am J Epidemiol* 1991;134:250–256.

58. Fine-Edelstein JS, Wolf PA, O'Leary DH, Poehlman H, Belanger AJ, Kase CS, D'Agostino RB. Precursors of extracranial carotid atherosclerosis in the Framingham Study. *Neurology* 1994;44:1046–1050.

59. O'Leary D, Polak JF, Kronmal RA, Kittner SJ, Bond MG, Wolfson SK Jr, Bommer W, Price TR, Gardin JM, Savage PJ, on behalf of the CHS Collaborative Research Group. Distribution and correlates of sonographically detected carotid artery disease in the cardiovascular health study. *Stroke* 1992;23:1752–1760.

60. Sridharan R. Risk factors for ischemic stroke: A case control analysis. *Neuroepidemiology* 1992;11:24–30.

61. Qizilbash N, Jones L, Warlow C, Mann J. Fibrinogen and lipid concentrations are risk factors for transient ischemic attacks and minor ischemic strokes. *BMJ* 1991;303: 605–609.

62. Kargman DE, Tuck C, Berglund LF, Gu Q, Boden-Albala B, Gan R, Roberts K, Hauser WA, Shea SC, Paik M, Ginsberg H, Sacco RL. High density lipoprotein: A potentially modifiable stroke risk factor: The Northern Manhattan Stroke Study. *Neuroepidemiology* 1996;15:20S.

63. Kargman DE, Tuck C, Berglund LF, Boden-Albala B, Lin IF, Paik M, Sacco RL. Elevated high density lipoprotein levels are more important in atherosclerotic ischemic stroke subtypes: The Northern Manhattan Stroke Study. *Ann Neurol* 1998;44: 442–443.

64. Benfante R, Yano K, Hwang LJ, Curb JD, Kagan A, Ross W. Elevated serum cholesterol is a risk factor for both coronary heart disease and thromboembolic stroke in Hawaiian Japanese men: Implications of shared risk. *Stroke* 1994;25:814–820.

65. Iso H, Jacobs DR, Wentworth D, Neaton JD, Cohen JD. Serum cholesterol levels and six-year mortality from stroke in 350,977 men screened from the Multiple Risk Factor Intervention Trial. *N Engl J Med* 1989;320:904–910.

66. Qizilbash N, Duffy SW, Warlow C, Mann J. Lipids are risk factors for ischemic stroke—overview and review. *Cerebrovasc Dis* 1992;2:127–136.

67. Prospective Studies Collaboration. Cholesterol, diastolic blood pressure, and stroke: 13,000 strokes in 450,000 people in 45 prospective cohorts. *Lancet* 1995;346:1647–1653.

68. Scandinavian Simvastatin Survival Study Group. Randomized trial of cholesterol lowering in 4,444 patients with coronary heart disease: The Scandinavian Simvastatin Survival Study (4S). *Lancet* 1994;344:1383–1389.

69. Hebert PR, Gaziano JM, Chan KS, Hennekens CH. Cholesterol lowering with statin drugs, risk of stroke, and total mortality: An overview of randomized trials. *JAMA* 1997;278:313–321.

70. Blauw GJ, Lagaay AM, Smelt AHM, Westendorp RGJ. Stroke, statins, and cholesterol: A meta-analysis of randomized, placebo-controlled, double-blind trials with HMG-CoA reductase inhibitors. *Stroke* 1997;28:946–950.

71. Sacks FM, Pfeffer MA, Moye LA, et al, for the Cholesterol and Recurrent Events Trial Investigators. The effects of pravastatin on coronary events after myocardial infarction in patients with average cholesterol levels. *N Engl J Med* 1996;335:1001–1009.

72. The Long-Term Intervention with Pravastatin in Ischemic Disease (LIPID) Study Group. Prevention of cardiovascular events and death with pravastatin in patients with coronary heart disease and a broad range of initial cholesterol levels. *N Engl J Med* 1998;339:1349–1357.

73. Blakenhorn DH, Selzer RH, Crawford DW, Barth JD, Liu CR, Lui CH, Mack WJ, Alaupovic P. Beneficial effects of colestipol-niacin therapy on the common carotid artery: Two- and four-year reduction of intama-media thickness measured by ultrasound. *Circulation* 1993;88:20–28.

74. Furberg CD, Adams HP, Applegate WB, Byington RP, Espeland MA, Hartwell T, Hunninghake DB, Lefkowitz DS, Probstfield J, Riley WA, Young B, for the Asymptomatic Carotid Artery Progression Study (ACAPS) Research Group. Effects of lovastatin on early carotid atherosclerosis and cardiovascular events. *Circulation* 1994;90:1679–1687.

75. Crouse JR, Byington RP, Bond MA, Espeland MA, Craven TE, Sprinkle JW, McGovern ME, Furberg CD. Pravastatin, lipids, and atherosclerosis in the carotid arteries (PLAC-II). *Am J Cardiol* 1995;75:455–459.

76. Solonen R, Nyyssonen K, Porkkala E, et al. Kuopio Atherosclerosis Prevention Study (KAPS): A population-based primary prevention trial of the effect of LDL lowering on atherosclerotic progression in carotid and femoral arteries. *Circulation* 1995;92:1758–1764.

77. Hodis HN, Mack WJ, LaBree L, et al. Reduction in carotid arterial wall thickness using lovostatin and dietary therapy: A randomized, controlled clinical trial. *Ann Intern Med* 1996;124:548–556.

78. Summary of the National Cholesterol Education Program (NCEP) Adult Treatment Panel II Report. *JAMA* 1993;269:3015–3023.

79. Higa M, Davanipour Z. Smoking and stroke. *Neuroepidemiology* 1991;10:211–222.

80. Gorelick PB, Rodin MB, Langenberg P, et al: Weekly alcohol consumption, cigarette smoking, and the risk of ischemic stroke: Results of a case control study at three urban medical centers in Chicago, Illinois. *Neurology* 1989;39:339–343.

81. Abbott RD, Yin Yin MA, Reed DM, Yano K. Risk of stroke in male cigarette smokers. *N Engl J Med* 1986;315:717–720.

82. Colditz GA, Bonita R, Stampfer MJ, et al: Cigarette smoking and risk of stroke in middle-aged women. *N Engl J Med* 1988;318:937–941.

83. Shinton R, Beevers G. Meta-analysis of relation between cigarette smoking and stroke. *Br Med J* 1989;298:789–794.

84. Howard G, Wagenknecht LE, Burke GL, Diez-Roux A, Evans GW, McGovern P, Nieto FJ, Tell GS, for the ARIC Investigators. Cigarette smoking and progression of atherosclerosis. *JAMA* 1998;279:119–124.

85. Sacco RL, Roberts JK, Boden-Albala B, Gu Q, Lin IF, Kargman DE, Berglund L, Hauser WA, Shea S, Paik M. Race-ethnicity and determinants of carotic atherosclerosis in a multi-ethnic population: The Northern Manhattan Stroke Study. *Stroke* 1997;27:929–935.

86. Mast H, Thompson JLP, Hin IF, Hofmeister C, Hartmann A, Marx P, Mohr JP, Sacco RL. Cigarette smoking as a determinant of high-grade carotid artery stenosis in Hispanic, African American, and caucasian patients with stroke or TIA. *Stroke* 1998; 29:908–912.

87. Heiss G, Sharrett AR, Barnes R, Chambless LE, Szklo M, Alzola C, and the ARIC Investigators. Carotid atherosclerosis measured by b-mode ultrasound in populations: Associations with cardiovascular risk factors in the ARIC study. *Am J Epidemiol* 1991;134:250–256.

88. O'Leary D, Polak JF, Kronmal RA, Kittner SJ, Bond MG, Wolfson SK Jr, Bommer W, Price TR, Gardin JM, Savage PJ, on behalf of the CHS Collaborative Research Group. Distribution and correlates of sonographically detected carotid artery disease in the cardiovascular health study. *Stroke* 1992;23:1752–1760.

89. Wolf PA, D'Agostino RB, Kannel WB, Bonita R, Belanger AJ. Cigarette smoking as a risk factor for stroke: The Framingham Study. *JAMA* 1988;259:1025–1029.

90. Kamachi I, Colditz GA, Stampfer MJ, Willett WC, Manson JE, Rosner B, et al. Smoking cessation and decreased risk of stroke in women. *JAMA* 1993;269:232–236.

91. Gorelick PB. Stroke prevention: Windows of opportunity and failed expectations—a discussion of modifiable cardiovascular risk factors and a prevention proposal. *Neuroepidemiology* 1997;16:163–173.

92. Prevention Services Task Force. *Guide to Clinical Prevention Services: Report to the U.S. Preventive Services Task Force.* Baltimore, Md: Williams & Wilkins, 1996: xcii, 953.

93. Gorelick PB. The status of alcohol as a risk factor for stroke. *Stroke* 1989;20: 1607–1610.

94. Camargo CA. Moderate alcohol consumption and stroke—the epidemiologic evidence. *Stroke* 1989;20:1611–1626.

95. Donahue RP, Abbott RD, Reed DM, Yano K. Alcohol and hemorrhagic stroke: The Honolulu Heart Study. *JAMA* 1986;255:2311–2314.

96. Henrich JB, Horwitz RJ. Evidence against the association between alcohol use and ischemic stroke risk. *Arch Int Med* 1989;149:1413–1416.

97. Abu-Zeid HAH, Choi NW, Maini KK, Hsu P, Nelson NA. Relative role of factors associated with cerebral infarction and cerebral hemorrhage. A matched pair case-control study. *Stroke* 1977;8:106–112.

98. Ben-Shlomo Y, Markowe H, Shipley M, Marmot MG. Stroke risk from alcohol consumption using different control groups. *Stroke* 1992;23:1093–1098.
99. Beghi E, Bolium G, Cosso P, Fiorelli G, Lorini C, Mandelli M, Bellini A. Stroke and alcohol intake in a hospital population: A case-control study. *Stroke* 1995;26: 1691–1696.
100. Sacco RL, Elkind M, Boden-Albala B, Lin I-F, Kargman DE, Hauser WA, Shea S, Paik M. The protective effect of moderate alcohol consumption on ischemic stroke. *JAMA* 1999;281:53–60.
101. Stampfer MJ, Colditz GA, Willett WA, et al: A prospective study of moderate alcohol consumption and the risk of coronary disease and stroke in women. *N Engl J Med* 1988;319:267–273.
102. Tanaka H, Ueda Y, Hayashi M, et al: Risk factors for cerebral hemorrhage and cerebral infarction in a Japanese rural community. *Stroke* 1982;13:62–73.
103. Truelsen T, Gronbaek M, Schnohr P, Boysen G. Intake of beer, wine, and spirits and risk of stroke—the Copenhagen City Heart Study. *Stroke* 1998;29:2467–2472.
104. Harmsen P, Rosengren A, Tsipogianni A, Wilhelmsen L. Risk factors for stroke in middle-aged men in Goteborg, Sweden. *Stroke* 1990;21:223–229.
105. Kono S, Ikeda M, Tokudome S, Nishizumi M, Kuratsune M. Alcohol and mortality: A cohort study of male Japanese physicians. *In J Epidemiol* 1986;15:527–532.
106. NIH Consensus Development Panel on Physical Activity and Cardiovascular Health. Physical activity and cardiovascular health. *JAMA* 1996;276:241–246.
107. Fletcher GF. Exercise in the prevention of stroke. *Health Reports* 1994;6:106–110.
108. Abbott RD, Rodriguez BL, Burchfiel CM, Curb JD. Physical activity in older middle-aged men and reduced risk of stroke: The Honolulu Heart Program. *Am J Epidemiol* 1994;139:881–893.
109. Kiely DK, Wolf PA, Cupples LA, Beiser AS, Kannel WB. Physical activity and stroke risk: The Framingham Study. *Am J Epidemiol* 1994;140:608–620.
110. Haheim LL, Holme I, Hjermann I, Leren P. Risk factors of stroke incidence and mortality: A 12-year follow-up of the Oslo Study. *Stroke* 1993;24:1484–1489.
111. Gillum RF, Mussolino ME, Ingram DD. Physical activity and stroke incidence in women and men—the NHANES I Epidemiologic Follow-up Study. *Am J Epidemiol* 1996;143:860–869.
112. Sacco RL, Gan R, Boden-Albala B, Lin IF, Kargman DE, Hauser WA, Shea S, Paik M. Leisure-time physical activity and ischemic stroke risk: The Northern Manhattan Stroke Study. *Stroke* 1998;29:380–387.
113. Wannamethee G, Shaper AG. Physical activity and stroke in British middle aged men. *BMJ* 1992;304:597–601.
114. Manson JE, Stampfer MJ, Willett WC, Colditz GA, Speizer FE, Hannekens CH. Physical activity and incidence of coronary heart disease and stroke in women. *Circulation* 1995;91 (suppl):5.
115. Lee IM, Hennekens CH, Berger K, Buring JE, Manson JE. Exercise and risk of stroke in male physicians. *Stroke* 1999;30:1–6.
116. Williams PT. High-density lipoprotein cholesterol and other risk factors for coronary heart disease in female runners. *N Engl J Med* 1996;334:1298–1303.
117. Nygard O, Vollset SE, Refsum H, et al. Total plasma homocysteine and cardiovascular risk profile—the Hordaland Homocysteine Study. *JAMA* 1995;274:1526–1533.
118. US Department of Health and Human Services. *Physical Activity and Health: A Report of the Surgeon General.* Atlanta, GA: US Department of Health and Human Services, Center for Disease Control and Prevention, National Center Chronic Disease Prevention and Health Promotion, 1996.

119. Department of Health and Human Services. *Healthy People 2000: National Health Promotion and Disease Prevention Objectives*. Washington, DC: Department of Health and Human Services, 1991; DHHS publication no. (PHS) 91-50213.

120. Takeya Y, Popper JS, Schmimizu Y, Kato H, Rhoads GC, Kagan A. Epidemiologic studies of coronary heart disease and stroke in Japanese men living in Japan, Hawaii and California. *Stroke* 1984;15:15–23.

121. Gillman MW, Cupples A, Millen B, Ellison RC, Wolf P. Inverse association of dietary fat with development of ischemic stroke in men. *JAMA* 1997;278:2145–2150.

122. Stampfer J, Rose G, Stamler R, et al. INTERSALT study findings: Public health and medical care implications. *Hypertension* 1989;14:570–577.

123. Ueland PM, Refsum H, Brattstrom L. Plasma homocysteine and cardiovascular disease. In: Francis RB, Jr., ed. *Atherosclerotic cardiovascular disease, hemostatis, and endothelial function*. New York: Marcel Dekker, 1992:183–236.

124. Boushey CJ, Beresford SAA, Omenn GS, Motulsky AG. A quantitative assessment of plasma homocysteine as a risk factor for vascular disease: Probable benefits of increasing folic acid intakes. *JAMA* 1995;274:1049–1057.

125. Giles WH, Croft JB, Greenlund KJ, Ford ES, Kittner SJ. Total homocyst(e)ine concentration and the likelihood of nonfatal stroke—results from the third National Health and Nutrition Examination Survey, 1988–1994. *Stroke* 1998;29:2473–2477.

126. Sacco RL, Roberts JK, Jacobs BS. Homocysteine as a risk factor for ischemic stroke: An epidemiological story in evolution. *Neuroepidemiology* 1998;17:167–173.

127. Selhub J, Jaques PF, Bostom AG, D'Agostino RB, Wilson PWF, Belanger AJ, O'Leary DH, Wolf PA, Schaefer EJ, Rosenberg IH. Association between plasma homocysteine concentration and extracranial carotid-artery stenosis. *N Engl J Med* 1995;332:286–291.

128. Jacobs BS, Sacco RL, Lui RC, Boden-Albala, Benson R, Pablos-Mendez A. Low dietary intake of vitamin B6 is associated with an increased risk of ischemic stroke. *Stroke* 1999;30:252.

129. Gillman MW, Cupples LA, Posner B, Ellison RC, Castelli W, Wolf P. Protective effects of fruits and vegtables on development of stroke in men. *JAMA* 1995;273:1113–1117.

130. Gey KF, Stahelin HB, Eichholzer M. Poor plasma status of carotene and vitamin C is associated with higher mortality from ischemic heart disease and stroke. *Clin Invest Med* 1993;71:3–6.

131. Khaw KT, Barrett-Connor E. Dietary potassium and stroke-associated mortality. *N Engl J Med* 1987;316:235–240.

132. Benson RT, Jacobs B, Boden-Albala B, Lui RC, Borawski JB, Rosengart AJ, Sacco RL. Vitamin E intake: A primary prevention measure in stroke. *Neurology* 1999;52:A146.

133. Diaz MN, Frei B, Vita JA, Keaney JF. Antioxidants and atherosclerotic heart disease. *N Engl J Med* 1997;282:408–416.

134. Dietary vitamin C, beta-carotene and 30-year risk of stroke: Results from the Western Electric Study. *Neuroepidemiology* 1997;16:69–77.

135. Abbott RD, Curb D, Rodriguez BL, Sharp DS, Burchfiell CM, Yano K. Effect of dietary calcium and milk consumption on risk of thromboembolic stroke in older middle-aged men: The Honolulu Heart Study. *Stroke* 1996;27:813–818.

136. Orenica AJ, Daviglus ML, Dyer AR, Shekelle RB, Stamler J. Fish consumption and stroke in Men: 30 year findings of the Chicago Western Electric Study. *Stroke* 1996;27:204–209.

137. Morris M, Manson J, Rosner B, Buring J, Willett W, Hennekens C. Fish consumption and cardiovascular disease in the Physician's Health Study: A prospective study. *Am J Epidemiology* 1995;142:166–175.

138. North American Symptomatic Carotid Endarterectomy Trial Collaborators. Beneficial effect of carotid endareterectomy in symptomatic patients with high-grade stenosis. *N Engl J Med* 1991;325:445–453.

139. Norris JW, Zhu CZ, Bornstein NM, Chambers BR. Vascular risks of a symptomatic carotid stenosis. *Stroke* 1991;22:1485–1490.

140. Barnett HJM, Taylor DW, Eliasziw M, Fox AJ, Ferguson GG, Haynes RB, et al. Benefit of carotid endarterectomy in patients with symptomatic moderate or severe stenosis. *N Engl J Med* 1998;339:1415–1425.

141. Pujia A, Rubba P, Spencer MP. Prevalence of extracranial carotid artery disease detectable by echo-Doppler in an elderly population. *Stroke* 1992;23:818–822.

142. Executive Committee for the Asymptomatic Carotid Atherosclerosis Study. Endarterectomy for asymptomatic carotid artery stenosis. *JAMA* 1995;273:1421–1428.

143. Hankey GJ, Slattery JM, Warlow CP. The prognosis of hospital-referred transient ischaemic attacks. *J Neurol Neurosurg Psychiat* 1991;54:793–802.

144. Feinberg WM, Albers GW, Barnett HJM, et al. Guidelines for the management of transient ischemic attacks. From the Ad Hock Committee on Guidelines for the Management of Transient Ischemic Attacks of the Stroke Council of the American Heart Association. AHA Medical/Scientific Statement:Special Report. 1994;1320.

145. Albers GW, Easton JD, Sacco RL, Teal P. Antithrombotic and thrombolytic therapy for ischemic stroke. *Chest* 1998;114:683S–698S.

146. Antiplatelet Trialists' Collaboration. Collaborative overview of randomised trials of antiplatelet therapy I: Prevention of death, myocardial infarction, and stroke by prolonged antiplatelet therapy in various categories of patients. *Br Med J* 1994;308:81–106.

147. Gorelick PB. Stroke prevention: An opportunity for efficient utilization of health care resources during the coming decade. *Stroke* 1994;25(1):220–224.

3

ALCOHOL AND STROKE

Jean-Marc Orgogozo and Serge Renaud

The mortality rate from coronary heart disease (CHD) and stroke has declined consistently since the 1970s in most industrialized countries.[1–3] In the former socialist economies of eastern Europe, such as Bulgaria, Hungary, Czechoslovakia, Poland, and Russia, the death rate from both causes increased during the same period. This concordance of trends for these two diseases suggests common causes that may be sensitive to the same preventive measures. The most important of these measures include careful control of arterial hypertension, avoidance of smoking, and proper diet. The MONICA project of WHO, with more than 40 centers in 20 countries, has produced data on mortality and risk factors for both CHD and stroke[4] revealing a significant correlation between cerebrovascular and CHD mortality (Fig. 3.1). These findings raise the questions of which intrinsic factors are common to CHD and stroke and which factors represent environmental influences that can be modified, such as the effects of alcohol.

Dietary habits, with their marked geographical and cultural diversity among ethnic groups, are among the most important influences. Alcohol and wine consumption may have the greatest impact on stroke risk, both positively and negatively. The effects of moderate alcohol consumption on the risk of stroke are still debated, but strong evidence exists for a protective effect on stroke of mild to moderate consumption, particularly of wine. However, the risk of cerebral hemorrhage increased markedly with the consumption of alcoholic beverages.[5,6]

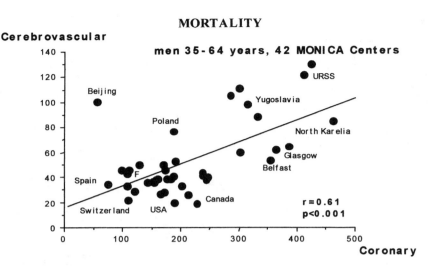

FIGURE 3.1. Relationship between cerebrovascular and coronary heart disease mortality in 42 MONICA centres. Adapted from WHO, World Health Statistics, 1989 (1994).

RELATION BETWEEN ALCOHOL CONSUMPTION AND CARDIOVASCULAR MORTALITY

Earlier studies of this relationship focused on deaths from ischemic heart disease, where the results favored a protective effect of moderate alcohol consumption.[7-13] A similar protective effect was later found for global mortality.[14-17] But some of the cohort studies found an increase in overall mortality proportional to alcohol consumption[18,19] beginning at rather low levels of consumption. These correlations tended to disappear after adjustment for major vascular risk factors (e.g., age, smoking, hypertension, hypercholesterolemia). Hypertension is induced by regular alcohol consumption,[20] but if separated from the rest of the analysis, the adverse relationship between alcohol and cardiovascular risk disappears, suggesting that alcohol-induced hypertension is the main determinant.[21]

Stroke mortality has been less well studied and was often included in global cardiovascular mortality. The first study specifically to address stroke mortality was one of *ecologic epidemiology* carried out by Saint-Léger and Cochrane in 1979.[22] They found a trend toward reduction of stroke mortality and a very significant reduction of cardiac mortality relating to wine consumption in the 18 countries they surveyed. The highly publicized paper by Renaud and de Lorgeril in 1992[23] on the "French Paradox," based on an ecologic survey of coronary heart disease mortality (but not specifically stroke) in 17 countries supported the finding that wine drinking exerts a dose-dependant protective effect on risk of stroke and CHD. These results were confirmed in a survey of 21 countries by Criqui and Ringel in 1994,[24] but the lower cardiovascular mortality associated with alcohol drinking, particularly wine, was partly counter-balanced by a proportional increase in the rate of fatal liver cirrhosis. Moreover, the only country with a lower CHD mortality than France was Japan, where the average wine consumption was extremely low at that time, a sort of "Japanese Paradox." Because ecologic epidemiology studies are sensitive to major confounders, they must be interpreted with caution.

The first large prospective study on alcohol drinking and mortality from various causes (Fig. 3.2)[15] found that alcohol consumption in the range of 10g per day decreased the risk of cerebrovascular mortality by approximately 20%, much less than for cardiovascular mortality. However, at a consumption of more than 25g of alcohol per day, the risk increased steadily, up to 50%–60%. The pattern of cerebrovascular response to alcohol drinking was very similar to that of mortality from all causes, that is, a J-shaped curve, while mortality from CHD continued to decrease with increasing amounts of alcohol, up to a certain threshold.[25] This upper limit was about 6 glasses a day in a study of 13,000 elderly male British physicians[17] and 2 glasses a day for women and 6 glasses a day for men in the 490,000 subjects enrolled in the Cancer Prevention Study II.[26] in Shang-

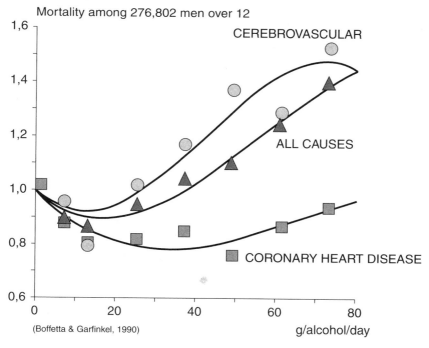

FIGURE 3.2. Mortality for cerebrovascular, coronary heart disease, and all causes in relation to the consumption of alcohol. Adapted from Boffetta and Garfinkel (1990).

hai, total mortality was reduced by 19% in 18,244 middle-aged men who consumed 1 to 14 drinks a week,[27] while those who consumed up to 28 drinks per week had a 36% reduction in CHD mortality. However, no reduction of stroke mortality was found at any level of alcohol consumption in this study.

In the Copenhagen Heart Study,[28] a follow-up for 10–12 years of 13,285 subjected aged 30 to 70 years showed that the incidence of cardiovascular mortality was reduced in proportion to the daily average consumption of wine, up to 3–5 glasses a day (RR = 0.51; 95% CI = 0.32–0.81), while no change in mortality was found in beer drinkers and an increased incidence was found at more than 2 glasses of spirits a day (RR = 1.34; 95% CI = 1.05–1.71). This study was the first to make a direct comparison of the effects of moderate wine consumption to that of beer and spirits. Earlier, Klatsky and Armstrong[29] had also shown some possible advantage of wine drinking against CHD mortality in the more then 123,000 subjects of the Kaiser Permanente study and later confirmed this finding for patients hospitalized for CHD.[30] Other studies showed the same protective effects for beer and spirits as for wine,[31] so that alcohol itself perhaps explains most of the protective role against CHD.

In an analysis of 30,014 men who volunteered for a health appraisal in Nancy, France, and were followed for 10–15 years,[32] a moderate intake of wine (2–5 glasses a day) was associated with a 24–30% reduction in all causes of death (RR = 0.70; 95% CI = 0.59–0.52 for 22–32g of alcohol per day; RR = 0.76; 95% CI = 0.66–0.87 for 33–54g/day). Heavy drinkers (more than 126g/day) had increased mortality compared to nondrinkers (RR = 1.37; 95% CI = 1.16–1.61).

Wine contains polyphenolic compounds, particularly flavonoids, gallic acid, and resveratrol, which may prevent ischemic cardiovascular diseases mainly through their antioxidant and antiaggregant properties.[33–37] This may explain the apparent superiority of wine drinking for cardiovascular protection in some studies, but healthier life styles in wine drinkers may explain at least part of this difference.[38] Binge drinking of beer increases the risk of fatal myocardial infarction.[39]

In summary, moderate consumption of alcoholic beverages is associated with a 20%–60% reduction in the risk of myocardial infarction and death. This was also observed after myocardial infarction in 5539 participants to the Physicians' Health Study,[40] and even recent consumption seems to have a protective effect.[41] Both these findings suggest that moderate alcohol consumption plays a role in the secondary prevention of large artery atherosclerotic disease.

RELATION BETWEEN DRINKING HABITS AND THE RISK OF STROKE

A number of studies have addressed specifically the relationship between alcohol (or wine) consumption and stroke. Early studies reported no association.[42,43] Accumulating evidence, however, suggests a global beneficial effect of moderate alcohol consumption against stroke, but the results are less impressive and less consistent than for ischemic heart disease. This might be due to the fact that fewer studies, with less subjects and less events per subjects, have addressed this point, thus yielding lower statistical power. Also, stroke is far less homogenous than myocardial infarction; in addition to the main dichotomy between ischemic and hemorrhagic strokes, ischemic strokes have subtypes that are possibly different in their response to alcohol. Also, stroke tends to occur much later in life than CHD, at an age at which the risk factors for atherosclerosis are no longer the same as for CHD.

Compared to studies of stroke mortality alone, studies of stroke mortality and morbidity are more informative because they help discriminate the different mechanisms of stroke and often allowed a more precise estimate of average alcohol consumption. In 1989[44] Camargo surveyed 62 studies published in English, and several others have been published since then, most to be found in the thorough reviews by Van Gijn et al. 1993[45] and Camargo in 1996.[46] The main studies are summarized below and/or presented in Tables 3.1 and 3.2.

TABLE 3.1. Relative Risks (or odds ratios—OR) of Stroke According to Alcohol Consumption in Epidemiology Studies; Case Control Studies, 1994–1999

STUDIES (YEAR) COUNTRY/SAMPLE NUMBER OF SUBJECTS[1]	ALCOHOL CONSUMPTION[1]	RELATIVE RISK OF STROKE (OR OR) (ADJUSTED VALUES WHENEVER AVAILABLE)		
		Ischemic	Hemorrhagic	All
Jamrozik et al[53]	Nondrinkers			1 (ref.)
(1994)	1–20 g/day			0.43
Australia	21–40			0.67
Population nested	41–60			0.55
N = 536/2620	>60			2.5
Caicoya et al[54]	Nondrinkers	1 (ref.)	1 (ref.)	1 (ref.)
(1999)	1–30 g/day	0.53	0.88	0.58
Spain	31–70	0.81	0.83	0.69
Population nested	71–140	1.16	0.56	0.80
N = 467/477	>140	5.05	6.24	3.22
		Men *Women*		*Men & Women*
Sacco et al[55]	Nondrinkers	1 (ref.) 1 (ref.)	NA[3]	1 (ref.)
(1999)	>1 drink/ month to	0.54 0.49		0.51
USA-Multiethnic	12 drinks/day[2]			
Ischemic strokes	3–4	0.72 0.23		0.58
N = 677/1139	≥5	1.33 5.35		1.63

[1]N/N: cases/controls.

[2]One standard glass = 10 to 12 grams of pure alcohol in most countries (Table 4).

[3]NA = not assessed.

TABLE 3.2. Relative Risk of Stroke (or Odds Ratios) of Stroke According to Alcoholic Consumption in Epidemiology Studies; Prospective Cohort Studies, 1986–1997

STUDIES (YEAR) COUNTRY/SAMPLE NUMBER OF SUBJECTS[1]	ALCOHOL CONSUMPTION[1]	RELATIVE RISK OF STROKE (OR OR) (ADJUSTED VALUES WHENEVER AVAILABLE)		
		Ischemic	Hemorrhagic	All
Stampfer et al.[67]	0	1 (ref.)	1 (ref.)	1 (ref.)
(1988), USA,	<1.5 g/day	0.7	2.4	0.9
women only,	1.5–4.9	0.4	2.9	0.6
N = 87,526	5.0–14.9	0.3	3.7	0.6
	15–25	0.5	2.6	0.5
	>25			1.2
Boffetta and	Nondrinkers			1 (ref.)
Garfinkel[15]	occasional			0.95
(1990), USA,	1 glass/day			0.8
men only,	2			0.98
N = 278,802	3			1.1
	4			1.3
	5			1.2
	6+			1.5
Klatsky et al.[68]	Nondrinkers	1 (ref.)	1 (ref.)	1 (ref.)
(1990), USA,	Ex-drinkers	0.9	1.4	1.0
N = 123,000	<1 glass/mouth	0.5	1.5	0.8
	<1 glass/day	0.5	1.6	0.8
	1–2 glasses/day	0.3	1.8	0.8
	3–5	0.4	1.3	0.7
	6+		4.7	1.4

Hansagi et al.[74]		Men Women	Men Women	Men Women
(1995), Sweden,	Nondrinkers	1 (ref.) 1 (ref.)	1 (ref.) 1 (ref.)	1 (ref.) 1 (ref.)
>42 years,	Ex-drinkers	1.5 3.3	0.9 —	1.2 2.3
N = 15,077	Occasional	2.0 0.6	0.8 0.7	1.7 0.6
	Binge/Intox.	1.5–1.8 0.6–1.0	0.8–0.9 0.6	1.3–1.5 0.4–0.8
	0–5 grams/day	1.3 0.6	0.8 0.7	1.2 0.6
	5–15	1.3 0.9	0.8 0.8	1.1 0.9
	>15	1.1 1.7	1.1 1.2	1.1 1.6

Wannamethee &	Never drinkers			1.8
Shaper[75] (1996),	Ex-drinkers			1.2
Great Britian,	Occasional			1 (ref.)
men only,	W-E: 1–2 drinks/day			0.7
N = 7,735	3–6			1.2
	>6			1.1
	Daily: 1–2			1.4
	3–6			1.0
	(heavy) >6			1.4
	Ex-heavy			1.3

(continued)

TABLE 3.2. continued

STUDIES (YEAR) COUNTRY/SAMPLE NUMBER OF SUBJECTS[1]	ALCOHOL CONSUMPTION[1]	RELATIVE RISK OF STROKE (OR OR) (ADJUSTED VALUES WHENEVER AVAILABLE)		
		Ischemic	Hemorrhagic	All
Camargo et al.[92] (1997), USA, male physicians, N = 22,071	<1 glass/week 1–6 >7			1 (ref.) 0.56 0.72
Thun et al.[26] (1997), USA, volunteers >30 years, N = 490,000	Glasses/day 0 <1 1 2–3 >4			stroke deaths 1 (ref.) 0.7 0.7 0.8 0.7
Truelsen et al.[73] (1998), Denmark, N = 13,329	Weekly units <1 1–7 (ref.) 8–14 15–21 22–41 ≥142	1.17 1 (ref.) 1.02 1.02 0.93 1.35		*Any* *Wine* 1.12 1 (ref.) 1 (ref.) 0.97 1.02 0.66 0.96 to 0.70 1.29

[1]N = number of subjects observed.

[2]One standard glass = 10 to 12 grams of pure alcohol in most countries (table 4).

The first case control studies, published in the 1980's, showed either a moderate increase in the risk of all strokes or no change in stroke risk associated with moderate alcohol consumption. For example, Herman et al.[47] analyzed the risk according to the level of alcohol intake and found no different between drinkers and nondrinkers at any lever.

Gill et al.[48,49] performed two studies based on the same 230 patients hospitalized consecutively for stroke, with 230 controls in the first study and 577 controls in the second, relating recent alcohol consumption and biological markers of chronic alcohol abuse with the occurrence of stroke. In the first comparison the controls were hospitalized in a surgery ward; they were randomized from a cohort of workers in the second. A standardized questionnaire was used to quantify alcohol consumption during the preceding months. After adjustment for high blood pressure, smoking, and anticoagulant treatment, the risk of stroke was halved (expressed as the odds ratio: OR = 0.5) in moderate drinkers (10–90g of alcohol a week) and increased (4-fold in the first study and 2-fold in the second) in heavy drinkers (more than 300g of alcohol a week). The ascending part of this J-shape curve was parallel to the levels of the main seric markers of heavy alcohol consumption but not to the mean red cell volume. These results were valid only for men, the number of women being too low in both studies. Unfortunately, only 20% of the cases had a computed tomography scan. A later study[50] found opposite differences in relative risk of stroke above 300g alcohol/week if the controls were medical patients (RR = 0.73) or people in the community (RR = 1.93), but none of the correlations was significant. This set of studies is quoted mainly to exemplify the sensitivity of case control studies to the choice of the controls: the resulting instability of results should be kept in mind for their interpretation.

Another interesting case control study[51] was based on 156 men less than 61 years of age admitted consecutively for an acute ischemic stroke, compared with 153 matched controls. Heavy drinking, defined as more than 300g of pure alcohol per week, was associated with a 4.45 higher relative risk of stroke compared to nondrinkers, with a large confidence interval (95% CI = 1.09–18.1). In light drinkers (up to 150 g/week) the risk, as assessed through odds ratio, was reduced by about half but also with a confidence interval that included unity (OR = 0.54; 95% CI = 0.28–1.05). No change in risk was found among moderate drinkers (150–300g/week). Due to the small sample size, these results would not have added much to already existing knowledge, except that on comparing regular drinkers (i.e., at least a drink 4 to 7 days a week) to irregular drinkers (i.e., 3 days a week or less), a much stronger negative association was found between light drinking and stroke in regular drinkers (OR = 0.12; 95% CI = 0.02–0.65) and a possible protection in moderate regular drinkers (OR = 055; NS), while intermittent drinking yielded no benefit.

Rodgers et al.[52] studied 364 cases of acute stroke compared with 364 community-based control subjects. The odds ratio for the risk of stroke for lifelong abstainers compared with subjects who had ever drunk regularly, particularly women (but not current heavy drinkers) was 2.36 (95% CI = 1.67–3.37). No relation was found between stroke and current nondrinkers (i.e., ex-drinkers). Hence, regular moderate drinking seems to be the most protective behavior.

A nested case control study was conducted on a population-based registry by Jamrozik et al.[53] in Australia. Of 536 strokes, each was matched for age and sex with up to 5 controls from the same geographic area. The usual drinking habits of the subjects were estimated from reported consumption during the preceding week. With univariate analysis, the main finding was a significantly lower incidence of all strokes (OR = 0.43; 05% CI = 0.32–0.58), of ischemic strokes, and of primary hemorrhage strokes associated with a consumption of 1–20g of alcohol per day during the previous week. Average consumptions of 21–40 and 41–60g per day were also associated with an apparent less marked risk reduction (OR = 0.67 and 0.55, respectively, NS), while consumption of more than

60g per day was associated with a 2.51 increase in risk of all strokes (95% CI = 1.33–4.74), rising to 6.71 (95% CI = 1.68–26.8) for first-ever strokes and to 5.88 (95% CI = 1.19–29.1) for cerebral hemorrhage (Table 1).

In Spain, Caicoya et al.[54] performed a careful analysis of risk factors in a consecutive series of strokes. Despite its relatively small size (cases = 467, controls = 477), this was the first study on alcohol to analyse separately cortical versus deep strokes and to find a similar pattern of correlation for the two categories. This suggests that an effect on large artery atherosclerosis may not be in the main determinant of the observed protection. This study was also one of the few to find a lower risk of hemorrhagic strokes associated with mild to moderate alcohol consumption (Table 3.1).

The latest, and so far the largest, case control study was conducted in northern Manhattan[55] on 667 cases of ischemic stroke in men and women of various ethnic groups compared with 1139 matched community controls. The results showed that an average consumption of up to 2 drinks a day, and even of 3 to 4 drinks a day of any alcoholic beverage, was associated with a significantly lower risk of ischemic stroke after adjustment for cardiac disease, hypertension, diabetes, current smoking, body mass index, and education (Table 3.1). This effect was observed in both sexes, at all ages, and in all ethnic groups. At excessive levels of consumption (7 or more drinks/day) there was an apparent increased risk.

Some earlier and smaller anecdotal series of case control studies[6,56,57] suggested an increased risk of hemorrhagic stroke with heavy alcohol consumption (acute or chronic), which might explain at least part of the net increase in stroke risk observed in alcohol abusers in some early studies. Studies on case series of "binge" drinking indicated that this behavior is associated with an increased risk of ischemic stroke, in particular "the next morning."[58–61] This has not been verified in formal epidemiology studies so far.[62] In young subjects, the risk is increased by a concomitant consumption of cigarettes.[61] Hypercoagulability induced by high blood alcohol content[56] or a rebound of hypercoagulability at withdrawal after temporary drinking[63] could explain this pattern of stroke occurrence, as well as cardiac sudden deaths in the same context.[64]

More important from the point of view of possible causality are the prospective epidemiologic cohort studies, which are less susceptible to biases and yield, in general, more reliable estimates of the correlations than case control studies. They therefore produce more convincing evidence of an association between drinking patterns and stroke, even if this evidence remains observational. A number of such studies reported results for all strokes. Among those controlling for confounding factors,[65–68] all found an elevated relative risk in the highest alcohol consumption categories, but the upper limits were open-ended in these studies, and no consistent definition of heavy drinking was established. So it is possible that the observed modest increase of risk for all stroke was due entirely to the excessive drinkers, who are at particular risk of cerebral hemorrhage. This was confirmed in most studies that separately analyzed ischemic and hemorrhagic strokes (Tables 3.2 and 3.3).

The Honolulu Heart Program[69] followed for 12 years a cohort of 8006 men of Japanese ancestry. Alcohol consumption was recorded at baseline and classified in four categories: none, mild (10–390g/month), moderate (420–1090g/month), and heavy (more than 1100g/month). The diagnosis of ischemic stroke was made clinically, but when there was suspicion of hemorrhage, radiologic examinations were made. Globally, no significant relation was found between alcohol consumption and ischemic strokes, but the relative risk of hemorrhagic stroke was 2.2 in mild drinkers, 2.9 in moderate drinkers, and 4.7 in heavy drinkers, com-

TABLE 3.3. Relative Risk of Stroke (or Odds Ratios) of Stroke According to Alcohol Consumption in Prospective Epidemiology Studies in Asians

STUDIES (YEAR) COUNTRY/SAMPLE NUMBER OF SUBJECTS[1]	ALCOHOL CONSUMPTION[1]	RELATIVE RISK OF STROKE			
		Ischemic		Hemorrhagic	All
Donahue et al.[69]	Nondrinker			1 (ref.)	1 (ref.)
(1986),	<1 glass*/day			2.3	1.2
Honolulu,	1–3			2.5	1.3
Japanese men,	>3			2.9	1.5
N = 8008					
Kono et al.[65]	Nondrinker			1 (ref.)	1 (ref.)
(1986), Japan,	Ex-drinker			1.0	2.3
men only	Occasional			1.2	1.1
(physicians),	<3.6 glasses/day			0.9	1.2
N = 5135	>3.6			1.6	1.7
		NHT[3]	*HT*[3]	*NHT*[3] *HT*[3]	NA[4]
Kiyohara et al.	Nondrinkers	1.05	1.39	1 1	
(1995), Japan,	1–33 g/day	1	1	1.37 2.06	
Age ≥ 40,	≥34 g/day	1.40	1.96	1.69 3.13	
N = 1621					
Yuan et al.[27]					(stroke deaths)
(1997), China,	0 glasses/week				1.0
men only,	1–28				1.02
45–64 years,	>29				1.65
N = 18,244					

[1]N = number of subjects observed.

[2]One standard glass = 10 to 12 grams of pure alcohol in most countries.

[3]NHT = non hypertensives; HT = hypertensives.

[4]NA = not available.

pared to nondrinkers. This increase of hemorrhagic risk was larger for sub-arachnoid hemorrhages (RR = 5.8) than for intracerebral hemorrhages (RR = 3.9). After adjustment, the authors concluded that these results were independent of high blood pressure, suggesting that a direct and causal relation existed between alcohol consumption and the risk of intracranial hemorrhage. Another analysis was performed later[70] on the 2946 men who were not lost at the end of 1988 and had reported a stable alcohol intake during the periods 1965 to 1968 and 1971 to 1974. A trend was found for lower rate of occurrence of fatal and nonfatal coronary heart disease with increasing alcohol consumption in all age subgroups but, differing from most previously published data, an insignificant but almost linear trend was found for higher risk of stroke events with increasing alcohol consumption in middle aged (51–64-year-old) men and a similar higher risk trend for light (1–14ml alcohol/day) and moderate (15–39ml/day) drinkers in elderly men (65 years and older). This was not found in elderly heavy drinkers (40ml/day and more). In all subgroups, the numbers of subjects and events were small.

In the Nurses Health Study, Stampfer et al.[67] analyzed data on 85,526 nurses aged 34–59, who were followed for four years. Their weekly alcohol consumption was recorded initially through a self-questionnaire of main dietary habits that had been earlier validated in a sample of 170 nurses. Even though only 66 ischemic and 28 hemorrhagic strokes occurred during the follow-up, the statistical calculations, with adjustment for vascular risk factors such as smoking, hypertension, age, and diabetes, showed that the risk of ischemic stroke was reduced by $\frac{2}{3}$ by mild alcohol consumption (between 5 and 14g/day) and halved by moderate consumption (15g or more/day). By contrast, the risk of meningeal hemorrhage was fourfold higher in the moderate drinkers, but overall a lower risk of all strokes was associated with moderate consumption (Table 3.2) since hemorrhagic strokes are much rarer than ischemic strokes in this age group.

This effect may not be present in all countries. Researchers in Japan found no reduction of stroke incidence in beer and spirit drinkers at any level of consumption.[71] In this study, stroke risk increased at any level of consumption in hypertensive patients, mainly due to an excess of cerebral hemorrhage.

In the first Copenhagen Heart Study,[72] an analysis was made of first stroke occurrence during 12 years of follow-up of 12,971 subjects aged 35 years and over in whom life-style risk factors had been recorded initially. A tendency was found for daily "moderate to heavy" alcohol intake to be associated with lower risk of stroke (OR = 0.86, NS), which was significant (OR = 0.79, 95% CI: 0.65–0.97) only in the subgroup of cigarette smokers, a group at much higher risk of stroke. With longer follow-up[73] a reduction of stroke incidence was associated only with moderate wine consumption and not with beer or spirit consumption. In 13,329 subjects of both sexes aged 45 to 84 years followed for 16 years, 833 first-ever strokes occurred that were related to various known risk factors and to average alcohol consumption. The reduction of stroke incidence was 33% to 41%, depending on the adjustments, in weekly wine drinkers and slightly less in daily wine drinkers (Table 3.2). Further studies in Europe have confirmed this lower risk of stroke in moderate drinkers but these studies did not discriminate between wine and other drinkers.[74,75]

The results of both case control and prospective epidemiologic studies can be summarized as follows: the risk of hemorrhagic stroke increases at least linearly, and possibly exponentially, as a function of alcohol consumption, independently of high blood pressure (which itself can be induced by chronic alcoholism). The relation between alcohol consumption and ischemic stroke is more complex: mild to moderate consumption is associated with a definite risk reduction in most studies, but heavy consumption is either associated with no change or with an increased risk (quadratic effect). This differs from myocardial infarction studies, in which the risk reduction is proportional to the daily amount ingested, including at levels qualifying as unsafe drinking and alcoholism.[29]

A likely explanation for the J- (or U-) shaped curve relationship between alcohol consumption and all strokes is that mild to moderate consumption decreases the risk of ischemic stroke without increasing the risk of cerebral hemorrhage, while at higher levels of consumption alcohol induced hemorrhages outnumber the ischemic strokes prevented. In other words, the risk/benefit balance is positive for light to moderate levels of consumption and becomes negative at a point above which the total number of strokes increases. What is not precisely known is the optimal level of consumption, at which the net risk reduction is maximum ("healthy drinking"). It is estimated to be between 1 and 4 glasses a day, and the point above which risk increases (the limit of "safe drinking") is estimated to be between 3 and 6 standard glasses a day. Because some alcohol-induced pathologies, such as liver cirrhosis[76] and digestive tract cancer, can be increased above a consumption of 3 standard glasses a day,[77] it is important to carefully weigh recommendations about what exactly are "healthy" and "safe" drinking. It may appear to vary in different countries because the definitions of standard units also differ (Table 3.4).

In the cohort of elderly British male doctors,[12] mortality from all causes and from ischemic heart disease were minimal at daily consumption of 2 and 3 standard glasses a day, respectively. An increase of alcohol deaths was observed above 4 glasses a day and an increase of deaths from all causes well above 6 glasses a day. This cohort comprised over 12,000 long-term survivors of about 40,000 men recruited in their early 50's, and initially enrolled to assess the hazards of cigarette smoking. The age range was 60 to 90 years; in men of this age group the main cause of mortality is cardiovascular, and censoring age groups below 60 largely eliminates most types of alcohol related mortality.

In young male military recruits in Sweden,[78] a linear increase was found in death rates from all causes (mostly accidents, violence, and suicide) with increasing alcohol consumption. In the Cancer Prevention Study II,[26] in which sub-

TABLE 3.4. Correspondance Between Standard Units (Drinks or Glasses) and Amount of Pure Alcohol in Various Countries

COUNTRY	STANDARD UNITS (IN GRAMS)	COUNTRY	STANDARD UNITS (IN GRAMS)
Australia	10 g	Italy	10 g
Canada	13.5 g	Japan	19.75 g
Denmark	12 g	Netherlands	9.9 g
Finland	11 g	New Zealand	10 g
France	12 g	Portugal	14 g
Hungary	17 g	Spain	10 g
Iceland	9.5 g	UK	8 g
Ireland	8 g	USA	12–14 g

jects were enrolled from age 30 and above, a 30% increase of breast cancer was found during the 9 years of follow-up in women having at least one drink daily (RR = 1.3, 95% CI = 1.1–1.6). However, mild alcohol consumption was globally associated with a substantial reduction in deaths due to all cardiovascular diseases and with a small reduction in overall mortality in middle-aged men and women. Mortality from all causes increased in heavy drinkers, particularly in those below 60 years of age without cardiovascular risk factors. In the middle-aged men of the Nancy study,[32] an increased risk of mortality (+37%) appeared only above an average consumption of 128g per day (10 French glasses), with a majority wine drinkers (70%). More direct evidence in favor of wine came from a study in Denmark[79] in which wine drinkers tended to have *less* cancers of the upper digestive tract, while even a moderate intake of beer or spirits increased this risk considerably.

By and large, almost all studies reporting potential benefits of moderate alcohol consumption on health and mortality indicate that these benefits are restricted to older subjects and that they increase with increasing age, at least in established market economies.[80] This should be viewed in conjunction with the recent observation that in people above 65 years of age, regular consumption of 3 to 4 glasses of wine a day is also associated with a marked reduction in the incidence of dementia and Alzheimer's disease.[81,82]

MECHANISMS OF THE EFFECTS OF ALCOHOL AND WINE ON STROKE

For a biological explanation of the effects of alcohol on atherosclerosis and on the hemostatic system that is relevant to the pathophysiology of the various types of ischemic and hemorrhagic stroke, the following observations have been made:[83]

1. A significant relationship exists between alcohol consumption and seric levels of HDL2 cholesterol, the main protective type against atherosclerosis, and also HDL3;[1,84–88] in addition, ethanol decreases the level of LDL cholesterol ("bad" cholesterol) when it is high.[89–91] This has been questioned in other studies.[92,93]

2. Ethanol stimulates liver microsomial oxidases, hence increasing synthesis of apolipoproteins A1 and A2, which contribute to the HDL levels.[94,95]

3. Ethanol has an antiplatelet effect, as evidenced by in vitro studies[96–101] and by a significant prolongation of bleeding time in volunteers.[102] The antiplatelet effect of alcohol is correlated with its protective effect against CHD.[23] However, this effect is only short lasting, and a rebound of platelet activation occurs one or two hours after an acute ingestion of alcohol[103] and after withdrawal in chronic alcoholics.[63] This rebound effect could be due to an increase in lipidic perodixides.[104] In vitro, ethanol enhances the anti-aggregating effect of both aspirin and prostacyclin in a dose-dependent manner.[105–107] In vivo, it potentiates the prolongation of bleeding time induced by aspirin.[108] In human studies, a relation was found between reported alcohol consumption and an increased fibronolytic activity in plasma,[109–112] with plasma t-PA production[113,114] a major factor of fibrinolytic in vivo, and also with urokinase-like plasminogen activator.[115]

Possible explanations for the difference between the effect of wine and of other alcoholic beverages in relation to cerebrovascular mortality seem to imply platelets. While an intake of alcohol is associated, within minutes, with a decrease in platelet aggregability,[97] it is followed hours later by a rebound effect, that is by an increased response of platelets to aggregation,[63] especially after an episode of drunkenness,[103] which can also be responsible for cardiac sudden death and ischemic stroke. It has been shown that the increased platelet aggregability following alcohol withdrawal is not observed after wine drinking, especially red wine.[116] This protection could be due to the antioxidant effects of the tannins (polyphenols) contained in wine.

CONCLUSION

Although cerebrovascular diseases present similarities with CHD, the effect of alcohol and wine drinking does not appear to be identical on both conditions. One possible reason is that stroke tends to occur later in life than CHD, at a time when high cholesterol no longer increases vascular risk, which may reduce the preventive effects of alcohol and wine on stroke due to large artery atherosclerosis. But the main difference is probably due to the opposite effects of alcohol on ischemic and hemorrhagic stroke. The risk reduction of ischemic stroke associated with mild to moderate consumption, particularly of wine, appears sim-

ilar to that found for myocardial infarction. On the contrary, the risk of intracranial hemorrhage increases linearly, and possibly exponentially, in proportion to
average alcohol consumption. This observation is consistent with the antithrombotic effects of alcohol, which may be beneficial at low doses but are definitely
harmful at high doses. The apparent risk reduction of ischemic stroke *observed*
in most prospective epidemiologic studies of healthy subjects (Table 3.2) is larger
than that *demonstrated* with any antiplatelet drug in trials of secondary prevention,[117] and no antiplatelet has ever worked in primary prevention. The very impressive relative stroke risk of 0.2 (an 80% reduction!) observed in moderate
drinkers versus nondrinkers in the SPAF I-III trials for patients with atrial fibrillation receiving aspirin for primary prevention[2] corresponds to a larger risk reduction than that achieved with anticoagulants in interventional studies.

A notable exception to these favorable observations concerns Asians, in whom
all studies have failed to show a reduced incidence of stroke mortality in moderate drinkers in Japan[65] and China[27] and in overall strokes in Honolulu,[69,70]
Japan,[71] and Taiwan.[118] Instead, most of these studies reported an increased risk
of stroke at high levels of consumption (Table 3.3), confirming earlier findings
from Japan.[119,120] This may be due to the higher proportion of hemorrhagic strokes
in Asians,[27,121] to their know higher prevalence of relative deficiency of the liver
aldehyde dehydrogenase,[122,123] a key enzyme for the degradation of alcohol, or to
both. In addition, the consumption of grape wine in Japan and China was almost
nil at the time of these studies.[27,71] So recommendations in favor of drinking alcohol or wine for health purposes in these populations may be particularly ill-advised.

Can it be concluded that moderate drinking is a valuable preventive measure
against ischemic stroke, at least in Caucasians? The weight of evidence is certainly in favor of a true protective effect, but its real magnitude cannot be measured precisely or even estimated because of the *observational,* not *experimental,*
nature of the available clinical evidence. Therefore, the influence of confounders
(biases) cannot be ruled out. In addition, the relation between alcohol and car-
dio vascular diseases is complex, and the following important issues remain to
be investigated before any inference as to the prevention of ischemic stroke can
be made:

1. The ratio between potential benefits and risks in younger subjects, especially women, at low risk of cardiovascular disease and even lower risk of
   ischemic stroke, but who may be at risk of intracranial hemorrhage, liver
   cirrhosis, and cancer and who may develop drinking problems.
2. The effects on subtypes of arterial vascular disease, e.g., large artery atherosclerosis[124] versus lacunar infarctions due to arteriolosclerosis.[54]
3. Confirmation of the apparently more positive effects of wine drinking, particularly red wine, compared to other alcoholic beverages,[73] which has been
   challenged.

4. The role of confounding socioeconomic,[125] health behaviour,[126] cultural, and dietary factors[38] on this apparent protection.

For instance, a study in Denmark found that wine drinking was associated with healthier dietary habits,[127] while, on the contrary, wine drinking was correlated with a high saturated fat diet in a study in Spain.[128] New analytical epidemiologic studies of prospective cohorts, including women and younger age groups, and assessment of potential confounders in more detail are necessary to resolve these questions. Randomized trials of primary or secondary prevention by moderate alcohol or wine consumption, the ultimate proof, may prove difficult, but not impossible, to accomplish. However, the weight of the epidemiologic and experimental data, which identified credible mechanisms by which alcohol and some constituents of red wine can be protective against ischemic cardiovascular disease, are strongly suggestive of a potential protection against the common types of ischemic stroke. The time has not yet come to recommend moderate and regular alcohol consumption for the primary or secondary prevention of stroke, but sufficient evidence exists to advise responsible moderate drinkers in the middle-aged and elderly groups not to change their habits.[81]

REFERENCES

1. Gaziano JM, Buring JE, Breslow JL, et al. Moderate alcohol intake, increased levels of high density lipoprotein and its subfractions, and decreased risk of myocardial infarction. *New Engl J Med* 1993;329:1829–1834.
2. Hart RG, Pearce LA, McBride R, et al., on behalf of the Stroke Prevention in Atrial Fibrillation (SPAF) Investigators. Factors associated with ischemic stroke during aspirin therapy in atrial fibrillation: Analysis of 2012 participants in the SPAF I-III clinical trials. *Stroke* 1999;30:1223–1229.
3. Thom TJ, Epstein FH. Heart disease, cancer and stroke mortality trends and their interrelations. An international perspective. *Circulation* 1994;90:574–582.
4. World Health Organization. *World Health Statistics Annual.* Geneva: World Health Organization, 1994.
5. Weisberg LA. Alcoholic intracerebral hemorrhage. *Stroke* 1988;19:1565–1569.
6. Montforte R, Estruch R, Graus F. High ethanol consumption as risk factor of intracerebral hemorrhage in young and middle-aged people. *Stroke* 1990;21:1529–1532.
7. Stason WB, Neff RK, Miettinen OS, et al. Alcohol consumption nonfatal myocardial infarction. *Am J Epidemiol* 1976;104:603–608.
8. Hennekens CH, Rosner B, Cole DS. Daily alcohol consumption and fatal coronary heart disease. *Am J Epidemiol* 1978;107:196–200.
9. Dyer AR, Stamler J, Paul O. Alcohol consumption and 17-year mortality in the Chicago Western Electric Company Study. *Prev Med* 1980;9:78–90.
10. Gordon T, Kannel WB. Drinking habits and cardiovascular disease: The Framingham Study. *Am Heart J* 1983;105:667–673.
11. Colditz GA, Branch LG, Lipnick RJ, et al. Moderate alcohol and decreased cardiovascular mortality in an elderly cohort. *Am Heart J* 1985;109:886–889.

12. Friedman LA, Kimball AW. Coronary heart disease mortality and alcohol consumption in Framingham. *Am J Epidemiol* 1987;124:481–489.
13. Moore RD, Pearson TA. Moderate alcohol consumption and coronary artery disease: A review. *Medicine* 1986;65:242–267.
14. Poikolainen K. Alcohol and mortality: A review. *J Clin Epidemiol* 1995;48:455–465.
15. Boffetta P, Garfinkel L. Alcohol drinking and mortality among men enrolled in an American Cancer Society prospective study. *Epidemiology* 1990;1:342–348.
16. Klatsky AL, Armstrong MA, Friedman GD. Alcohol and mortality. *Ann Intern Med* 1992;117:646–654.
17. Doll R, Peto R, Hall E, et al. Mortality in relation to consumption of alcohol: 13 years' observations on male British doctors. *BMJ* 1994;309:911–918.
18. Blackwelder WC, Yano K, Roads GG. Alcohol and mortality: The Honolulu Heart Study. *Am J Med* 1980;68:164–169.
19. Kozarevic DJ, Vojvodic N, Dawber T. Frequency of alcohol consumption and morbidity and mortality: The Yugoslavia Cardiovascular Disease Study. *Lancet* 1980; 1:613–616.
20. Witteman JCM, Willett WC, Stampfer MJ, et al. The relation of moderate alcohol consumption and increased risk of hypertension in women. *Am J Cardiol* 1990; 65:633–637.
21. Taylor JR, Coomes T, Anderson D, et al. Alcohol, hypertension and stroke. *Alcohol Clin Exp Res* 1984;3:283–286.
22. Saint-Léger AS, Cochrane AL, Moore W. Factors associated with cardiac mortality in developed countries with particular reference to the consumption of wine. *Lancet* 1979;1:1017–1020.
23. Renaud S, De Lorgeril M. Wine, alcohol, platelets, and the French paradox for coronary heart disease. *Lancet* 1992;339:1523–1526.
24. Criqui MH, Ringel BL. Does diet or alcohol explain the French paradox? *Lancet* 1994;344:1719–1723.
25. Rimm EB, Giovannucci EL, Willett WC, et al. Prospective study of alcohol consumption and risk of coronary disease in men. *Lancet* 1991;338:464–468.
26. Thun MJ, Peto R, Lopez AD, et al. Alcohol consumption and mortality among middle-aged and elderly U.S. adults. *N Engl J Med* 1997;337:1705–1714.
27. Yuan JM, Ross RK, Gao YT, et al. Follow up study of moderate alcohol intake and mortality among middle aged men in Shangai, China. *BMJ* 1997;314:18–23.
28. Gronbaeck M, Deis A, Sorensen TIA, et al. Mortality associated with moderate intakes of wine, beer or spirits, *BMJ* 1995;310:1165–1169.
29. Klatsky AL, Amstrong MA, Friedman GD. Relations of alcoholic beverage use to subsequent coronary artery disease hospitalization. *Am J Cardiol* 1986;58:710–714.
30. Klatsky AL. Red wine, white wine, liquor, beer and risk for coronary artery disease hospitalization. *Am J Cardiol* 1997;80:416–419.
31. Rimm EB, Klatsky A, Grobbee D, et al. Review of moderate alcohol consumption and reduced risk of coronary heart disease: Is the effect due to beer, wine or spirits. *BMJ* 1996;312:731–736.
32. Renaud SC, Gueguen R, Schenker J, et al. Alcohol and mortality in middle-aged men from eastern France. *Epidemiology* 1998;9(2):184–188.
33. Hertog MG, Feskens EJ, Hollman PC, et al. Dietary antioxidant flavonoids and risk of coronary heart disease. *Lancet* 1993;342:1007–1011.
34. Frankel EN, Kanner J, German JB, et al. Inhibition of oxidation of human low-density lipoprotein by phenolic substances in red wine. *Lancet* 1993;341:454–457.

35. Frankel EN, Waterhouse AL, Kinsella JE. Inhibition of human LDL oxidation by resveratrol. *Lancet* 1993;341:1103–1104.
36. Pace-Asciak CR, Hahn S, Diamandis P, et al. The red wine phenolics trans-resveratrol and quercetin block human platelet aggregation and eicosanoid synthesis: Implication for protection against coronary heart disease. *Clin Chim Acta* 1995;235: 207–219.
37. Teissedre PL, Frankel EN, Waterhouse AL, et al. Inhibition of in vitro human LDL oxidation by phenolic antioxidants from grapes and wines. *J Sci Food Chem* 1996; 70:55–61.
38. Rimm EB. Alcohol consumption and coronary heart disease: Good habits may be more important than just good wine. *Am J Epidemiol* 1996;143:1094–1098.
39. Kauhanen J, Caplan GA, Goldberg DE, et al. Beer binging and mortality: Results from the Kuopio ischemic heart disease risk factor study, a prospective population based study. *BMJ* 1997;315:846–851.
40. Muntwyler J, Hennekens CH, Buring JE, et al. Mortality and light to moderate alcohol consumption after myocardial infarction. *Lancet* 1998;352:1882–1885.
41. Jackson R, Scragg R, Beaglehole R. Does recent alcohol consumption reduce the risk of acute myocardial infarction and coronary death in regular drinkers? *Am J Epidemiol* 1992;819–824.
42. Klatsky AL, Friedman GD, Siegelaub AB. Alcohol and mortality: A ten-year Kaiser Permanente experience. *Ann Intern Med* 1981;95:139–145.
43. Paganini-Hill A, Ross RK, Henderson BE. Postmenopausal oestrogen treatment and stroke: A prospective study. *BMJ* 1988;297:519–522.
44. Camargo CA. Moderate alcohol consumption and stroke: The epidemiologic evidence. *Stroke* 1989;20:1611–1626.
45. Van Gijn J, Stampfer MJ, Wolfe C, et al. The association between alcohol and stroke. In: Verschuren PM, ed. *Health Issues Related to Alcohol Consumption*. Ilsi Press, 1993:43–79.
46. Camargo CA. Case-control and cohort studies of moderate alcohol consumption and stroke. *Clin Chim* 1996;246:107–119.
47. Herman B, Shmitz PIM, Leyten ACM. Multivariate logistic analysis of risk factors for stroke in Tilburg, The Netherlands. *Am J Epidemiol* 1983;118:514–525.
48. Gill JS, Zezulka V, Shipley MI, et al. Stroke and alcohol consumption. *N Engl J Med* 1986;315:1041–1046.
49. Gill JS, Shipley MJ, Gill SK, et al. A community case-control study of alcohol consumption in stroke. *Int J Epidemiol* 1988;3:542–547.
50. Ben-Shlomo Y, Markovwe H, Shipley M, et al. Stroke risk from alcohol consumption using different control groups. *Stroke* 1991;1093–1098.
51. Palomäki H, Kaste M. Regular light-to-moderate intake of alcohol and the risk of ischemic stroke: Is there a benefit? *Stroke* 1993;24:1828–1832.
52. Rodgers H, Aitken PD, French JM, et al. Alcohol and stroke: A case-control study of drinking habits past and present. *Stroke* 1993;24:1473–1477.
53. Jamrozik K, Phil D, Broadhurst J, et al. The role of lifestyle factors in the etiology of stroke: A population-based case-control study in Perth, Western Australia. *Stroke* 1994;25:51–59.
54. Caicoya M, Rodriguez T, Corrales C, et al. Alcohol and stroke: A community case-control study in Asturias, Spain. *J Clin Epidemiol* 1999;52:677–684.
55. Sacco RL, Elkind M, Boden-Albala B, et al. The protective effect of moderate alcohol consumption on ischemic stroke. *JAMA* 1999;281:53–60.

56. Hillbom M, Kaste M. Alcohol intoxication: A risk factor for primary subarachnoid hemorrhage. *Neurology* 1982;32:706–711.
57. Calandre L, Arnal C, Fernandez Ortega J. Risk factors for spontaneous hematomas: Case-control study. *Stroke* 1986;17:1126–1128.
58. Hillbom M, Kaste M. Ethanol intoxication: A risk factor for ischemic brain infarction. *Stroke* 1983;14:694–698.
59. Lindegard B, Hillbom M. Associations between brain infarction, diabetes and alcoholism: Observations from the Gothenburg population cohort study. *Acta Neurol Scand* 1987;75:195–200.
60. Hillbom M, Kaste M. Alcohol abuse and brain infarction. *Ann Med* 1990; 22:347–352.
61. Hillbom M, Haapaniemi H, Juvela S, et al. Recent alcohol consumption, cigarette smoking, and cerebral infarction in young adults. *Stroke* 1995;26:40–45.
62. Gorelick PB, Redin MB, Langenberg P, et al. Is acute alcohol ingestion a risk factor for ischemic stroke? Results of a controlled study in middle-aged and elderly stroke patients at three urban centers. *Stroke* 1987;18:359–364.
63. Fink R, Hutton RA. Changes in the blood platelets of alcoholics during alcohol withdrawal. *J Clin Pathol* 1983;36:337–340.
64. Peterson B. Analysis of the role of alcohol in mortality, particularly sudden unwitnessed death, in middle-aged men in Malmö, Sweden. *Alcohol* 1988;23:259–263.
65. Kono S, Ikeda M, Tokudome S, et al. Alcohol and mortality: A cohort study of male Japanese physicians. *Int J Epidemiol* 1986;15:527–532.
66. Boysen G, Nyboe J, Appleyard M, et al. Stroke incidence and risk factors for stroke in Copenhagen, Denmark. *Stroke* 1988;19:1345–1353.
67. Stampfer MJ, Colditz GA, Willet WC, et al. A prospective study of moderate alcohol consumption and the risk of coronary disease and stroke in women. *N Engl J Med* 1988;319:267–273.
68. Klatsky AL, Armstrong MA, Friedman GD. Risk of cardiovascular mortality in alcohol drinkers, ex-drinkers and non-drinkers. *Am J Cardiol* 1990;l66:1237–1242.
69. Donahue RP, Abbott RD, Reed DM, et al. Alcohol and hemorrhage stroke: The Honolulu Heart Program. *JAMA* 1986;255:2311–2314.
70. Goldberg RJ, Burchfield CM, Reed DM, et al. A prospective study of the health effects of alcohol consumption in middle-aged and elderly men: The Honolulu Program. *Circulation* 1994;89:651–659.
71. Kiyohara Y, Kato I, Iwamoto H, et al. The impact of alcohol and hypertension on stroke incidence in a general Japanese population: The Hisayama Study. *Stroke* 1995;26:368–372.
72. Lindenstrom E, Boysen G, Nyboe J. Risk factors for stroke in Copenhagen, Denmark. *Neuroepidemiology* 1993;12:37–42.
73. Truelsen T, Gronbaek M, Schnohr P, et al. For the Copenhagen City Heart Study. Intake of beer, wine and spirits and risk of stroke. *Stroke* 1998;29:2467–2472.
74. Hansagi H, Romelsjo A, Gerhardsson de Verdier M, et al. Alcohol consumption and stroke mortality: 20-year follow-up of 15,077 men and women. *Stroke* 1995;26(10): 1768–1773.
75. Wannamethee SG, Shaper AG. Patterns of alcohol intake and risk of stroke in middle-aged British men. *Stroke* 1996;27:1033–1039.
76. Norton R, Batey R, Dwyer T, et al. Alcohol consumption and the risk of alcohol related cirrhosis in women. *BMJ* 1987;295:80–82.
77. Popham RE, Schmidt W. The biomedical definition of safe alcohol consumption: A crucial issue for the researcher of the drinker. *Br J Addict* 1978;73:233–235.

78. Andreasson S, Allebeck P, Rosmelsjö A. Alcohol and mortality among young men: Longitudinal study of Swedish conscripts. *BMJ* 1998;226:1021–1025.
79. Gronbaek M, Becker U, Johansen D, et al. Population based cohort study of the association between alcohol intake and cancer of the upper digestive tract. *BMJ* 1998; 317:844–847.
80. Murray CJ, Lopez AD. Global mortality, disability, and the contribution of risk factors: Global burden of disease study. *Lancet* 1997;349:1436–1442.
81. Orgogozo JM, Dartigues FJ, Lafon S, et al. Wine consumption and dementia in the elderly: A prospective community study in the Brodeaux area. *Rev Neurol* 1997: 153(3):185–192.
82. Lemeshow S, Letenneur L, Dartigues JF, et al. Illustration of analysis taking into account complex survey considerations: The association between wine consumption and dementia in the PAQUID study. *Am J Epidemiol* 1998;148:298–306.
83. Hillbom M, Numminen H. Alcohol and stroke: Pathophysiologic mechanisms. *Neuroepidemiology* 1998;17:281–287.
84. Fraser GE, Anderson JT, Foster N, et al. The effect of alcohol on serum high density lipoprotein (HDL). *Atherosclerosis* 1983;46:275–286.
85. Thornton J, Symes C, Heaton K. Moderate alcohol intake reduces bile cholesterol saturation and raises HDL cholesterol. *Lancet* 1983;1:819–821.
86. Taskinen RM, Nikkilä EA, Välimäki M, et al. Alcohol-induced changes in serum lipoproteins and their metabolism. *Am Heart J* 1987;113:458–464.
87. Contaldo F, D'Arrigo E, Carandente V, et al. Short-term effects of moderate alcohol consumption on lipid metabolism and energy balance in normal men. *Metabolism* 1989;38:166–171.
88. Suh I, Shaten BJ, Cutler JA, et al. Alcohol use and mortality from coronary heart disease: The role of high-density lipoprotein cholesterol: The Multiple Risk Factor Intervention Trial Research Group. *Ann Intern Med* 1992;116:881–887.
89. Castelli WP, Doyle JT, Gorden T, et al. Alcohol and blood lipids: The Cooperative Lipoprotein Phenotyping Study. *Lancet* 1977;2:153–155.
90. Masarei JRL, Puddey IB, Rouse IL, et al. Effects of alcohol consumption on serum lipoprotein: Lipid and apolipoprotein concentrations. Results from an intervention study in healthy subjects. *Atherosclerosis* 1986;60:79–87.
91. Suzukawa M, Ishikawa T, Yoshida H, et al. Effects of alcohol consumption on antioxidant content and susceptibility of low-density-lipoprotein to oxidative modification. *J Am Coll Nutr* 1994;13:237–242.
92. Camargo CA Jr, Hennekens CH, Gaziano JM, et al. Prospective study of moderate alcohol consumption and mortality in US male physicians. *Arch Intern Med* 1997; 157:79–85.
93. Enas AE. Alcohol and cardiovascular mortality in US physicians: Is there a modifier effect by low-density lipoprotein? *Arch Intern Med* 1997;157:1769–1770.
94. Camargo CA, Williams PT, Vranizan KM, et al. The effect of moderate alcohol intake on serum apolipoproteins AI and AII: A controlled study. *JAMA* 1985;253:2854–2857.
95. Branchi A, Rovellini A, Tornella C, et al. Association of alcohol consumption with HDL subpopulations defined by apolipoprotein A-I and apolipoproteins I and apolipoproteins A-II content. *Eur J Clin Nutr* 1997;51:362–365.
96. Davis JW, Philips PE. The effect of ethanol on human platelet aggregation in vitro. *Atherosclerosis* 1970;11:473–477.
97. Haut MJ, Cowan DH. The effect of ethanol on hemostatic properties of human blood platelets. *Am J Med* 1974;56:22–33.

98. Fenn CG, Littleton JM. Inhibition of platelet aggregation by ethanol in vitro shows specificity for aggregating agent used and is influenced by platelet lipid composition. *Thromb Haemost* 1982;48:49–53.

99. Rand ML, Packham MA, Kinlouigh-Rathbone RL, et al. Effects of ethanol on pathways of platelet aggregation in vitro. *Thromb Haemost* 1988;59:383–387.

100. Rubin R. Ethanol interferes with collagen-induced platelet activation by inhibition of arachidonic acid mobilization? *Arch Biochem Biophys* 1989;270:99–113.

101. Benistant C, Rubin R. Ethanol inhibits thrombin-induced secretion by human platelets at a site distinct from phospholipase C or protein kinase C. *Biochem J* 1990; 269–289.

102. Elmer O, Göransson G, and Zoucas E. Impairment of primary hemostasis and platelet function after alcohol ingestion in man. *Hemostasis* 1984;14:223–228.

103. Hillbom M, Kangasaho M, Kaste M, et al. Acute ethanol ingestion increases platelet reactivity: Is there a relationship to stroke? *Stroke* 1985;16:19–23.

104. Cederbaum AI. Introduction: Role of lipid peroxidation and oxidative stress in alcohol toxicity. *Free Rad Biol Med* 1989;7:537–539.

105. Landolfi R, Steiner M. Ethanol raises prostacyclin in vivo and in vitro. *Blood* 1984;64:679–682.

106. Mehta P, Mehta J, Lawson D, et al. Ethanol stimulates prostacyclin biosynthesis by human neutrophils and potentiates anti-platelet aggregatory effects of prostacyclin. *Thromb Res* 1987;48:653–661.

107. Jakubovski JA, Vaillancourt R, Deykin D. Interaction of ethanol, prostacyclin, and aspirin in determining human platelet reactivity in vitro. *Arteriosclerosis* 1988;8: 436–441.

108. Deykin D, Janson P, McMahon I. Ethanol potentiation of aspirin-induced prolongation of the bleeding time. *N Engl J Med* 1982;306:852–854.

109. Meade TW, Chakrabarti R, Haines AP, et al. Characteristics affecting fibrinolytic activity and plasma fibrinogen concentrations. *BMJ* 1979;1:153–156.

110. Pikaar NA, Wedel M, van der Beek EJ, et al. Effects of moderate alcohol consumption on platelet aggregation, fibrinolysis and blood lipids. *Metabolism* 1987;6:538–543.

111. Smokovitis A, Kokolis N, Ploumis T. Enhancement of plasminogen activator activity in the gastric wall after chronic ethanol consumption. *Alcohol* 1991;8:17–20.

112. Hendriks HFJ, Veenstra J, Velthuis-te Wierick EJM, et al. Effect of moderate dose of alcohol with evening meal on fibronolytics factors. *BMJ* 1994;308:1003–1006.

113. Laug WE. Ethyl alcohol enhances plasminogen activator secretion by endothelial cells. *JAMA* 1983;250:772–776.

114. Ridker PM, Vanghan DE, Stampfer MJ, et al. Association of moderate alcohol consumption and plasma concentration of endogenous tissue-type plasminogen activator. *JAMA* 1994;272:929–933.

115. Sumi H, Hamada H, Tsushima H, et al. Urokinase-like plasminogen activator increased in plasma after alcohol drinking. *Alchol* 1988;23:33–43.

116. Ruf JC, Berger JL, Renaud S. Platelet rebound effect of alcohol withdrawal and wine drinking in rats: Relation to tanins and lipid peroxidation. *Arterioscler Thromb Vasc Biol* 1995;1:140–144.

117. Antiplatelet Trialist's Collaboration. Collaborative overview of randomized trials of antiplatelet therapy. I: Prevention of death, myocardial infarction and stroke by prolonged antiplatelet therapy in various categories of patients. *BMJ* 1994;308:81–106.

118. Lee TK, Huang ZS, Ng SK, et al. Impact of alcohol consumption and cigarette smoking on stroke among the elderly in Taiwan. *Stroke* 1995;26:790–794.

119. Okada H, Horibe H, Ohno Y, Hayakawa N, and Aoki N. A prospective study of cerebrovascular disease in Japanese rural communities: Akabane and Asahi, part I: Evaluation of risk factors in the occurrence of cerebral hemorrhage and thrombosis. *Stroke* 1976;7:599–607.
120. Tanaka H, Ueda Y, Hayashi M, Date C, Baba T, Yamashita H, Shoji H, Tanaka Y, Owada K, and Detels R. Risk factors for cerebral hemorrhage and cerebral infarction in a Japanese rural community. *Stroke* 1982;13:62–73.
121. Ueda K. Hasuo Y, Kiyohara Y, et al. Intracerebral hemorrhage in a Japanese community, Hisayama: Incidence, changing pattern during long-term follow-up, and related factors. *Stroke* 1982;13:62–73.
122. Ohmori T, Koyama T, Chen CC, et al. The role of aldehyde dehydrogenase isozyme variance in alcohol sensitivity, drinking habits formation and the development of alcoholism in Japan, Taiwan and the Philippines. *Prog Neuropsychopharmacol Biol Psychiatr* 1986;10:229–235.
123. Chen CCC, Hwu HG, Yeh EK, et al. Aldehyde dehydrogenase deficiency, flush patterns and prevalence of alcoholism: An interethnic comparison. *Acta Med Okayama* 1991;45:409–416.
124. Bogousslavsky J, Van Melle G, Despland PA, et al. Alcohol consumption and carotid atherosclerosis in the Lausanne Stroke Registry. *Stroke* 1990;21:715–720.
125. Wannamethee SG and Shaper AG. Socioeconomic status within social class and mortality: A prospective study in middle-aged British men. *Int J Epidemiol* 1997:26: 532–541.
126. Pekkanen J, Tuomilheto J, Uutela A, et al. Social class, health behaviour and mortality among men and women in eastern Finland. *BMJ* 1995;311:589–593.
127. Tjonneland A, Gronbaek M, Stripp C, et al. Wine intake and diet in a random sample of 48763 Danish men and women. *Am J Nutr* 1999;69:49–54.
128. Artalejo FR, Guallar-Castillon P, Gautierrez F, et al. Socio-economic level, sedentary lifestyle, and wine consumption as possible explanations for geographic distribution of cerebrovascular disease in Spain. *Stroke* 1997;28:922–928.

4

LIPIDS AND STROKE

E. John Nasrallah and Harold P. Adams, Jr.

After making remarkable advances in preventing and curing infectious diseases that killed millions of people, modern medicine now is attacking the chronic diseases that have become more prominent as life expectancy has increased. Heart disease and stroke rank first and second, respectively, as causes of death in the world.[1] Annually, approximately 750,000 Americans have a stroke or recurrent stroke, and 150,000 of these persons die.[2] During the last 30 years, the incidence of and mortality from stroke declined in the United States, Canada, Australia, and Western Europe.[3] These declines probably were, in part, secondary to improved treatment of hypertension. However, other countries of the world have not seen a decrease in the frequency of stroke, and rates have increased in eastern Europe. Now, the declines in North America and Europe have stopped, and the number of persons who are having strokes is increasing around the world. The number of strokes will grow considerably during the next 50 years simply as a result of the increasing age of the population.[4] The economic consequences of stroke are huge in terms of both health care costs and losses in productivity. In costs of human suffering, the effects of stroke are even greater. Thus, measures to prevent stroke have huge implications for society. A number of factors that increase the risk of stroke have been identified, and measures to control these factors have the potential to lessen the likelihood of a potentially disabling or fatal brain injury. This chapter examines one of the modifiable risk factors for ischemic stroke—elevated serum cholesterol. Recently, Gorelick estimated that up to 100,000 strokes could be avoided annually in the United States if hypercholesterolemia were treated better.[5]

Certain recurrent themes are worth noting at the outset. Although atherosclerosis is the major underlying arterial disease leading to ischemic stroke, the magnitude of the association between a high serum cholesterol value and stroke is much weaker than that between an elevated cholesterol level and coronary artery disease. Part of the problem in confirming a strong relationship between hypercholesterolemia and stroke relates to the heterogenous nature of stroke. In addition, a low level of serum cholesterol increases the risk of hemorrhagic stroke, whereas hypercholesterolemia probably increases the risk of ischemic stroke. Still, despite the apparent weakness of a cause-and effect relationship, evidence is mounting that the 3-hydroxy-3-methylyglutaryl (HMG) coenzyme A (CoA) reductase inhibitors are effective in lowering the overall risk of ischemic stroke without a concomitant increase in intracranial hemorrhage.

The term *stroke* encompasses a number of vascular diseases of the brain. Because of the heterogenous nature of stroke, some of the associations between risk factors and cerebrovascular events are not as clear as for heart disease. Approximately 80% of strokes involve an arterial occlusion leading to a focal area of infarction (ischemic stroke), while the remaining strokes are due to a rupture of an intracranial vessel (hemorrhagic stroke). Some conditions that predispose to brain hemorrhage differ from those that increase the risk of ischemic stroke. For example, vascular malformations, aneurysms, and bleeding diatheses are etiologies of intracranial hemorrhage, while ischemic stroke can be secondary to a large number of vascular diseases, including embolism from the heart, prothrombotic states, nonatherosclerotic vasculopathies, and atherosclerosis. In addition, rather than a solitary disease, ischemic stroke should be considered a symptom of a vascular occlusive process that may result from a diverse range of underlying causes.

ATHEROSCLEROSIS AND STROKE

Despite the large number of causes of stroke, atherosclerosis is recognized as the leading cause of brain ischemia.[6] Atherosclerosis preferentially affects both major intracranial and extracranial arteries and also involves deep penetrating vessels that perfuse the brain. The most common sites for involvement include the middle portion of the basilar artery, the origin and distal segment of the vertebral artery, the proximal segment of the middle cerebral artery, the intracranial portion of the internal carotid artery, and the origin of the internal carotid artery at the bifurcation. The latter is the most common location. The sites for severe atherosclerosis differ among ethnic groups. The origin of the internal carotid artery is the most common site for persons of European ancestry, while the intracranial arteries are more commonly implicated in persons of African or Asian background.[7–9] A reappraisal of small vessel (lacunar) disease indicates that the underlying pathology usually is an atheroma rather than lipohyalinosis. Atherosclerotic disease of the aorta and its major brachiocephalic branches is being increasingly recognized as a frequent cause of stroke in the elderly. Advanced aortic atherosclerosis is also an important risk factor for cerebral ischemia as a complication of major cardiovascular procedures. Atherosclerotic coronary artery disease indirectly leads to stroke. Cerebral embolism is a complication of acute myocardial infarction, especially when the anterior wall is affected. Ischemic heart disease leads to atrial fibrillation, a well-known risk factor for cardioembolic stroke. Long-standing ischemic heart disease also leads to embolism from an intracardiac thrombus that develops in an akinetic ventricular segment or from an ischemic cardiomyopathy.

Atherosclerosis is an arterial disease that evolves over a lifetime. The first changes of atherosclerosis can be found in youths and young adults. The disease gradually progresses over an individual's life to become symptomatic and the cause of an ischemic stroke. Two major theories for the development and maturation of atherosclerosis have been advanced—the lipid hypothesis and the injury–healing hypothesis.[6] The lipid hypothesis postulates that an elevated blood level of cholesterol can initiate the atherosclerotic process by accumulating in endothelial cells. The injury–healing hypothesis proposes that the initial event is a disruption to the vascular endothelium by any number of potential assailants, including mechanical shear stress, toxins, homocysteine, viruses, and immunologic mediators. Rather than two independent processes, the lipid and injury–healing mechanisms probably are synergistic.

THE GENESIS OF THE ATHEROMATOUS PLAQUE

The first stage in the formation of an atheroma is the development of a fatty streak characterized by the adhesion of monocytes to the endothelium and their subsequent migration to subendothelial portions of the arterial wall. The monocytes become tissue macrophages that develop a foamy appearance by accumulating intracellular lipids. Fatty streaks appear in the aorta and other major arteries as early as late childhood or adolescence. Subsequently, some fatty streaks, especially those located at vascular bifurcations or sites of turbulence, develop into fibrous plaques. These plaques usually are seen in middle-aged or older adults. The fibrous cap of the plaque consists of foam cells, transformed smooth muscle cells, lymphocytes, and a connective tissue matrix. The core of the plaque includes cellular debris, free extracellular lipid, and cholesterol crystals. An intact endothelial lining covers the luminal surface of the plaque. The plaque insidiously enlarges over decades, secondary to the elaboration of cytokines and growth factors released by endothelial cells, platelets, macrophages, and smooth muscle cells. These factors promote migration of smooth muscle cells from the adventitial surface of the artery. The smooth muscle cells accumulate in the intimal-medial portions of the artery. Areas of calcification can occur in the plaque. Growth of the plaque leads to constriction of the vascular lumen (arterial stenosis), which, in turn, leads to diminution of flow and turbulence of the circulating blood. The turbulence and sluggish flow promote activation of platelets and clotting factors, which, in turn, promote thrombosis or growth of the arterial lesion.

Subsequently, an unstable atheromatous plaque can become acutely symptomatic by developing discontinuities of the endothelial surface (ulceration), by fracturing of the fibrous cap, or by incipient intraplaque hemorrhage.[10,11] Both ulceration and rupture result in acute clot formation by exposing the highly thrombogenic subendothelial surface. Pieces of atherosclerotic debris (cholesterol embolism) can be released from a complex, highly ulcerated plaque and embolize to distal vascular beds. The intramural hemorrhage can cause sudden arterial occlusion, while the fracture of the plaque disrupts the endothelium and leads to thrombosis.

Fracture (or rupture) of an atherosclerotic plaque is now recognized as a leading cause of acute coronary artery thrombosis and myocardial infarction. Based on a pathological evaluation of carotid endarterectomy specimens, Carr et al.[12] found that symptomatic patients had significantly higher rates of plaque rupture, thinning of the fibrous cap, infiltration of the fibrous cap with foam cells, and intraplaque fibrin deposition than did asymptomatic patients. They concluded that fracture of the atherosclerotic plaque could be as important in promoting thrombosis of the carotid artery as it is in thrombosis of the coronary arteries.

THE COURSE OF ATHEROSCLEROSIS

Atherosclerotic disease becomes symptomatic in different vascular territories at different ages. In general, coronary artery disease becomes symptomatic approximately one decade before the appearance of symptoms of cerebrovascular atherosclerosis. This clinical phenomenon is confirmed by post-mortem studies that show that the aorta and coronary arteries are involved before the peripheral and cerebrovascular arteries. Recent evidence suggests that advanced atherosclerotic disease of the aorta is a significant cause of stroke.[13] Thus, stroke secondary to atherosclerosis can occur even when the cerebrovascular arteries do not show advanced changes.

The course of atherosclerosis is not uniform between persons. Some individuals have accelerated atherosclerosis while others may never have symptoms from the arterial disease despite living to an advanced age. Epidemiologic studies have identified several factors that accelerate the course of atherosclerosis. Some factors that predict advanced atherosclerosis are not modifiable, including age, sex, ethnicity, and family history. Atherosclerosis is more common in older persons, men, African Americans, and among those who have first-degree relatives who have had coronary artery disease or stroke. Inherited disorders, such as familial hyperlipoproteinemia, also may be implicated. Other conditions that can be controlled or treated, such as arterial hypertension, diabetes mellitus, and smoking, also promote atherosclerosis and ischemic stroke. Some conditions, such as hypertension and smoking, are potent risk factors for several types of stroke, including intracranial hemorrhage. On the other hand, until recently, the role of elevated blood lipids, or cholesterol, on the frequency of stroke was less clear. Now, recent data have clarified the critical importance of elevated levels of cholesterol in promoting premature cerebrovascular atherosclerosis.

INTERACTIONS BETWEEN CHOLESTEROL AND ATHEROSCLEROSIS

Elevated serum cholesterol has been recognized as a potent risk factor for myocardial infarction.[14–17] Below the age of 60, the incidence of coronary artery disease increases dramatically with rising levels of total serum cholesterol. A majority of persons who have a myocardial infarction before the age of 60 have abnormalities of serum lipids. For example, Genest et al.[18] studied levels of lipoproteins in men with a mean age of 50 with angiographically documented coronary artery disease; levels of total cholesterol, low density lipoprotein (LDL) cholesterol, and apolipoprotein B were significantly increased compared to controls. An elevated level of cholesterol or LDL now is recognized as the single most important forecaster of premature coronary artery disease. The Lyon Diet Heart Study found that each 1 mmol/L increase in total cholesterol was associated with an 18% to 28% increase in the risk of recurrent myocardial ischemia.[19]

The definition of elevated serum total cholesterol that portends an increased risk of ischemic events has changed; in the past, a total serum cholesterol greater than 6.20 mmol/L (240 mg/dl) was considered high. Now, a level above 5.17 mmol/L (200 mg/dl) is considered as elevated. Although it is a potent risk factor for myocardial infarction in men or women under the age of 60, above this age the relationship between ischemic heart disease and total serum cholesterol wanes. However, the association between abnormalities of lipoprotein subfractions, particularly, low concentrations of high-density lipoprotein (HDL) cholesterol, and coronary artery disease persists among older persons. Aronow[20] noted a relationship for new coronary events and high serum total cholesterol and triglyceride levels and low HDL cholesterol in older women.

Because lipids are insoluble in blood, they are incorporated into protein-lipid complexes called lipoproteins. A lipoprotein consists of a core of lipid surrounded by a coat of proteins, cholesterol, and phospholipids. The lipoproteins include chylomicrons, very low-density lipoprotein (VLDL) cholesterol, LDL cholesterol, and HDL cholesterol. Each lipoprotein subfraction has a specific function in the overall system of cholesterol and lipid metabolism. Because cholesterol must be packaged in these lipoproteins to be transported in the blood, the measured "total" cholesterol represents the sum of the cholesterol contained in each of the subfractions. Since each of the different lipoproteins plays distinct roles in cholesterol transport and accumulation in tissues versus removal from tissues, measurement of the proportions of lipoproteins is the most specific way to assess the risk for vascular disease.

Chylomicrons serve as the vehicle of transport of dietary triglycerides and cholesterol from the intestine to the liver. The chylomicrons are modified and taken up by the liver cells. Cholesterol delivery from the liver to other tissues is accomplished by VLDL cholesterol that is changed by intravascular enzymes into LDL cholesterol. LDL cholesterol is the predominant lipoprotein in the blood and accounts for approximately two-thirds of the total cholesterol level. Cells, including those in the arterial wall, bind LDL cholesterol, and it is subsequently oxidized by macrophages. Oxidized LDL cholesterol enters the endothelium and promotes the accumulation of foam cells in the arterial wall. Hypercholesterolemia is associated with endothelial cell dysfunction and arterial stiffness.[21] Oxidized LDL cholesterol also can promote vasoconstriction by reducing the stores of nitric oxide in the endothelium. HDL cholesterol is the smallest lipoprotein. Its role as a protectant against atherosclerosis may relate to its property of transporting lipids from peripheral sources in the body to the liver, where the cholesterol can be metabolized. HDL cholesterol also protects LDL cholesterol from oxidation and thus limits the deleterious actions of the oxidized form of LDL cholesterol. HDL cholesterol also helps arterial constriction by activating endothelial production of prostacyclin.

ROLE OF LIPOPROTEINS

Lipoprotein α is a variant of LDL cholesterol,[22] and its role in the development of atherosclerosis is controversial. Some studies suggest that elevations of lipoprotein α are associated with an increased risk of coronary artery disease,[15,18,23,24] but there is no evidence that this is a potent risk factor for either atherosclerosis or thrombosis. At present, the atherogenic role of lipoprotein α appears to be most closely related to concentrations of LDL cholesterol.

A number of lipoprotein abnormalities lead to elevation of blood lipids. Some are inherited while others are secondary to medication or acquired diseases. Familial hypercholesterolemia, in particular type II-a hyperlipoproteinemia, is implicated as an important risk factor for premature coronary artery atherosclerosis.[25,26] Among the medications that lead to hyperlipidemia are diuretics, beta-blockers, and androgens. Estrogens can lower blood lipids by reducing lipoproteins. Obesity, diets high in saturated fats and cholesterol, physical inactivity, alcohol consumption, diabetes mellitus, liver disease, and renal disease also promote elevations of cholesterol or lipoproteins. Lipid disorders that are characteristic of non–insulin dependent diabetes mellitus (low HDL cholesterol, high LDL cholesterol, high triglycerides, and high apolipoprotein β levels) are predictive of cardiovascular events among this group of patients.[27,28] Both total cholesterol and HDL cholesterol levels change with advancing age and may be part of the natural aging process.[29]

ROLE OF CHOLESTEROL

Elevated LDL cholesterol correlates with increased risk of coronary artery disease, while elevated HDL cholesterol appears to be cardioprotective.[30] A serum LDL cholesterol level >3.30 mmol/L (130 mg/dl) is generally considered too high, while a serum HDL cholesterol <0.87 mmol/L (35 mg/dl) is usually considered too low. The ratio of total cholesterol to HDL cholesterol is the best predictor of and correlates with the risk of coronary artery disease for persons up to the age of 80; the desired ratio is >1:5. For example, the risk of heart disease is increased by a factor of 1.6 among men and 1.8 among women aged 75–79 when the ratio is <1:4. Still, the predictive value of total cholesterol or the lipoprotein fractions is low in forecasting cardiovascular events in the very elderly. The Leiden 85-plus study showed that although cardiovascular disease is a leading cause of death among persons older than 80 years, the rates of cardiac events were similar among patients with low, medium, and high levels of total cholesterol.[31]

Because of the strong relationship of hypercholesterolemia and ischemic heart disease, lowering total serum cholesterol and increasing HDL cholesterol are critical in managing patients at risk of myocardial infarction. Because of the strong interactions between coronary artery disease and ischemic cerebrovascular disease, patients with ischemic stroke, particularly those with carotid disease, should be considered at high risk for myocardial infarction.[32–35] For example, patients with stroke followed for five years in the Northern Manhattan Stroke Study were twice as likely to die of cardiac disease as from recurrent stroke.[36] Thus, even if elevated total cholesterol and LDL cholesterol levels are not associated with an increased stroke risk, the implicit high risk of coronary artery disease mandates their treatment in patients with stroke.[6] Treatment of hypercholesterolemia is called for regardless of the patient's age or the presence of other risk factors for atherosclerosis—if for no other reason, to prevent myocardial infarction or cardiac death.

INTERACTIONS BETWEEN CHOLESTEROL AND STROKE

The epidemiologic data regarding the relationship between serum levels of cholesterol and the risk of stroke are controversial.[37] Early clinical studies generally ignored the lipoprotein subfractions and attempted to correlate total cholesterol with the risk of stroke, regardless of type. The results were contradictory due to differences in geographic location, ethnicity, age, sex, and demographic characteristics of subjects and because of differences in study design, and some included all strokes, irrespective of the type.[38]

The Prospective Studies Collaboration performed a large meta-analysis based on more than 45 studies and did not find a correlation between serum cholesterol levels and the risk of stroke.[39] However, they did not differentiate ischemic from hemorrhagic stroke. Some studies used data of doubtful value collected from death certificates or hospital records and looked only at fatal cerebrovascular events, while three-quarters of all strokes in this meta-analysis consisted of only fatal stroke cases.[39]

Because of the diverse nature of stroke, it is difficult to establish a cause-and-effect relationship from a single risk factor, unlike that of elevated cholesterol in atherosclerosis.[38] Some studies included all ischemic strokes, regardless of cause, yet arterial dissection and vasculitis have little association with the traditional risk factors for stroke. Also, stroke from large artery atherosclerosis must be differentiated from cardioembolism and lacunar stroke. In a case control study, Hachinski et al.[40] found a strong correlation between total serum cholesterol and stroke when patients with lacunar or cardioembolic events were excluded.

In addition, the shared risk of coronary artery disease and cerebrovascular disease may dilute any association between cholesterol and stroke, and high-risk patients often die prematurely of heart disease. In a study of cholesterol as a risk factor for heart disease and stroke among men of Japanese ancestry living in Hawaii, a strong positive relationship was found between total cholesterol level and ischemic stroke.[41] The rates of stroke were similar to those of men of European heritage, but the Hawaiian men had very low rates of symptomatic coronary artery disease. The absence of cardiac events during a long period of observation allowed the demonstration of a strong correlation between serum cholesterol levels and ischemic stroke.

THE ROLE OF ELEVATED LIPIDS IN STROKE

Recent data support the relationship of elevated lipids as a risk factor for ischemic stroke.[40,42] Blood levels of total and LDL cholesterol and triglycerides were significantly elevated, and those of HDL cholesterol significantly reduced in patients with atherothrombotic strokes or transient ischemic attack (TIA).

An association among high levels of lipoprotein α and LDL cholesterol and low levels of HDL cholesterol in ischemic stroke was also reported.[24] Levey et al.[43] found an association between a low serum HDL cholesterol level and severe carotid atherosclerosis among persons younger than 50 who underwent carotid endarterectomy. Patients with stroke secondary to large artery atherosclerosis had higher total cholesterol levels than did those with lacunar strokes.

The Northern Manhattan Stroke Study[36] found that patients with levels of 35 to 50 mg/dl (0.875–1.25 mmol/L) of HDL cholesterol had a 0.81% stroke risk compared to those with levels of <35 mg/dl (0.875 mmol/L). Those with levels of HDL >50 mg/dl (1.25 mmol/L) had a stroke risk of only 0.39. The benefit was greatest for lowering the risk of large artery atherosclerosis.

A large clinical trial evaluating the benefit of treatment for hypertension, the Systolic Hypertension in the Elderly Program, revealed that low HDL cholesterol is associated with an increased risk of TIA and ischemic stroke.[44] A study in Australia had similar results: a 36% reduction in the risk for stroke was noted for each 1 mmol/L (40 mg/dl) increase in HDL cholesterol.[45] The influence of concentrations of total cholesterol, HDL cholesterol, and triglycerides was evaluated in 19,698 men and women enrolled in the Copenhagen City Heart Study.[46,47] The investigators were able to correlate an increased risk of nonhemorrhagic stroke only among patients with total cholesterol levels greater than 8 mmol/L (240 mg/dl); no relationships to the incidence of stroke were seen at lower levels. On the other hand, they found a strong protective effect from HDL cholesterol concentrations; the relative risk was 0.53 (95% CI 0.34–0.83). For each 1 mmol/L (90 mg/dl) increase in triglyceride concentration, the relative risk of stroke rose by 1.12 (95% CI 1.07–1.16). Based on an overview of 10 trials, Qizilbash[37] found a strong association between elevations of serum total cholesterol and the risk of ischemic stroke. A total cholesterol >5.50 mmol/L (220 mg/dl) predicted a relative risk of 1.31 (95% CI 1.11–1.54) of stroke compared to persons with lower levels.

The data on the relationship between serum cholesterol levels and the risk of stroke among women are even less clear than the data among men. Women have a lower risk for coronary artery disease and carotid atherosclerosis than men.[48] At all ages, the incidence of stroke is higher in men than in women. Even among patients with symptomatic atherosclerosis of the extracranial internal carotid artery, women have a better prognosis than do men. With a lower risk for stroke and fewer strokes among women, along with generally lower levels of cholesterol, establishing a cause and effect relationship in women can be difficult. Bostrom et al.[49] found that an elevated lipoprotein α was a strong independent predictor of cerebrovascular disease in women. The Framingham Study also found a strong association between total cholesterol values and coronary artery disease in women under the age of 70, but no relationship to stroke mortality could be found.[50] Both stroke and myocardial infarction are relatively uncommon among women under the age of 55, and the relative risk from an increased cholesterol concentration may be somewhat exaggerated. For older women, no association could be ascribed. The lack of relationship may be because ischemic stroke among older women is most commonly secondary to atrial fibrillation and large artery atherosclerosis appears to be a less common factor. Lindenstrom et al.[47] found similar effects from cholesterol and triglycerides on stroke risk among men and women.

The information about the role of elevated lipoprotein α levels and the likelihood of stroke is mixed. Markus et al.[51] found no relationship between lipoprotein α concentrations and TIA, stroke, or carotid atherosclerosis. Nguyen et al.[52] found that lipoprotein α was a weak risk factor for cerebrovascular disease in men and not a significant forecaster of stroke in women. Similarly, Dutch and American studies could not find a relationship between lipoprotein α levels and stroke.[53,54] Conversely, a Japanese study showed that elevated lipoprotein α levels were accompanied by an increased risk of atherothrombotic strokes, especially among patients under the age of 50.[55] Christopher et al.[56] found that elevated lipoprotein α levels are an important risk factor for the development of ischemic stroke among persons aged less than 40 years. Further research is required to evaluate the role of lipoprotein α as a risk factor for ischemic stroke.

Differentiating hemorrhagic from ischemic stroke is important because of the U-shaped relationship described between total serum cholesterol value and stroke.[57–60] While an elevated serum cholesterol value is associated with an increased risk for ischemic stroke, a low level of total cholesterol predicts an increased risk for intracerebral hemorrhage.[61,62] Brain hemorrhage probably is the only major cause of mortality that is correlated with a low serum total cholesterol value.[61] Yano et al.[59] found that the relative risk of intracerebral hemorrhage was 2.55 (95% CI 1.58–4.12) among men with a total cholesterol under 4.72 mmol/L (189 mg/dl) compared to higher levels. The relationship persisted even when controlled for age, blood pressure, tobacco use, and alcohol consumption. The Multiple Risk Factor Intervention Trial (MRFIT) found that the risk of intracerebral hemorrhage was inversely related to serum total cholesterol.[57] The trial evaluated the frequency of vascular events among 350,977 men aged 35–57 years (90.1% white and 6.4% African American) in the United States. The rate of intracranial hemorrhage was three times higher among men whose serum total cholesterol was below 4.14 mmol/L (160 mg/dl) than among men with higher levels. This association was observed despite considerable competition from cardiovascular disease in the study—cardiac mortality was 60.5/10,000, while deaths secondary to hemorrhagic stroke occurred at a rate of 2.36/10,000 and ischemic stroke at a rate of 2.62/10,000. Ibibarren et al.[63] described similar results involving 61,576 persons aged 40–89 years who lived in California. Serum total cholesterol levels below 4.62 mmol/L (178 mg/dl) increased the risk of hemorrhagic stroke among men older than 65 by a rate of 2.7 (5% CI 1.4–5.0) compared to similarly aged men with higher values. A parallel, but not statistically significant, trend was noted among elderly women. No association between hemorrhage and total cholesterol levels could be found among younger men or women. The inverse association between serum total cholesterol and intracranial hemorrhage has been confirmed by Japanese studies. Konishi et al.[60] reported that the mean total cholesterol level among patients with cerebral hemorrhage was 4.10 mmol/L (164 mg/dl); with lacunar infarction it was 4.61 mmol/L

(177 mg/dl); and with cortical infarction it was 4.99 mmol/L (200 mg/dl). The Eastern Stroke and Coronary Heart Disease Collaborative Research Group found the risk of hemorrhagic stroke increased by a rate of 1.27 (0.84–1.91) with each decrease of total cholesterol of 0.6 mmol/L (22 mg/dl).[65] Hemorrhagic stroke is a leading cause of death in Japan, but its incidence has dropped in recent years.[58] This decline has been attributed to shifts in the Japanese diet. With increased intake of animal fats and rising serum cholesterol levels, the frequency of brain hemorrhage has fallen, while the incidence of myocardial infarction has risen in Japan.[64]

Serum Cholesterol Level as a Prognostic Factor after Stroke

Dyker et al.[66] performed a retrospective study on outcomes of 977 patients with acute stroke. They found that higher concentrations of serum total cholesterol were associated with a lower mortality after stroke regardless of stroke type, patient age, or vascular territory. The relative hazard was 0.91 for each 1 mmol/L (40mg/dl) increase in cholesterol. The significance of this finding has not been established. It is possible that patients with low serum cholesterol had more serious co-morbid diseases and may have had some element of malnutrition prior to their cerebrovascular event.[67] The elevated cholesterol may represent inflammation after stroke.[68] A negative interaction in relation to atrial fibrillation also has been proposed.[69] Additional information about the importance of this finding is needed.

Interactions Between Serum Cholesterol Levels and Carotid Intima-Media Thickness and Atherosclerosis

The severity of atherosclerosis, including the extent detected by ultrasound, in the carotid artery is strongly associated with risk of severe coronary artery disease.[70–72] In particular, the extent of atherosclerotic disease in other circulations can be predicted by the severity of intimal-medial thickness (IMT) in the common carotid artery and proximal internal carotid artery.[73,74] In one study, the relative risk for myocardial infarction increased by a rate of 2.2 (95% CI 1.4–3.6) for each 0.03 mm increase in carotid IMT. The relationships are found in both men and women.[71] Thus, an association between lipid levels and carotid artery atherosclerosis should not be surprising. The prevalence and severity of atherosclerotic plaques of the internal carotid artery are significantly correlated with elevated total cholesterol or lowered HDL cholesterol values, especially at younger ages.[43,75] Sacco et al.[36] also found a relationship between high LDL cholesterol concentrations and the thickness of carotid artery plaques in African Americans, Hispanics, and whites. The relationship was strongest among Hispanic patients. Gronholde[76] found that LDL cholesterol concentrations are the best predictor of the extent of atherosclerosis of the carotid artery detected by ultrasound. Grotta et al.[77] reported that an elevated level of LDL cholesterol was a strong predictor of progressing carotid stenosis. Hodis et al.[78] found that progression of IMT in the carotid artery wall is strongly associated with levels of triglyceride-rich lipoproteins.

Evaluation of Serum Cholesterol in Patients with Stroke

Aull et al.[79] reported that lipid and lipoprotein levels among patients with TIA or stroke often are unreliable if they are measured after 48 hours but within several days following the neurologic event. They recommended delaying assessments of blood lipid concentrations for several weeks after stroke. Mendez et al.[80] reported similar results and concluded that important lipoprotein abnormalities can be missed during the first days after stroke. The reported magnitude in the drop of both total cholesterol and LDL cholesterol was approximately 10% at 24 hours and 25% at seven days compared to samples measured three months after stroke. However, Kargman et al.[81] did not find changes in lipoprotein α, total cholesterol, HDL cholesterol, LDL cholesterol, or triglycerides by serial measurements during the first weeks after stroke.

Treatment of Elevations of Serum Cholesterol and Prevention of Stroke

General measures

Measures aimed at lowering LDL cholesterol, triglycerides, or lipoprotein α, halting oxidation of LDL cholesterol, and increasing HDL cholesterol may slow the progression of atherosclerosis and reduce the risk of myocardial infarction, vascular death, and ischemic stroke.[82–85] Success in modification of risk factors, however, including total cholesterol levels, is hard to achieve among persons at high risk for stroke.[86] The choices include modification in diet and lipid-lowering medications. In addition, weight control, increased exercise, reduced alcohol consumption, and control of concomitant diseases, such as diabetes mellitus, are part of the strategy to lower blood lipids.

Evidence is strong that a traditional Western diet, which includes consumption of large amounts of saturated and animal fats, plays a role in fostering development of atherosclerosis. It is unclear whether the amount of fats or types of fats consumed is the critical factor.[87] A very low-fat diet has been recommended to reduce total cholesterol levels. Still, data are lacking about the efficacy of a very low-fat diet in preventing either myocardial infarction or stroke.[87] A surprising report from the Framingham Heart Study noted the lowest risk of stroke among those men who consumed the largest amounts of saturated and monounsaturated fats.[88] The report by Gillman et al.[88] is buttressed by an autopsy-based study from Greenland that found a significant interaction between high levels of polyunsaturated fatty acids and the occurrence of fatal hemorrhagic stroke.[89] Considerable additional research is needed to define the value of a severe restriction in dietary fats in the prevention of ischemic stroke. The possibility of an increase in a risk for hemorrhagic stroke with a low fat diet needs to be considered. Some carbohydrates may have positive effects and others have negative effects on HDL cholesterol levels.[90] Thus, dietary measures to treat hypercholesterolemia may require more than changes in consumption of saturated fats.

A diet similar to that consumed in eastern Asia, which includes high consumption of vegetables, carbohydrates, and fish with limited meat, has been advocated. The traditional Japanese diet, which involves consumption of large amounts of polyunsaturated fats and fatty acids, has not shown a reduction in the risk of stroke despite low levels of serum cholesterol.[91] However, other parts of the traditional Japanese diet, including the consumption of large amounts of salt, may contribute to the high risk of stroke in that country. Recently, a Mediterranean-style diet has been shown to be superior to a prudent Western-type diet in reducing cardiovascular events.[19] The Mediterranean diet substitutes vegetable oils, in particular olive oil, for animal fats and usually limits the amount of meat consumption. It also emphasizes consumption of fish, vegetables, fruit, and wine. Diets high in consumption of fresh fruits and vegetables have been shown to lower the risk of stroke. While these diets' effects are ascribed to increased ingestion of potassium and antioxidant vitamins, a concomitant lowering of dietary fats also may play a role.

Modest alcohol consumption can reduce the risk of coronary artery disease, possibly because of its effects on blood lipids, particularly an increase in HDL cholesterol.[92] Similar beneficial effects from consumption of modest amounts of alcohol, particularly wine, may reduce the risk of ischemic stroke.[93] Still, consumption of large of amounts of alcohol has other health implications, including hemorrhagic stroke, liver disease, and the possibility of increasing serum lipids. Alcohol abuse and binge alcohol consumption also predispose to ischemic stroke. A patient who drinks approximately one glass of wine per day does not need to change his or her practice. Wine may be more protective against stroke than either beer or distilled spirits.[94] However, a patient who does not consume alcohol should not be encouraged to start drinking in order to reduce the likelihood of a stroke. At present, alcohol consumption should not be viewed as a method to reduce the risk of stroke.

Estrogen is reported to be protective against the development of coronary artery disease and atherosclerosis in premenopausal women.[48] Estrogen supplementation in women does lower LDL cholesterol and increase HDL cholesterol levels. However, despite an 11% drop in LDL cholesterol and 10% rise in HDL cholesterol concentrations, the benefit of estrogen treatment in reducing cardiovascular events and stroke has not been demonstrated.

The levels of total cholesterol, LDL cholesterol, and HDL cholesterol that should prompt initiation of a lipid-lowering medication are not easy to establish.[95,96] Poor compliance with dietary recommendations may lower the threshold at which it is necessary to start medications. On the other hand, dietary modifications are cheaper and more physiologic than medications. It would seem prudent to start medication when an individual has a total cholesterol level >6.20 mmol/L (240 mg/dl), an LDL cholesterol level >3.30 mmol/L (130 mg/dl), or an HDL cholesterol level <0.87 mmol/L (35 mg/dl).

Traditional medications to lower cholesterol

Before the development of the statins, the treatment of hyperlipidemia included adminstration of cholestyramine, colestipol, nicotinic acid, gemfibrozil, or clofibrate. Despite their usefulness in lowering serum levels of total cholesterol, the benefit of these agents in lowering the risk of stroke has not been established.[97,98] Cholestyramine and colestipol have been used for approximately 40 years and were the primary medications used to lower LDL cholesterol before the development of the statins. These anion exchange resins act primarily within the intestine to sequester bile acids. A decline in the concentration of bile acids leads to an increased hepatic conversion of cholesterol into bile acids. Clinical studies have shown that cholestyramine and colestipol can lower LDL cholesterol levels by approximately 6% to 20% and raise HDL cholesterol levels by approximately 2% to 3%. Regrettably, cholestyramine can increase serum levels of triglycerides. The daily doses of cholestyramine and colestipol are approximately 8–24 grams and 10–30 grams, respectively. These agents can cause gastrointestinal side effects, including constipation. Many patients do not tolerate these medications, and their role has become secondary following the introduction of the statins. The monthly costs of these medications are approximately US$80 to $200.

The primary mechanism of action of nicotinic acid (niacin) on lipids is reduction in the production of VLDL cholesterol. It indirectly reduces LDL cholesterol and triglyceride levels by 20% to 25% and 20% to 50%, respectively. Simultaneously, HDL cholesterol levels are increased by 25% to 50%. In clinical trials, nicotinic acid has reduced cardiovascular mortality and nonfatal myocardial infarction, but no information is available about its effectiveness in preventing stroke. Nicotinic acid is a potent vasodilator that can lead to marked flushing of the skin, which many patients cannot tolerate. While this symptom is bothersome and often leads to halting treatment, it is not life threatening. The administration of aspirin in conjunction with nicotinic acid can lessen the problem of skin flushing. Other side effects include gastritis, hepatitis, elevated serum glucose, and an increased serum uric acid. The usual daily dose of nicotinic acid for lowering cholesterol is 2 to 3 grams. It is inexpensive, the monthly cost being approximately $8.

Gemfibrozil and clofibrate increase lipoprotein lipase activity. These medications are metabolized by the liver and excreted from the kidneys. They reduce triglyceride levels by 20% to 70%, but their effect on LDL-cholesterol levels is modest. These agents can increase HDL cholesterol levels approximately 10% to 20%. In clinical trials, these agents have shown no major benefit in reducing either cardiac death or myocardial infarction. Conversely, they have been associated with an increased rate of nonvascular death and a trend toward an increased risk of stroke.[98] The mechanism that leads to a clofibrate-related increase in risk of fatal stroke is not known.[98] Most side effects of these agents are gastrointestinal and include an increased risk of gallstones. The usual daily dose of gemfibrozil is 1200 mg, and the monthly cost is approximately $10.

HMG-CoA reductase inhibitors

These agents (the statins) suppress 3-hydroxy-3-methylglutaryl (HMG) coenzyme A (CoA) reductase, the rate-limiting step in the hepatic biosynthesis of cholesterol. At present, six statin agents (atorvastatin, cerivastatin, fluvastatin, lovastatin, pravastatin, and simvastatin) are available. They vary in their pharmacodynamic properties, including solubility. Pravastatin is the most hydrophilic, and simvastatin is the most lipophilic. All six agents reduce LDL cholesterol levels by approximately 20% to 40% and increase HDL cholesterol levels by approximately 5% to 10%. In addition, atorvastatin, pravastatin, and simvastatin also can reduce levels of triglycerides. Pravastatin may allow for increased stability of the fibrous cap of an atheroma.

These agents also appear to have antiatherogenic effects over and above their capacity to lower atherogenic lipoproteins.[99,100] Statins lessen the inflammatory, thrombogenic, and proliferative properties of atherosclerotic plaque, which reduces the likelihood of plaque rupture.[101,102] The Multicentre Anti-Atheroma Study reported that administration of simvastatin improved the morphology of arterial walls.[101] The statins also appear to improve endothelial function, affect inflammatory reactions, decrease platelet thrombus formation, and improve fibrinolytic activity.[99–101,103] They also affect fibrinogen concentrations and levels of C-reactive protein, which is a marker of inflammation.[104,105] Kaesemeyer et al.[106] reported that pravastatin reduces platelet aggregation and causes vasodilation through activation of endothelial nitric oxide synthase independently of its cholesterol-lowering properties. In a small, randomized, diet-controlled study, Anderson et al.[107] found that cholesterol-lowering medications improved endothelium-dependent vasomotion. These features may explain some of the efficacy of the statins in reducing the risk of myocardial infarction and ischemic stroke.

Clinical trials have shown that the addition of a statin to other medical therapies can lessen the likelihood of fatal or nonfatal myocardial infarction.[17,108] They also have reduced the need for cardiovascular interventions, including bypass grafting and angioplasty.[108] The agents can reduce the risk of an acute coronary event among asymptomatic men and women with average cholesterol values.[109] They are effective in both men and women and regardless of the presence of hypertension or diabetes mellitus.[110] The Long-Term Intervention with Pravastatin in Ischemic Disease (LIPID) Study Group found a 24% reduction in death from coronary artery disease and a 22% decline in overall mortality with treatment with pravastatin among a group of patients with symptomatic coronary artery disease and a wide range of cholesterol levels.[111]

Clinical trials have tested the usefulness of the statins in slowing the progression or reversing the growth of atherosclerotic plaques in the internal carotid artery. These studies have recruited asymptomatic patients and those with a history of symptomatic coronary artery disease, but they have not included patients who had a history of stroke or TIA. MacMahon et al.[112] noted that pravastatin reduced the development of carotid atherosclerosis among persons with ischemic heart disease and a broad spectrum of cholesterol levels. During the four-year study, the investigators noted an increase in mean thickness of the carotid artery wall of by 0.048 mm in the placebo-treated group and a decrease of 0.014 mm in the pravastatin-treated group. The Asymptomatic Carotid Artery Progression Study tested the effects of lovastatin on changes of IMT among asymptomatic patients with mild carotid artery plaques and elevated total cholesterol.[113] All patients received low-dose aspirin. By three years, the trial found a modest regression in IMT among those treated with lovastatin and a modest progression of plaques in the placebo-treated group. Concomitantly, the trial found a significant reduction of vascular events among the treated patients. Hodis et al.[114] also found that lovastatin reduced IMT among patients with preintrusive atherosclerosis of the carotid artery. The Kuopio Atherosclerosis Prevention Study found that pravastatin slowed the progression of carotid atherosclerotic plaques; responses were greater among patients who smoked.[115]

Several studies have examined the usefulness of the statins in reducing the incidence of ischemic stroke among patients with elevated cholesterol and a history of coronary artery disease (Table 4.1). In general, the use of statins has been shown to lower the risk of stroke by approximately 30%.[17,17,42,101,106–118] Several meta-analyses examined the cumulative results of clinical trials for the effectiveness of statins in preventing stroke; all yielded similar results.[98,119–124] The degree of benefit in preventing thrombotic stroke with treatment with the statins was greater in the meta-analyses because the number of cerebrovascular events was small in each of the individual trials.[125] In addition, most of the trials focused on prevention of cardiac events, with prevention of stroke a secondary goal. In the meta-analyses, the reduction in the risk of stroke with statin therapy was 24% to 31% (95% CI 8%–41%, $p = .001$). The similarity of the results of these analyses is due in large part to their mutual inclusion of the three largest trials, which accounted for approximately 90% of all strokes.[126–128] The other studies included in these analyses examined the influence of the statins on the progres-

TABLE 4.1. Reduction in Rates of Stroke: Clinical Trials of HMG-Co A Reductase Inhibitors

STUDY	AGENT	PATIENT GROUP	TREATMENT GROUP		CONTROL GROUP	
			TOTAL	STROKES	TOTAL	STROKES
WOSCOPS	Pravastatin	Primary[1]	3302	46	3293	51
4 S	Simvastatin	Secondary[2]	2221	75	2223	102
CARE	Pravastatin	Secondary	2081	54	2078	78
LIPID	Pravastatin	Secondary	4512	171	4502	198
ACAPS	Lovastatin	Primary	460	0	459	2
KAPS	Pravastatin	Primary	224	2	223	4

[1]Primary = patients without symptomatic coronary artery disease.
[2]Secondary = patients with symptomatic coronary artery disease.
WOSCOP = West of Scotland Coronary Prevention Study,[128] 4 S = Scandinavian Simvastatin Survival Study,[126] CARE = Cholesterol and Recurrent Events[108,127] LIPID = Long-term Intervention with Pravastatin in Ischaemic Disease,[111] ACAPS = Asymptomatic Carotid Artery Progression Study,[113] KAPS = Kuopio Atherosclerosis Prevention Study.[115]

sion of carotid artery atherosclerosis and either enrolled a limited number of subjects or followed them for short periods of time. The meta-analyses revealed similar reductions in total cholesterol level (approximately 20%) and LDL cholesterol level (30%) and increases in HDL cholesterol level (5%). The results of the meta-analyses provide conclusive evidence that the statins do lower the risk of ischemic stroke among persons with heart disease. The likelihood is high that these agents will be equally effective among persons with symptomatic cerebrovascular atherosclerosis.

The Scandinavian Simvastatin Survival Study enrolled 4,444 patients with a history of angina pectoris or myocardial infarction.[126] Patients received a lipid-lowering diet and either simvastatin or a placebo, and they were followed for a median period of 5.4 years. The primary purpose of the study was to test total mortality, and stroke data were evaluated in a post-hoc analysis. Men accounted for 81% of the subjects, and 51% were older than 60. These numbers are important when looking at the effects of the medication on stroke because these patients were at high risk for large artery atherosclerosis. Use of simvastatin was associated with a 25% and 35% reduction in total cholesterol and HDL cholesterol levels, respectively. HDL cholesterol levels increased by 8%. There was a 30% reduction in the risk of death in the treatment group (95% CI 15%–44%, $p = 0.0003$), due largely to fewer cardiac deaths. Fatal or nonfatal strokes occurred in 70 simvastatin-treated and 98 placebo-treated patients (relative risk 0.70–95%, CI 0.52–0.96, $p = .024$). The beneficial effects of treatment were discernible at one year and persisted throughout the follow-up period.

The West of Scotland Coronary Prevention Study (WOSCOPS) was a primary prevention trial that studied the ability of pravastatin to prevent cardiovascular events among 6595 men aged 45 to 64 who had a mean plasma cholesterol level of 7.0 ± 0.6 mmol/L (272 ± 23 mg/dl).[128] The men received a placebo or pravastatin at 40 mg/day and were followed for a mean of 4.9 years. Pravastatin lowered total cholesterol levels and LDL cholesterol levels by 20% and 26%, respectively. This study noted significant declines in myocardial infarction and cardiovascular death, but an 11% reduction in stroke risk did not reach statistical significance.

The LIPID study, whose data were not included in the meta-analyses, tested pravastatin (40 mg/day) or placebo for up to 6.1 years in 9014 patients who were 31 to 75 years old.[111] The patients had a history of symptomatic heart disease and initial total cholesterol of 4.00–7.00 mmol/L (155–271 mg/dl). A relative reduction in risk of death from ischemic heart disease of 24% was found. The trial also noted a 19% reduction in the risk of stroke among patients treated with pravastatin 40 mg/day.

In a placebo-controlled study, the Cholesterol and Recurrent Events (CARE) Trial, investigators noted that pravastatin lowered total cholesterol by 20%, LDL cholesterol by 32%, and triglycerides by 14% among a group of 4159 patients with a history of myocardial infarction and an average total cholesterol (total cholesterol <240 mg dl).[108,127] This was the first study that included stroke as a prespecified endpoint. The primary endpoint of the study, coronary artery disease–related death or myocardial infarction, was reduced by 24% among the pravastatin-treated patients. During the follow-up, strokes were diagnosed among 52 subjects treated with pravastatin and 76 persons given placebo, a 32% reduction (95% CI 4%–52%). The reduction in either stroke or TIA was 27%. There were too few strokes of each stroke subtype to make any inference about the efficacy of pravastatin on these subtypes, but there were fewer events with treatment in all subgroups. Importantly, pravastatin had benefit despite concomitant use of antithrombotic medications in both arms of the study: approximately 83% of the patients were taking aspirin daily. The mean total serum cholesterol level reached 4.32 mmol/L (167 mg/dl) among the pravastatin-treated patients, which is very close to the cut-off of 4.14 mmol/L (160 mg/dl), below which increased risks for hemorrhage were noted by the MRFIT study.[57] Still, the investigators did not note an increase in risk of hemorrhagic stroke with treatment.[127]

Lewis et al.[129] tested the usefulness of pravastatin in the prevention of recurrent ischemic events among 576 postmenopausal women with a history of myocardial infarction who had normal levels of total and LDL cholesterol. Pravastatin at 40 mg per day reduced coronary events by 46% compared to placebo. While the number of strokes in both arms of the study was small, a 56% reduction in the rate of stroke was seen with pravastatin treatment. In a subgroup analysis, the same investigators found that pravastatin reduced the absolute incidence of stroke from 7.3% to 4.5% (2.9% reduction, [CI 0.3%–4.5%], relative risk reduction of approximately 40%) among persons older than 65.[130] This analysis is important because this age group represents the population at greatest risk for stroke. The relative risk reduction with pravastatin was as great as that seen with some of the medications that are given to prevent stroke in high-risk older persons.

Currently, trials are testing the ability of atorvastatin to prevent recurrent brain ischemic events among persons with stroke or TIA. Taken together, these studies and the meta-analyses reveal several important points. First, with the exception of WOSCPOS, the individual studies show a fairly consistent reduction of approximately 30% in the risk of stroke. This risk reduction became apparent within 12 to 18 months after starting treatment. The magnitude in and the timing of the reduction in the risk of stroke are comparable to the statins' ability to lessen the risk of myocardial infarction and cardiac death. In general, the trials demonstrate that the statins are well tolerated, and the frequency of serious adverse experiences with treatment was not higher than that among the placebo-treated patients. The studies, which included measures to discriminate hemorrhagic stroke from ischemic stroke, did not show an increase in brain hemorrhage.

Overall, the HMG-CoA reductase inhibitors are relatively safe.[110] Some have questioned whether the HMG-CoA reductase inhibitors may increase the risk of violent death.[123] Current data are insufficient to establish such a relationship. Experimental models in rodents have suggested that lipid-lowering drugs, including the HMG-CoA reductase inhibitors, may cause cancer.[131] Still, clinical data are limited. One trial, the Cholesterol and Recurrent Events Study, reported that 12 cases of breast cancer were reported in the treatment group versus one case in the placebo-treated patients.[108] The absolute numbers are small and the confidence intervals for these data are very wide, so further study will be needed to determine if the association is solid. The other clinical trials testing the statins have not reported high rates of malignancies. At present, no significant increase in risk of cancer can be ascribed to the use of the statins.[123]

The most important adverse experiences from the HMG-CoA reductase inhibitors include hepatotoxicity, myopathy, dyspepsia, and skin eruption. Approximately 1% of patients develop elevated blood levels of liver enzymes, which usually are asymptomatic. The hepatic side effects are more common in persons who also regularly consume alcohol or who are taking other medications that may affect the liver. Still, because of the risk of hepatic adverse experiences, patients who are taking a statin should have a transaminase level measured approximately six weeks and three months after starting treatment and approximately every six months thereafter. A threefold rise in transaminase should prompt discontinuance or a lowering of the dosage of the statin. A myopathy complicating the use of a statin usually presents with marked generalized weakness and myalgias. Serum levels of creatine kinase are markedly elevated in these patients.

In severe cases, rhabdomyolysis and myoglobinuria may be detected. This complication can occur with the administration of any of the agents, but the risk of a myopathy increases if the patient also is using cyclosporin, gemfibrozil, or nicotinic acid. The cause of myopathic complication is not clear.

These medications are expensive.[132] The monthly costs range from $50 to more than than $200. Still, pharmacoeconomic studies have demonstrated that the statins are cost-effective because of their ability to reduce cardiovascular morbidity and mortality. The cost-effectiveness of the statins is significantly greater when the costs of stroke care are included.[133]

CONCLUSIONS

The impact of elevated blood levels of cholesterol on the incidence of stroke is smaller than its influence on coronary artery disease. Accumulating evidence indicates that it is an important risk factor for ischemic stroke, especially due to large artery atherosclerosis and cardioembolism secondary to ischemic heart disease.[82,96] Because a large percentage of persons living in North America have elevated serum cholesterol values, the potential for public health benefit is substantial from modification of this risk factor. Robust evidence is available indicating that the use of statins reduces the risk of ischemic stroke and lessens the progression of extracranial carotid artery disease in adults who do or do not have symptomatic coronary artery disease. These agents also dramatically lower the risk of serious cardiac events. Therefore, statin therapy has the potential to help lower the risk of ischemic events (myocardial infarction and recurrent stroke) among patients with an asymptomatic carotid stenosis, TIA, or prior ischemic stroke. The agents should be prescribed to patients with concomitant symptomatic coronary artery disease and cerebrovascular atherosclerosis. The usefulness of these agents in persons who have had a stroke but show no evidence of coincident coronary artery disease is uncertain. Clinical trials are testing the efficacy of the agents in such a situation. The role of the statins in treatment of patients with stroke not secondary to atherosclerosis is unknown. While the use of the statins should be tied to dietary modifications and control of other risk factors, the role of the other cholesterol-lowering medications has become secondary. Their use should be restricted to those patients who cannot take the statins or as possible adjuncts to the HMG-CoA reductase inhibitors.

Looking further ahead, additional research in the role of lipids in the course of cerebrovascular disease is needed. Among the issues is the possible relationship between intracranial hemorrhage and low cholesterol values. In addition, the revolution in neurogenetics provides the opportunity to identify those individuals with particular genetic polymorphisms that could interact with factors such as dietary cholesterol to place a person at very high risk for stroke.

REFERENCES

1. Bonita R, Stewart A, Beaglehole R. International trends in stroke mortality: 1970–1985. *Stroke* 1990;21:989–992.
2. Broderick J, Brott T, Kothari R, et al. The Greater Cincinnati/Northern Kentucky Stroke Study: Preliminary first-ever and total incidence rates of stroke among blacks. *Stroke* 1998;29:415–421.
3. May DS, Kittner SJ. Use of Medicare claims data to estimate national trends in stroke incidence, 1985–1991. *Stroke* 1994;25:2343–2347.
4. Sudlow CL, Warlow CP. Comparing stroke incidence worldwide: What makes studies comparable? *Stroke* 1996;27:550–558.
5. Gorelick PB. Stroke prevention: Windows of opportunity and failed expectations? A discussion of modifiable cardiovascular risk factors and a prevention proposal. *Neuroepidemiology* 1997;16:163–173.
6. Yatsu FM, Fisher M. Atherosclerosis: Current concepts on pathogenesis and interventional therapies. *Ann Neurol* 1989;26:3–12.
7. Bogousslavsky J, Barnett HJ, Fox AJ, Hachinski VC, Taylor W. Atherosclerotic disease of the middle cerebral artery. *Stroke* 1986;17:1112–1120.
8. Feldmann E, Daneault N, Kwan E, et al. Chinese–white differences in the distribution of occlusive cerebrovascular disease. *Neurology* 1990;40:1541–1545.
9. Wityk RJ, Lehman D, Klag M, Coresh J, Ahn H, Litt B. Race and sex differences in the distribution of cerebral atherosclerosis. *Stroke* 1996;27:1974–1980.
10. Lafont A, Libby P. The smooth muscle cell: Sinner or saint in restenosis and the acute coronary syndromes? *J Am Coll Cardiol* 1998;32:283–285.
11. Fisher M, Blumenfeld AM, Smith TW. The importance of carotid artery plaque disruption and hemorrhage. *Arch Neurol* 1987;44:1086–1089.
12. Carr S, Farb A, Pearce WH, Virmani R, Yao JS. Atherosclerotic plaque rupture in symptomatic carotid artery stenosis. *J Vasc Surg* 1996;23:755–765.
13. Lehmann ED, Hopkins KD, Gosling RG. Atherosclerosis in the ascending aorta and risk of ischaemic stroke. *Lancet* 1995;346:589–590.
14. Goode GK, Miller JP, Heagerty AM. Hyperlipidaemia, hypertension, and coronary heart disease. *Lancet* 1995;345:362–364.
15. Maher VM, Brown BG, Marcovina SM, Hillger LA, Zhao XQ, Albers JJ. Effects of lowering elevated LDL cholesterol on the cardiovascular risk of lipoprotein(α). *JAMA* 1995;274:1771–1774.
16. Geurian KL. The cholesterol controversy. *Ann Pharmacother* 1996;30:495–500.
17. Kashyap ML. Cholesterol and atherosclerosis: A contemporary perspective. *Ann Acad Med Singapore* 1997;26:517–523.
18. Genest JJ, McNamara JR, Ordovas JM, et al. Lipoprotein cholesterol, apolipoprotein A-I and B and lipoprotein α abnormalities in men with premature coronary artery disease. *J Am Coll Cardiol* 1992;19:792–802.
19. de Lorgeril M, Salen P, Martin JL, Monjaud I, Delaye J, Mamelle N. Mediterranean diet, traditional risk factors, and the rate of cardiovascular complications after myocardial infarction: Final report of the Lyon Diet Heart Study. *Circulation* 1999;99:779–785.
20. Aronow WS. Prevalence of heart disease in older women in a nursing home. *Journal of Womens Health* 1998;7:1105–1112.
21. Wilkinson IB, Cockcroft JR. Cholesterol, endothelial function and cardiovascular disease. *Curr Opin Lipidol* 1998;9:237–242.

22. Lip GY, Jones AF. Lipoprotein α and vascular disease: thrombogenesis and athero-genesis. *QJM* 1995;88:529–539.
23. Craig WY, Bostom AG. Lipoprotein α. concentration and risk of atherothrombotic disease. *JAMA* 1995;274:1198–1199.
24. Pedro-Botet J, Senti M, Nogues X, et al. Lipoprotein and apolipoprotein profile in men with ischemic stroke. Role of lipoprotein(α), triglyceride-rich lipoproteins, and apolipoprotein E polymorphism. *Stroke* 1992;23:1556–1562.
25. Rubba P, Mercuri M, Faccenda F, et al. Premature carotid atherosclerosis: Does it occur in both familial hypercholesterolemia and homocystinuria? Ultrasound assessment of arterial intima-media thickness and blood flow velocity. *Stroke* 1994;25:943–950.
26. Goldbourt U, Neufeld HN. Genetic aspects of arteriosclerosis. *Arteriosclerosis* 1986;6:357–377.
27. Niskanen L, Turpeinen A, Penttila I, Uusitupa MI. Hyperglycemia and compositional lipoprotein abnormalities as predictors of cardiovascular mortality in type 2 diabetes: A 15-year follow-up from the time of diagnosis. *Diabetes Care* 1998;21:1861–1869.
28. Laakso M, Lehto S. Epidemiology of risk factors for cardiovascular disease in diabetes and impaired glucose tolerance. *Atherosclerosis* 1998;137 Suppl:S65–S73.
29. Abbott RD, Sharp DS, Burchfiel CM, et al. Cross-sectional and longitudinal changes in total and high-density-lipoprotein cholesterol levels over a 20–year period in elderly men: The Honolulu Heart Program. *Ann Epidemiol* 1997;7:417–424.
30. Ballantyne CM, Herd JA, Dunn JK, Jones PH, Farmer JA, Gotto AM Jr. Effects of lipid lowering therapy on progression of coronary and carotid artery disease. *Curr Opin Lipidol* 1997;8:354–361.
31. Weverling-Rijnsburger AW, Blauw GJ, Lagaay AM, Knook DL, Meinders AE, Westendorp RG. Total cholesterol and risk of mortality in the oldest old. *Lancet* 1997;350:1119–1123.
32. Wilterdink JL, Furie KL, Easton JD. Cardiac evaluation of stroke patients. *Neurology* 1998;51:S23–S26.
33. Chimowitz MI, Poole RM, Starling MR, Schwaiger M, Gross MD. Frequency and severity of asymptomatic coronary disease in patients with different causes of stroke. *Stroke* 1997;28:941–945.
34. Love BB, Grover-McKay M, Biller J, Rezai K, McKay CR. Coronary artery disease and cardiac events with asymptomatic and symptomatic cerebrovascular disease. *Stroke* 1992;23:939–945.
35. Chimowitz MI, Mancini GB. Asymptomatic coronary artery disease in patients with stroke. Prevalence, prognosis, diagnosis, and treatment. *Stroke* 1992;23:433–436.
36. Sacco RL, Roberts JK, Boden-Albala B, et al. Race-ethnicity and determinants of carotid atherosclerosis in a multiethnic population: The Northern Manhattan Stroke Study. *Stroke* 1997;28:929–935.
37. Qizilbash N. Are risk factors for stroke and coronary disease the same? *Curr Opin Lipidol* 1998;9:325–328.
38. Stoy NS. Stroke and cholesterol: 'enigma variations'? *J R Coll Physicians Lond* 1997;31:521–526.
39. Prospective Studies Collaboration. Cholesterol, diastolic blood pressure, and stroke: 13,000 strokes in 450,000 people in 45 prospective cohorts. *Lancet* 1995;346:1647–1653.
40. Hachinski V, Graffagnino C, Beaudry M, et al. Lipids and stroke: a paradox resolved. *Arch Neurol* 1996;53:303–308.

41. Benfante R, Yano K, Hwang LJ, Curb JD, Kagan A, Ross W. Elevated serum cholesterol is a risk factor for both coronary heart disease and thromboembolic stroke in Hawaiian Japanese men. Implications of shared risk. *Stroke* 1994;25:814–820.

42. Gorelick PB, Schneck M, Berglund LF, Feinberg W, Goldstone J. Status of lipids as a risk factor for stroke. *Neuroepidemiology* 1997;16:107–115.

43. Levy PJ, Olin JW, Piedmonte MR, Young JR, Hertzer NR. Carotid endarterectomy in adults 50 years of age and younger: A retrospective comparative study. *J Vasc Surg* 1997;25:326–331.

44. Davis BR, Vogt T, Frost PH, et al. Risk factors for stroke and type of stroke in persons with isolated systolic hypertension: Systolic Hypertension in the Elderly Program Cooperative Research Group. *Stroke* 1998;29:1333–1340.

45. Simons LA, McCallum J, Friedlander Y, Simons J. Risk factors for ischemic stroke: Dubbo Study of the elderly. *Stroke* 1998;29:1341–1346.

46. Boysen G, Lindenstrom E. Cholesterol and risk of stroke. *Lancet* 1996;347:762

47. Lindenstrom E, Boysen G, Nyboe J. Influence of total cholesterol, high density lipoprotein cholesterol, and triglycerides on risk of cerebrovascular disease: The Copenhagen City Heart Study. *BMJ* 1994;309:11–15.

48. Thomas JL, Braus PA. Coronary artery disease in women: A historical perspective. *Arch Intern Med* 1998;158:333–337.

49. Bostom AG, Gagnon DR, Cupples LA, et al. A prospective investigation of elevated lipoprotein α detected by electrophoresis and cardiovascular disease in women. The Framingham Heart Study. *Circulation* 1994;90:1688–1695.

50. Emond MJ, Zareba W. Prognostic value of cholesterol in women of different ages *Journal of Womens Health* 1997;6:295–307.

51. Markus HS, Kapadia R, Sherwood RA. Relationship between lipoprotein α and both stroke and carotid atheroma. *Ann Clin Biochem* 1997;34:360–365.

52. Nguyen TT, Ellefson RD, Hodge DO, et al. Predictive value of electrophoretically detected lipoprotein(α) for coronary heart disease and cerebrovascular disease in a community-based cohort of 9936 men and women. *Circulation* 1997;96:1390–1397.

53. Ridker PM, Stampfer MJ, Hennekens CH. Plasma concentration of lipoprotein α. and the risk of future stroke. *JAMA* 1995;273:1269–1273.

54. van Kooten F, van Krimpen J, Dippel DW, Hoogerbrugge N, Koudstaal PJ. Lipoprotein α in patients with acute cerebral ischemia. *Stroke* 1996;27:1231–1235.

55. Shintani S, Kikuchi S, Hamaguchi H, Shiigai T. High serum lipoprotein α levels are an independent risk factor for cerebral infarction. *Stroke* 1993;24:965–969.

56. Christopher R, Kailasanatha KM, Nagaraja D, Tripathi M. Case-control study of serum lipoprotein α. and apolipoproteins A-I and B in stroke in the young. *Acta Neurol Scand* 1996;94:127–130.

57. Iso H, Jacobs DRJ, Wentworth D, Neaton JD, Cohen JD. Serum cholesterol levels and six-year mortality from stroke in 350,977 men screened for the multiple risk factor intervention trial. *N Engl J Med* 1989;320:904–910.

58. Reed D, Jacobs DRJ, Hayashi T, et al. A comparison of lesions in small intracerebral arteries among Japanese men in Hawaii and Japan. *Stroke* 1994;25:60–65.

59. Yano K, Reed DM, MacLean CJ. Serum cholesterol and hemorrhagic stroke in the Honolulu Heart Program. *Stroke* 1989;20:1460–1465.

60. Konishi M, Iso H, Komachi Y, et al. Associations of serum total cholesterol, different types of stroke, and stenosis distribution of cerebral arteries: The Akita Pathology Study. *Stroke* 1993;24:954–964.

61. Puddey IB. Low serum cholesterol and the risk of cerebral haemorrhage. *Atherosclerosis* 1996;119:1–6.
62. Thrift AG, McNeil JJ, Forbes A, Donnan GA. Risk factors for cerebral hemorrhage in the era of well-controlled hypertension. Melbourne Risk Factor Study. MERFS. Group. *Stroke* 1996;27:2020–2025.
63. Iribarren C, Jacobs DR, Sadler M, Claxton AJ, Sidney S. Low total serum cholesterol and intracerebral hemorrhagic stroke: Is the association confined to elderly men? The Kaiser Permanente Medical Care Program. *Stroke* 1996;27:1993–1998.
64. Shimamoto T, Iso H, Iida M, Komachi Y. Epidemiology of cerebrovascular disease: Stroke epidemic in Japan. *J Epidemiol* 1996;6:S43–S47.
65. Eastern Stroke and Coronary Heart Disease Collaborative Research Group. Blood pressure, cholesterol, and stroke in eastern Asia. *Lancet* 1998;352:1801–1807.
66. Dyker AG, Weir CJ, Lees KR. Influence of cholesterol on survival after stroke: Retrospective study. *BMJ* 1997;314:1584–1588.
67. Hutchesson A, Martin S. Influence of cholesterol on survival after stroke. Regression to the mean may have been a factor. *BMJ* 1997;315:1158.
68. Socin HV. Influence of cholesterol on survival after stroke: Cholesterol may be marker of inflammation. *BMJ* 1997;315:1159.
69. Marini C, Di Napoli M, Carolei A. Influence of cholesterol on survival after stroke: Effect of cholesterol on prognosis may rely on negative association with atrial fibrillation. *BMJ* 1997;315:1159.
70. Craven TE, Ryu JE, Espeland MA, et al. Evaluation of the associations between carotid artery atherosclerosis and coronary artery stenosis: A case-control study. *Circulation* 1990;82:1230–1242.
71. Wofford JL, Kahl FR, Howard GR, McKinney WM, Toole JF, Crouse JR. Relation of extent of extracranial carotid artery atherosclerosis as measured by B-mode ultrasound to the extent of coronary atherosclerosis. *Arterioscler Thromb* 1991;11:1786–1794.
72. Hodis HN, Mack WJ, LaBree L, et al. The role of carotid arterial intima-media thickness in predicting clinical coronary events. *Ann Intern Med* 1998;128:262–269.
73. O'Leary DH, Polak JF, Kronmal RA, Manolio TA, Burke GL, Wolfson SK, Jr. Carotid-artery intima and media thickness as a risk factor for myoardial infarction and stroke in older adults. *N Engl J Med* 1999;340:14–22.
74. Burke GL, Evans GW, Riley WA, et al. Arterial wall thickness is associated with prevalent cardiovascular disease in middle-aged adults: The Atherosclerosis Risk in Communities. ARIC. Study. *Stroke* 1995;26:386–391.
75. Micieli G, Cavallini A, Bosone D, Poli M, Nappi G. Carotid artery atherosclerosis and risk factors for stroke in a selected population of asymptomatic men. *Funct Neurol* 1998;13:27–35.
76. Gronholdt MM. Ultrasound and lipoproteins as predictors of lipid-rich, rupture-prone plaques in the carotid artery. *Arterioscler Thromb Vasc Biol* 1999;19:2–13.
77. Grotta JC, Yatsu FM, Pettigrew LC, et al. Prediction of carotid stenosis progression by lipid and hematologic measurements. *Neurology* 1989;39:1325–1331.
78. Hodis HN, Mack WJ, Dunn M, Liu C, Selzer RH, Krauss RM. Intermediate-density lipoproteins and progression of carotid arterial wall intima-media thickness. *Circulation* 1997;95:2022–2026.
79. Aull S, Lalouschek W, Schnider P, Sinzinger H, Uhl F, Zeiler K. Dynamic changes of plasma lipids and lipoproteins in patients after transient ischemic attack or minor stroke. *Am J Med* 1996;101:291–298.

80. Mendez I, Hachinski V, Wolfe B. Serum lipids after stroke. *Neurology* 1987;37:507–511.
81. Kargman DE, Tuck C, Berglund L, et al. Lipid and lipoprotein levels remain stable in acute ischemic stroke: The Northern Manhattan Stroke Study. *Atherosclerosis* 1998;139:391–399.
82. Summary of the second report of the National Cholesterol Education Program. NCEP. Expert Panel on Detection, Evaluation, and Treatment of High Blood Cholesterol in Adults. Adult Treatment Panel II). *JAMA* 1993;269:3015–3023.
83. Levine GN, Keaney JFJ, Vita JA. Cholesterol reduction in cardiovascular disease. Clinical benefits and possible mechanisms. *N Engl J Med* 1995;332:512–521.
84. Perry IJ. Primary prevention of stroke. *N Engl J Med* 1996;334:1138.
85. Wolf PA, Belanger AJ, D'Agostino RB. Management of risk factors. *Neurol Clin* 1992;10:177–191.
86. Joseph LN, Babikian VL, Allen NC, Winter MR. Risk factor modification in stroke prevention: The experience of a stroke clinic. *Stroke* 1999;30:16–20.
87. Gaziano JM, Manson JE. Diet and heart disease. The role of fat, alcohol, and antioxidants. *Cardiol Clin* 1996;14:69–83.
88. Gillman MW, Cupples LA, Millen BE, Ellison RC, Wolf PA. Inverse association of dietary fat with development of ischemic stroke in men. *JAMA* 1997;278:2145–2150.
89. Pedersen HS, Mulvad G, Seidelin KN, Malcom GT, Boudreau DA. N-3 fatty acids as a risk factor for haemorrhagic stroke. *Lancet* 1999;353:812–813.
90. Hudson CN. Are there good and bad carbohydrates for HDL cholesterol? *Lancet* 1999;353:1029–1030.
91. Seino F, Date C, Nakayama T, et al. Dietary lipids and incidence of cerebral infarction in a Japanese rural community. *J Nutr Sci Vitaminol* 1997;43:83–99.
92. Gaziano JM, Buring JE. Alcohol intake, lipids and risks of myocardial infarction. *Novartis Foundation Symposium* 1998;216:86–95.
93. Sacco RL, Eikind M, Boden-Albala B, et al. The potential effect of moderate alcohol consumption on ischemic stroke. *JAMA* 1999;281:53–60.
94. Truelsen T, Gronbaek M, Schnohr P, Boysen G. Intake of beer, wine, and spirits and risk of stroke. *Stroke* 1998;29:2467–2472.
95. Grover S. Gambling with cardiovascular risk: picking the winners and the losers. *Lancet* 1999;353:254.
96. Durrington PN, Prais H, Bhatnagar D, et al. Indications for cholesterol-lowering medication: Comparison of risk-assessment methods. *Lancet* 1999;353:278–281.
97. Rosendorff C. Statins for prevention of stroke. *Lancet* 1998;351:1002–1003.
98. Atkins D, Psaty BM, Koepsell TD, Longstreth WTJ, Larson EB. Cholesterol reduction and the risk for stroke in men. A meta-analysis of randomized, controlled trials. *Ann Intern Med* 1993;119:136–145.
99. Vaughan CJ, Murphy MB, Buckley BM. Statins do more than just lower cholesterol. *Lancet* 1996;348:1079–1082.
100. Farnier M, Davignon J. Current and future treatment of hyperlipidemia: The role of statins. *Am J Cardiol* 1998;82:3J–10J.
101. Delanty N, Vaughan CJ. Vascular effects of statins in stroke. *Stroke* 1997;28:2315–2320.
102. Williams JK, Sukhova GK, Herrington DM, Libby P. Pravastatin has cholesterol-lowering independent effects on the artery wall of atherosclerotic monkeys. *J Am Coll Cardiol* 1998;31:684–691.
103. Rosenson RS, Tangney CC. Antiatherothrombotic properties of statins: Implications for cardiovascular event reduction. *JAMA* 1998;279:1643–1650.

104. Strandberg RE, Vanhanen H, Tikkanen MJ. Effect of statins on C-reactive protein in patients with coronary artery disease. *Lancet* 1999;353:118–119.
105. Wierzbicki AS, Lumb PJ, Semra YK, Crook MA. Effect of atorvastatin on plasma fibrinogen. *Lancet* 1998;351:569–570.
106. Kaesemeyer WH, Caldwell RB, Huang J, Caldwell RW. Pravastatin sodium activates endothelial nitric oxide synthase independent of its cholesterol-lowering actions. *J Am Coll Cardiol* 1999;33:234–241.
107. Anderson TJ, Meredith IT, Yeung AC, Frei B, Selwyn AP, Ganz P. The effect of cholesterol-lowering and antioxidant therapy on endothelium-dependent coronary vasomotion. *N Engl J Med* 1995;332:488–493.
108. Sacks FM, Pfeffer MA, Moye LA, et al. The effect of pravastatin on coronary events after myocardial infarction in patients with average cholesterol levels: Cholesterol and Recurrent Events Trial investigators. *N Engl J Med* 1996;335:1001–1009.
109. Downs JR, Clearfield M, Weis S, et al. Primary prevention of acute coronary events with lovastatin in men and women with average cholesterol levels: Results of AFCAPS/TexCAPS. Air Force/Texas Coronary Atherosclerosis Prevention Study. *JAMA* 1998;279:1615–1622.
110. Rifkind BM. Clinical trials of reducing low-density lipoprotein concentrations. *Endocrinol Metab Clin North Am* 1998;27:585–595.
111. The Long-Term Intervention with Pravastatin in Ischaemic Disease. LIPID. Study Group. Prevention of cardiovascular events and death with pravastatin in patients with coronary heart disease and a broad range of initial cholesterol levels. *N Engl J Med* 1998;339:1349–1357.
112. MacMahon S, Sharpe N, Gamble G, et al. Effects of lowering average of below-average cholesterol levels on the progression of carotid atherosclerosis: Results of the LIPID Atherosclerosis Substudy. LIPID Trial Research Group. *Circulation* 1998; 97:1784–1790.
113. Furberg CD, Adams HP Jr., Applegate WB, et al. Effect of lovastatin on early carotid atherosclerosis and cardiovascular events: Asymptomatic Carotid Artery Progression Study. ACAPS. Research Group. *Circulation* 1994;90:1679–1687.
114. Hodis HN, Mack WJ, LaBree L, et al. Reduction in carotid arterial wall thickness using lovastatin and dietary therapy: A randomized controlled clinical trial. *Ann Intern Med* 1996;124:548–556.
115. Salonen R, Nyyssonen K, Porkkala E, et al. Kuopio Atherosclerosis Prevention Study. KAPS): A population-based primary preventive trial of the effect of LDL lowering on atherosclerotic progression in carotid and femoral arteries. *Circulation* 1995;92: 1758–1764.
116. Spence JD. Statins for prevention of stroke. *Lancet* 1998;352:909
117. Fey RE. Statins for prevention of stroke. *Lancet* 1998;352:144–145.
118. Wallis EJ, Ramsay LE, Yeo WW, Jackson PR. Statins for prevention of stroke. *Lancet* 1998;352:909–910.
119. Blauw GJ, Lagaay AM, Smelt AH, Westendorp RG. Stroke, statins, and cholesterol: A meta-analysis of randomized, placebo-controlled, double-blind trials with HMG-CoA reductase inhibitors. *Stroke* 1997;28:946–950.
120. Blauw GJ, Lagaay AM, Westendorp RG. Statins for prevention of stroke. *Lancet* 1998;352:144.
121. Bucher HC, Griffith LE, Guyatt GH. Effect of HMGcoA reductase inhibitors on stroke: A meta-analysis of randomized, controlled trials. *Ann Intern Med* 1998;128: 89–95.

122. Crouse JR, Byington RP, Hoen HM, Furberg CD. Reductase inhibitor monotherapy and stroke prevention. *Arch Intern Med* 1997;157:1305–1310.
123. Hebert PR, Gaziano JM, Chan KS, Hennekens CH. Cholesterol lowering with statin drugs, risk of stroke, and total mortality: An overview of randomized trials. *JAMA* 1997;278:313–321.
124. Crouse JR, Byington RP, Furberg CD. HMG-CoA reductase inhibitor therapy and stroke risk reduction: An analysis of clinical trials data. *Atherosclerosis* 1998;138: 11–24.
125. Papadakis JA, Mikhailidis DP, Winder AF. Lipids and stroke: neglect of a useful preventive measure?. *Cardiovasc Res* 1998;40:265–271.
126. Randomised trial of cholesterol lowering in 4444 patients with coronary heart disease: The Scandinavian Simvastatin Survival Study. 4S). *Lancet* 1994;344:1383–1389.
127. Plehn JF, Davis BR, Sacks FM, et al. Reduction of stroke incidence after myocardial infarction with pravastatin: The Cholesterol and Recurrent Events. CARE. Study. *Circulation* 1999;99:216–223.
128. Shepherd J, Cobbe SM, Ford I, et al. Prevention of coronary heart disease with pravastatin in men with hypercholesterolemia: West of Scotland Coronary Prevention Study Group. *N Engl J Med* 1995;333:1301–1307.
129. Lewis SJ, Sacks FM, Mitchell JS, et al. Effect of pravastatin on cardiovascular events in women after myocardial infarction: The Cholesterol and Recurrent Events. CARE. trial. *J Am Coll Cardiol* 1998;32:140–146.
130. Lewis SJ, Moye LA, Sacks FM, et al. Effect of pravastatin on cardiovascular events in older patients with myocardial infarction and cholesterol levels in the average range: Results of the Cholesterol and Recurrent Events. CARE. trial. *Ann Intern Med* 1998;129:681–689.
131. Newman TB, Hulley SB. Carcinogenicity of lipid-lowering drugs. *JAMA* 1996;275: 55–60.
132. Jacobson TA, Schein JR, Williamson A, Ballantyne CM. Maximizing the cost-effectiveness of lipid-lowering therapy. Arch Intern Med 1998;158:1977–1989.
133. Szucs TD. Pharmaco-economic aspects of lipid-lowering therapy: Is it worth the price? *Eur Heart J* 1998;19 Suppl M:M22–M28.

5

HYPERTENSION

Philip A. Wolf

In 1973, Sir George Pickering wrote, "It has been known for over a century that high arterial pressure lessens life expectancy and for half that time that in most patients the raised pressure and its consequences constitute the disease (essential hypertension)".[1] The prevalence of hypertension in the United States, defined by the Joint National Committee on Prevention, Detection, Evaluation, and Treatment of High Blood Pressure as ≥140 mm Hg systolic or ≥90 mm Hg diastolic, is high.[2] Hypertension is present in 38% of persons aged 50 to 59 and 71% of those aged 80 and above, and it is a potent risk factor for the development of cardiovascular disease, particularly stroke.[3] The relationship of hypertension to cardiovascular disease and specifically to "apoplexy" has long been known.[4] While hypertension, cerebral hemorrhage, and the miliary aneurysms of Charcot and Bouchard have been closely related for more than 50 years, the link to ischemic stroke was made more recently.[5,6] In fact, it has only been in the past 30 years that epidemiologic study has confirmed the role of elevated blood pressure in stroke.[7] Hypertension is now known to be the most prevalent and powerful risk factor for stroke. It is also one of the most treatable conditions predisposing to stroke. What had been accepted as normal or average blood pressure (at a given age) is now considered to be much higher than ideal or optimal as far as stroke or cardiovascular disease risk is concerned. In older adults, particularly in persons above aged 65, in whom stroke occurs most frequently, the systolic component of blood pressure has been shown to be no less important than the diastolic. Both systolic and diastolic pressures increase with age from childhood into middle adult years. By age 60, while the systolic pressure continues to rise, the diastolic pressure has already reached a plateau and has begun to fall. With advancing age the diastolic continues to decline. In these older persons, aged 60 years and above, the level of risk of cardiovascular disease, particularly stroke, is directly related to the level of the systolic component, even in the presence of normal diastolic pressure.

The availability of a large number of potent antihypertensive agents makes it possible to control virtually all hypertension. At the same time, a host of randomized clinical trials has shown such treatment is safe and effective. In the past, physicians were cautioned not to reduce blood pressure to normal levels for fear of *precipitating* stroke. Although some still advocate only moderate reduction of elevated pressure, most experts favor vigorous control of elevated blood pressure. With accumulating data, the target level has been gradually lowered. Now, a normal blood pressure of systolic <140 mm Hg and diastolic <90 mm Hg (or lower) is considered to be the optimal blood pressure level for stroke prevention.[2]

ETIOLOGY OF STROKE

Unlike myocardial infarction, in which atherosclerosis of the coronary arteries is the underlying disease process, stroke is heterogenous; approximately 85% is due to infarction and the remainder to hemorrhage (half intracerebral and half subarachnoid). With the exception of embolism from a cardiac source, most brain infarctions result from occlusion of large and small arteries to the brain. Hypertension is the most common potent risk factor for noncardioembolic ischemic stroke, and reduction of elevated blood pressure clearly prevents stroke regardless of infarct subtype. Much of the observational data presented is based on the study of stroke in the general population sample at Framingham, Massachusetts. After 40 years of follow-up, stroke occurred in 718 persons—312 in men and 406 in women. Incidence increased with age, approximately doubling in each successive decade above age 55. The most common type, accounting for approximately 60% of all stroke cases, has been called atherothrombotic brain infarction (ABI) and includes infarction resulting from large vessel atherothrombosis, lacunar infarction, and infarct of undetermined cause; embolic stroke from a known cardiac source was excluded.

HYPERTENSION AND RISK OF STROKE

Among stroke risk factors, hypertension is clearly preeminent and is of importance for all stroke types, infarction as well as hemorrhage. Using the systolic blood pressure levels in the most recent classification of hypertension (sixth report of the Joint National Committee on Prevention, Detection, Evaluation, and Treatment of High Blood Pressure), the incidence of nonembolic ischemic stroke in Framingham (ABI) was approximately 3 times greater in persons with definite hypertension ($\geq 160/\geq 95$ mm Hg) than in normotensives.[7] Hypertension made a powerful and significant *independent* contribution to the incidence of ABI, even after age and other pertinent risk factors had been taken into account.

While the incidence of stroke is increased in hypertensives, the dichotomy of hypertensive and normotensive obscures the powerful, graded, direct relationship that exists between increasing level of blood pressure and increasing incidence of stroke. Using the systolic blood pressure categories of the JNC VI, stroke incidence increased with increasing levels of systolic pressure from normal (<130 mm Hg systolic) through high normal (130–139 mm Hg systolic), mild hypertension (140–159 mm Hg systolic), moderate hypertension (160–179 mm Hg systolic), to severe hypertension (≥ 180 mm Hg systolic) (Figure 5.1).[8] This was true in both sexes and in all age categories, including the elderly, aged 75 to 84 years. There was no evidence women tolerated hypertension better than men or that hypertension was unimportant in the elderly.

Furthermore, although the incidence rate of stroke was greatest at the upper levels of blood pressure, most stroke events occurred in persons with moderate

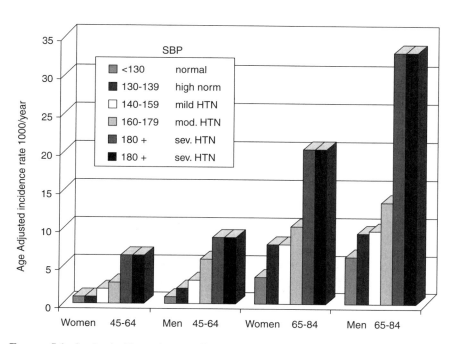

FIGURE 5.1. Stroke incidence by systolic blood pressure. *Source*: Joseph LN, Kase CS, Beiser AS, Wolf PA. Mild Blood Pressure Elevation and Stroke: The Framingham Study. *Stroke* 1998;29(1):277.

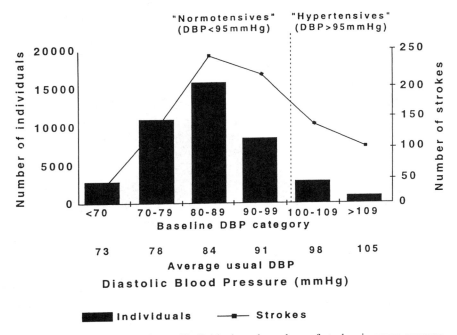

FIGURE 5.2. Absolute numbers of individuals and numbers of strokes in seven prospective observational studies, subdivided by baseline diastolic blood pressure (DBP) category (405,000 individuals and 843 strokes in total). Approximately 80% of all strokes occurred among the 95% of individuals classified as "normotensive" (usual DBP <95 mm Hg). Reprinted from MacMahon S, Rodgers A. The epidemiological association between blood pressure and stroke: implications for primary and secondary prevention. *Hyperten Res* 1994;17(suppl 1):523–532. Used by permission.

and "normotensive" diastolic blood pressure levels (Figure 5.2).[9] Similarly, for systolic blood pressure, most stroke events occurred in persons at high normal, mild, and moderate hypertension levels. Among subjects aged 65 to 84 years, after 40 years of follow-up in Framingham, only 19% of strokes occurred in those with severe hypertension (Figure 5.3).[8] This was true for stroke due to hemorrhage or ischemia. More than two-thirds (69%) of all strokes occurred at systolic blood pressure levels between 130 mm Hg and 179 mm Hg.

CONTROL OF HYPERTENSION AND STROKE PREVENTION

Following clinical observation of patients with treated and untreated hypertension with prospective epidemiologic study, it is apparent that level of blood pressure is related to incidence of stroke, and this is true for severe, moderate, and mild hypertensives.[10] Analysis of nine major prospective studies that included 420,000 individuals with a mean 10-year follow-up, the evidence clearly showed

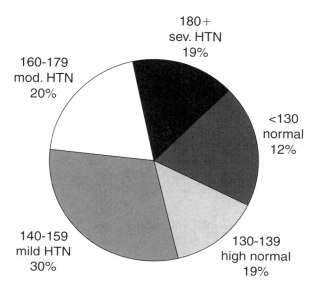

FIGURE 5.3. Percent of stroke by systolic blood pressure in subjects aged 65–84 years. *Source*: Joseph LN, Kase CS, Beiser AS, Wolf PA. Mild blood pressure elevation and stroke: The Framingham Study. *Stroke* 1998;29(1):277.

a graded relationship between diastolic pressure and stroke and coronary heart disease (CHD) incidence. There was no threshold level below which risk gradients were flat. For every 7.5 mm Hg diastolic pressure increase, there was a 46% increase in stroke incidence and a 29% increase in CHD.[10] Matching these findings derived from observational studies, an analysis of 14 treatment trials with a total of 37,000 hypertensive subjects showed reduction of blood pressure in hypertensives reduced stroke incidence.[11] The average diastolic blood pressure was reduced by 5.8 mm Hg and was associated with a corresponding reduction in stroke incidence of 42%. This observed reduction in stroke closely approximated what had been expected from the prospective observational studies. These findings should put to rest the concern that reduction of blood pressure in hypertensives precipitates stroke.

The 14% decrease in CHD rates was, however, considerably less than what might be expected. The explanation for the lesser effect on CHD incidence may relate to the adverse influence on electrolyte, glucose, and lipid metabolism of the thiazide diuretics that were the mainstay of treatment in most of the trials and on the relatively lesser importance of hypertension to CHD (where blood lipid levels are key) than stroke. It is important to note that these substantial and significant reductions in stroke incidence occurred during the course of the trials. In these studies, the duration of blood pressure reduction was brief, from two to five years, suggesting interruption of a precipitating factor rather than interfering with atherogenesis.[11] Presumably, more prolonged blood pressure control would have both effects.

These trials were conducted in younger individuals, generally below the age of 65, and physicians were hesitant to reduce the blood pressures of elderly hypertensives. In the Swedish Trial in Old Patients with Hypertension (STOP), 1627 patients, aged 65 to 84 years (mean age 78 years), with elevated systolic (180–230 mm Hg) and diastolic (>90 mm Hg) blood pressure levels were randomized to treatment (thiazide diuretic and beta-blockers) and placebo groups.[12] Blood pressure was reduced, on average, 20/8 mm Hg. The trial was stopped after 2.1 years, with a 47% reduction in stroke incidence. Cardiovascular events were 40% lower and deaths 43% lower in the treatment group. A number of other trials of antihypertensives in elderly persons with mild diastolic hypertension also demonstrated the benefit and safety of this treatment in elderly persons.[13–15]

ISOLATED SYSTOLIC HYPERTENSION

Traditionally, greater importance has been ascribed to the diastolic than the systolic blood pressure level, and while most clinical trials of hypertension treatment have classified subjects by the diastolic level, evidence for the ascendancy of the diastolic component of the blood pressure over the systolic is lacking.[16] With advancing age, systolic blood pressure continues to rise into the 70s, while diastolic pressures peak in the early 50s, then decline. In the elderly, isolated systolic hypertension, that is, blood pressure levels ≥160 mm Hg systolic and <90 mm Hg diastolic, becomes highly prevalent: approximately 25% of persons above age 80 are affected.[17] Although common, it is not innocuous. In Framingham, men 65 to 84 years of age with isolated systolic hypertension had approximately a 2-fold increased risk of stroke and women had a 1.5-fold increase in stroke risk.[18] Since isolated systolic hypertension is a consequence of reduced elasticity of the great arteries, it has been suggested that the arterial rigidity per se, rather than the systolic blood pressure, was responsible for the increased stroke rate. However, data from Framingham showed the risk of stroke was increased in persons with isolated systolic hypertension, even after the arterial rigidity was taken into account, and incidence of stroke rose in direct relation to the level of systolic pressure.[18] Furthermore, in two large clinical trials, reduction of increased systolic blood pressure levels was followed by a 40% to 50% reduction in stroke incidence rates.[19,20] It had been assumed that reduction of blood pressure would be difficult to achieve, hazardous in terms of side effects, and unwarranted on the basis of available data. The Systolic Hypertension in the Elderly Program (SHEP) was a double-blind, placebo-controlled trial involving 4736 persons of an average age of 72 years with systolic blood pressure levels of 160 mm Hg. or greater and diastolic pressures below 90 mm Hg.[19] In the treatment group, where blood pressure reduction averaged 11/4 mm Hg, there was a 37% reduction in stroke and a 27% reduction in MI and coronary death after 4.6 years of follow-up. The magnitude of the benefit was probably an underestimate of the impact of treatment on disease outcomes since, by the end of the SHEP trial, 44% of patients assigned to the placebo group were no longer receiving randomized treatment. These findings have enormous importance because two-thirds of all individuals with hypertension above the age of 65 years have isolated systolic hypertension. Of course, the majority of strokes occur in this age group.

It is clear from the SHEP trial and from the European Working Party on Hypertension in the Elderly (EWPHE) study that antihypertensive medication was well tolerated by the elderly.[13] SHEP demonstrated that reduction of pressure was accomplished with relative ease. Approximately half were controlled with chlorthalidone (a thiazide diuretic) alone, which was well tolerated, as evidenced by a 90% compliance rate in the active treatment group at five years. Contrary to the fears of clinicians, the treatment group did not experience greater syncope, confusion, falls, or depression.[19]

More recently, the Systolic Hypertension in Europe (Syst-Eur) trial, a double-blind, randomized trial in 4695 elderly persons with systolic hypertension, compared the antihypertensive agent nitrendipine to placebo. After a median two years of follow-up, a 42%, (95% CI -60 to -17), $p = 0.003$ reduction in stroke incidence was found.[20] Nitrendipine, a dihydropyridine calcium channel blocker, was the antihypertensive drug used (an angiotensin-converting enzyme, then a thiazide diuretic could be added) and was quite effective in stroke prevention. Total coronary events declined by 26% ($p = 0.03$), but cardiovascular mortality and all causes of mortality were not significantly reduced. However, concerns have been raised that certain calcium channel blockers increase rates of myocardial infarction.[21,22] The treatment of choice for control of hypertension is generally considered to be a diuretic, a beta-blocker, or both.[2] Because increased blood pressure is the most powerful risk factor for stroke, and because the benefits of treatment occur so promptly, control of increased blood pressure, systolic as well as diastolic, is the cornerstone of stroke prevention.

OPTIMAL BLOOD PRESSURE

The optimal level to which elevated blood pressure should be reduced for stroke prevention remains unknown, but it is clearly lower than had been previously thought. Fears that overzealous blood pressure reduction would reduce cerebral blood flow in persons with cerebral atherosclerosis and precipitate stroke have not been borne out. Despite the evidence that careful and sustained reduction of elevated blood pressure prevents stroke, less than vigorous control has been advocated by some.[23] In a highly regarded textbook of geriatric medicine, the author states "Although advocated as a possible ideal, there is therefore no need to 'normalize' the blood pressure to a diastolic below 90 or a systolic below 160 mm Hg in order to produce at least some benefit. A more modest reduction of pressure may constitute a desirable compromise between benefit and adverse effects of treatment for some patients."[23] The major concern expressed is that vigorous treatment of hypertension in the elderly might precipitate stroke or produce serious adverse effects. These specific effects of treatment include hypokalemia, hyponatremia, and increased rates of dementia, depression, faints, falls, and fractures. The occurrence of these adverse effects was systematically monitored in the treated groups and did not occur in these large trials of isolated systolic hypertension in the elderly.[19,20]

On the basis of an analysis of a number of clinical trials and meta-analyses, for stroke prevention, the recommended target for systolic pressure is less than 125 mm Hg. and the diastolic pressure less than 85 mm Hg (Figure 5.4).[24] To address this question, the Hypertension Optimal Treatment (HOT) trial randomly

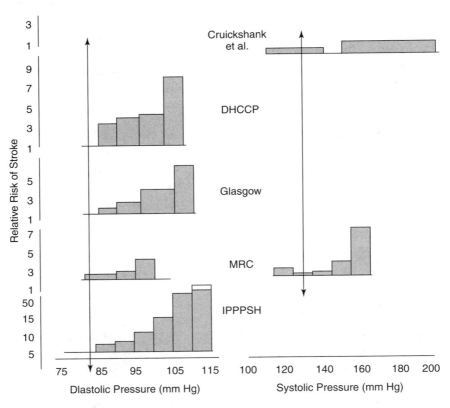

Figure 5.4. Relative risks of stroke according to blood pressure during treatment for hypertension in eight studies and meta-analyses. The arrows indicate the levels of treated systolic and diastolic blood pressure associated with the lowest risks of stroke. Reprinted from Fletcher AE, Bulpitt CJ. How far should blood pressure be lowered? *N Engl J Med.* 1992;326:251–254. Used by permission.

assigned 18,790 patients, aged 50–80 years (mean 61.5 years) with diastolic blood pressures between 100 mm Hg and 115 mm Hg (mean 105 mm Hg), to goals of one of three diastolic pressure ranges.[25] One-third was allocated to the target pressure ≤90 mm Hg, one-third to ≤85 mm Hg, and one-third ≤80 mm Hg. Diastolic pressure was reduced by 20.3 mm Hg, 22.3 mm Hg, and 24.3 mm Hg in these target groups, respectively. The lowest incidence of major cardiovascular events occurred at a mean achieved diastolic level of 82.6 mm Hg and at a mean systolic pressure of 138.5 mm Hg. For stroke, the lowest risk was below 80 mm Hg diastolic and 142.2 mm Hg systolic. However, the small differences in blood pressure reduction in the three target groups made it difficult to recognize significant differences in event rates in the three groups, and for stroke these differences were not statistically significant. Statistical significance was reached only for the end point "all myocardial infarction" (p for trend = 0.05, relative risk = 1.37, 95% CI 0.99–1.91) comparing the group whose target was ≤90 mm Hg vs. ≤80 mm Hg. In the subgroup of 1501 patients with diabetes mellitus, greater reduction in the diastolic pressure was associated with an approximately 30% relative risk reduction in stroke, although these effects also were not statistically significant. This issue of target blood pressure levels has yet to be definitively resolved and is still under study.

CHOICE OF ANTIHYPERTENSIVE DRUGS

Concern about the expense of antihypertensive medication is real, but for stroke, most trials have demonstrated approximately a 40% relative risk reductions with inexpensive agents—thiazide diuretics, beta-blockers, and hydralazine. The optimal drugs and combinations of drugs for specific patients is currently being intensively studied in many large scale trials, with more than 100,000 patients already randomized.[21]

SUBGROUPS OF HYPERTENSIVE PATIENTS INCLUDING STROKE RISK PROFILE

Type 2 diabetics experience an increase in microvascular and macrovascular disease incidence, including stroke.[26] To determine if tight control of blood pressure could reduce these cardiovascular complications, 1148 hypertensive type 2 diabetics were recruited. They were randomized to either an angiotensin converting enzyme inhibitor (captopril) or a beta-blocker (atenolol) and to two levels of blood pressure control. Of the patients, 758 were allocated to a tight control of blood pressure group (goal <150/<85 mm Hg) and 390 to a less-tight control group (<180/105 mm Hg).[27] Reductions in all the cardiovascular endpoints occurred in the tight control group compared to the less-tight control group. A 44% relative risk reduction of stroke was seen after 8.4 years of median follow-up. Neither antihypertensive agent was superior, either in terms of the benefit or absence of harm. It thus seems likely the marked increase in stroke and other micro- and macrovascular complications of type 2 diabetes mellitus may be significantly reduced by tight control of the frequently associated elevated blood pressures.[28]

Among asymptomatic persons with elevated blood pressure, it would be helpful to be able to identify those at greatly increased risk of stroke. At any given blood pressure level, the presence of associated risk factor abnormalities exerts a powerful influence on stroke risk. For example, a 70-year-old man with a systolic blood pressure of 120 mm Hg may have several times the risk of stroke of someone with a systolic pressure of 180 mm Hg who is free of other risk factor abnormalities.[29] In persons with high normal blood pressure or mild systolic hypertension and few associated stroke risk factors, control might be accomplished with hygienic measures, such as weight loss, increase in dietary potassium, reduction in dietary sodium, moderation of alcohol consumption, and promotion of moderate physical activity. Of course, these measures can also be advocated for most people. Persons with higher blood pressure levels and those with associated cardiovascular disease, cigarette smoking, or, particularly, diabetes mellitus will undoubtedly require medication to achieve blood pressure control.

In order to select those persons at greatest risk of developing cardiovascular disease and stroke, a risk profile was developed based on 36 years of follow-up data from Framingham.[29] Using information collected during a complete history and physical examination, including an electrocardiogram (ECG), probability of stroke may be determined. Using a separate table for men and women, stroke probability is determined by a point system based on age, systolic blood pressure, antihypertensive therapy use, presence of diabetes, cigarette smoking, history of cardiovascular disease [coronary heart disease (CHD) or cardiovascular heart failure (CHF)], and electrocardiogram (ECG) abnormalities [left ventricular hypertrophy (LVH) or atrial fibrillation (AF)]. It is apparent that in persons at varying levels of blood pressure, the probability of stroke varies across a wide range. Probability rises with increased systolic blood pressure (120 mm Hg and 180 mm Hg are shown) depending on the presence of other abnormalities in the risk profile (Figure 5.5).[29] This risk profile provides a quantitative determination of probability of stroke relative to what is average for a man of this age. The realization that the probability of stroke is increased several-fold may help the patient and physician to more fully appreciate the need for serious risk factor management.

PREVENTIVE IMPLICATIONS

The recent demonstration of the benefits of treatment and control of hypertension in stroke prevention in the elderly with diastolic or isolated systolic hyper-

Probability of Stroke %

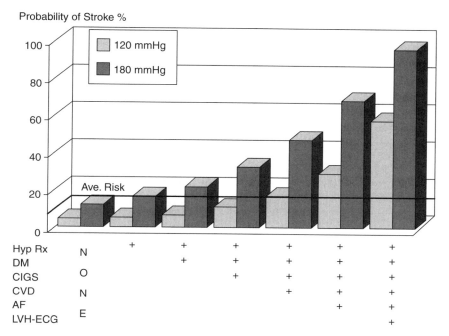

FIGURE 5.5. Probability of stroke during 10 years in men aged 70 years at two systolic blood pressure levels: impact of other risk factors. Hyp Rx = antihypertensive therapy; DM = diabetes mellitus; Cigs = cigarette smoking; CVD = previously diagnosed coronary heart disease, cardiac failure, or intermittent claudication; AF = atrial fibrillation; LVH-ECG = left ventricular hypertrophy by electrocardiogram. *Source*: Wolf PA, D'Agostino RB, Belanger AJ, Kannel WB. Probability of stroke: A risk profile from the Framingham Study. *Stroke* 1991;22:312–318.

tension suggests that considerable progress remains to be achieved. Recently, it has been estimated that of the 50 million hypertensives in the United States, only 32.5 million were aware of its presence and 24.5 million were being treated. Unfortunately, only 10.5 million hypertensives had their blood pressure controlled, leaving nearly 40 million either unaware, untreated, or treated but uncontrolled. Because clinical trial data suggest an approximately 40% reduction in stroke incidence, even with short-term treatment trials (i.e., less than 5 years), a great deal of stroke prevention could be achieved by blood pressure control. It has been estimated that nearly 250,000 new strokes could be prevented each year by such efforts. In light of the end of the decline in stroke mortality, it is imperative that such preventive efforts be redoubled. Effective programs to detect, treat, and control hypertension, particularly in those at greatest risk of stroke, those above age 65 years, hold promise that stroke incidence and mortality may be reduced still further. When these measures are combined with a long-term, sustained program of risk factor modification, such as cigarette smoking cessation, the tools for achieving further substantial reduction in death and disability from stroke are already available.

REFERENCES

1. Pickering G. In: Laragh JH, ed. *Hypertension Manual: Mechanisms, Methods, Management*, New York: Yorke Medical Books, 1973.
2. JNC-VI: The sixth report of the Joint National Committee on prevention, detection, evaluation, and treatment of high blood pressure. *Arch Intern Med.* 1997;157: 2413–2446.
3. *Morbidity & Mortality: 1998 Chartbook on Cardiovascular, Lung and Blood Diseases.* National Institutes of Health, National Heart, Lung, and Blood Institute. October, 1998.
4. Janeway TC. A clinical study of hypertensive cardiovascular disease. *Arch Intern Med.* 1913;12:755.
5. Russell RWR. Observations on intracerebral aneurysms. *Brain* 1963;86:425.
6. Cole FM, Yates PO: The occurrence and significance of intracerebral microaneurysms. *J Pathol Bacteriol* 1967;93:393.
7. Kannel WB, Wolf PA, Verter J, McNamara PM. Epidemiologic assessment of the role of blood pressure in stroke. The Framingham Study. *JAMA.* 1970;214(2):301–310.
8. Joseph LN, Kase CS, Beiser AS, Wolf PA. Mild blood pressure elevation and stroke: The Framingham Study. *Stroke* 1998;29(1):277.
9. MacMahon S, Rodgers A. The epidemiological association between blood pressure and stroke: Implications for primary and secondary prevention. *Hypertens Res.* 1994; 17(suppl I):S23–S32.
10. MacMahon S, Peto R, Cutler J, Collins R, Sorlie P, Neaton J, Abbott R, Godwin J, Dyer A, Stamler J. Blood pressure, stroke, and coronary heart disease. Part 1: Prolonged differences in blood pressure: Prospective observational studies corrected for the regression dilution bias. *Lancet* 1990;335(8692):765–774.
11. Collins R, Peto R, MacMahon S, Hebert P, Fiebach NH,. Eberlein KA, Godwin J, Qizilbash N, Taylor JO, Hennekens CH. Blood pressure, stroke, and coronary heart disease. Part 2: Short-term reductions in blood pressure: Overview of randomised drug trials in their epidemiological context. *Lancet* 1990;335(8693):827–838.
12. Dahlof B, Lindholm LH, Hansson L, Schersten B, Ekbom T, Wester PO. Morbidity and mortality in the Swedish Trial in Old Patients with Hypertension (STOP-Hypertension. *Lancet* 1991;338(8778):1281–1285.
13. Amery A, Birkenhager W, Brixko P, Bulpitt C, Clement D, Deruyttere M, De Schaepdryver A, Dollery C, Fagard R, Forette F, et al. Mortality and morbidity results from the European Working Party on High Blood Pressure in the Elderly trial. *Lancet* 1985;1(8442):1349–1354.
14. Coope J, Warrender TS. Randomised trial of treatment of hypertension in elderly patients in primary care. *Brit Med J Clin Res Ed* 1986;293(6555):1145–1151.
15. MRC Working Party. Medical Research Council trial of treatment of hypertension in older adults: principal results. *BMJ* 1992;304(6824):405–412.
16. Rutan GH, McDonald RH, Kuller LH: A historical perspective of elevated systolic vs diastolic blood pressure from an epidemiological and clinical trial viewpoint. *J Clin Epidemiol* 1989;42:663–673.
17. Wilking SV, Belanger A, Kannel WB, D'Agostino RB, Steel K: Determinants of isolated systolic hypertension. *JAMA* 1988;260:3451–3455.

18. Kannel WB, Wolf PA, McGee DL, Dawber TR, McNamara P, Castelli WP. Systolic blood pressure, arterial rigidity, and risk of stroke: The Framingham Study. *JAMA* 1981;245(12):1225–1229.

19. SHEP Cooperative Research Group. Prevention of stroke by antihypertensive drug treatment in older persons with isolated systolic hypertension. Final results of the Systolic Hypertension in the Elderly Program (SHEP. *JAMA* 1991;265(24):3255–3264.

20. Staessen JA, Fagard R, Thijs L, Celis H, Arabidze GG, Birkenhager WH, Bulpitt CJ, de Leeuw PW, Dollery CT, Fletcher AE, Forette F, Leonetti G, Nachev C, O'Brien ET, Rosenfeld J, Rodicio JL, Tuomilehto J, Zanchetti A. Randomised double-blind comparison of placebo and active treatment for older patients with isolated systolic hypertension: The Systolic Hypertension in Europe (Syst-Eur. Trial Investigators. *Lancet* 1997;350(9080):757–764.

21. Fletcher AE, Bulpitt CJ. How far should blood pressure be lowered? *N Engl J Med* 1992;326(4):251–254.

22. Estacio RO, Jeffers BW, Hiatt WR, Biggerstaff SL, Gifford N, Schrier RW. The effect of nisoldipine as compared with enalapril on cardiovascular outcomes in patients with non-insulin-dependent diabetes and hypertension. *N Engl J Med* 1998;338(10): 645–652.

23. Cutler JA. Calcium-channel blockers for hypertension—uncertainty continues. *N Engl J Med* 1998;338(10):679–681.

24. Evans JG. The prevention of stroke. In: Evans JG, Williams TF, eds. Oxford Textbook of Geriatric Medicine. New York: Oxford University Press, 1992:329–334.

25. Hansson L, Zanchetti A, Carruthers SG, Dahlof B, Elmfeldt D, Julius S, Menard J, Rahn KH, Wedel H, Westerling S. Effects of intensive blood-pressure lowering and low-dose aspirin in patients with hypertension: Principal results of the Hypertension Optimal Treatment (HOT. randomised trial. HOT Study Group. *Lancet* 1998; 351(9118):1755–1762.

26. Manson JE, Colditz GA, Stampfer MJ, Willett WC, Krolewski AS, Rosner B, Arky RA, Speizer FE, Hennekens CH. A prospective study of maturity-onset diabetes mellitus and risk of coronary heart disease and stroke in women. *Arch Int Med* 1991; 151(6):1141–1147.

27. Turner R, Holman R, Stratton I, et al. Tight blood pressure control and risk of macrovascular and microvascular complications in type 2 diabetes: UKPDS 38. UK Prospective Diabetes Study Group. *BMJ* 1998;317(7160):703–713.

28. Orchard T. Diabetes: A time for excitement—and concern. Hopeful signs exist that the ravages of diabetes can be tamed. *BMJ* 1998;317(7160):691–692.

29. Wolf PA, D'Agostino RB, Belanger AJ, Kannel WB. Probability of stroke: A risk profile from the Framingham Study. *Stroke* 1991;22(3):312–338.

6

ATRIAL FIBRILLATION

David Sherman

Atrial fibrillation (AF) is an important cause of ischemic stroke. It represents the most common arrhythmia in the general population and is particularly relevant as a focus for stroke prevention considering its growing prevalence and the effectiveness of strategies for stroke prevention. About 15% of patients suffering ischemic stroke have associated AF, but the percentage rises with age, so that by age 80 more than 30% of ischemic stroke patients have associated AF.[1] The evidence is overwhelming that more than two-thirds of these strokes can be prevented with appropriate preventive therapy.

Accurate estimates of the number of individuals in the population with AF are difficult to obtain. In the United States almost certainly three million people have AF. Estimates must be continually increased because of the striking association of AF with advancing age. The median age of the population with documented AF is 75 years. Because the elderly population is increasing each year, the number of individuals with AF and exposed to its attendant stroke risk is also increasing. The contention that estimates are low is supported by the observation that many patients with AF are unaware of their arrhythmia until it is documented in a medical evaluation. Many patients have paroxysmal AF, especially early in the course of the arrhythmia, and most bouts of AF in patients with paroxysmal AF are unrecognized by the patient. Symptoms of palpitations, lightheadedness, or dyspnea may be absent in some patients with AF, making them oblivious to the presence of this potentially devastating cardiac irregularity. This fact is painfully apparent when one finds that more than one-third of patients with stroke and AF were unaware of the arrhythmia until the occurrence of a major cardioembolic stroke.[2,3] Thus, population screening for AF before the occurrence of a stroke is an important public health priority, especially in the elderly but otherwise healthy population at greatest risk for development of this arrhythmia.

Epidemiologic evidence of the importance of AF as a risk factor for stroke led to the formulation of hypotheses as to potential prevention strategies. The Framingham study, for example, showed that the risk of stroke in a population with AF is five to six times that of a comparable population without AF. Patients with AF and associated mitral stenosis had a seventeen-fold increase in risk of stroke or embolus.[4] This difference in risk observed in AF subpopulations illustrates an important principle in the management of patients with AF, namely, that the risk of stroke can vary widely depending on associated cardiovascular conditions.

The clinical and radiologic features of a cardioembolic stroke due to AF are not highly specific. Unfortunately, most strokes associated with AF are unheralded by more benign cerebrovascular events, such as transient ischemic attacks (TIA). Quite the opposite is the case, in that strokes from a left atrial embolus tend to be large and disabling with a higher mortality than strokes from other sources.[5–7] Stroke onset is more often sudden, with maximal deficit immediately. Any arterial territory can be involved, but the middle cerebral artery is the commonest site of embolization. Cortical strokes from middle cerebral artery branch embolic occlusions are suggestive of a cardioembolic source. In the vertebrobasilar territory, posterior cerebral artery occlusions and "top of the basilar" strokes should raise suspicion of a potential cardiac source of embolus.[8] Large subcortical strokes, "lagoons" rather than "lacunes," may be due to embolic occlusion of the small penetrating arteries arising from the proximal middle cerebral artery and demand investigation for a cardiac source of embolus rather than assuming their location dictates a small artery occlusive mechanism. As noted, antecedent TIAs in the same arterial territory are uncommon with cardiogenic emboli. A somewhat increased probability of a seizure or transient loss of consciousness exists at stroke onset with a cardiogenic embolus.[9,10] The lack of specificity of these clinical features dictates that appropriate diagnostic studies be done to explore other etiologic possibilities, such as significant carotid atherosclerotic disease that might warrant consideration of endarterectomy.

The radiological features of a stroke related to a cardiogenic embolus from AF are generally what one might expect based on the anatomic observations outlined above. Characteristic findings with computerized tomography (CT) or magnetic resonance imaging (MRI) are cortical or large subcortical infarcts in the middle or posterior cerebral artery territories. Also suggestive are multiple cortical infarcts in different arterial territories. The "dense middle cerebral artery" sign is indicative of an occlusion, usually embolic, of the middle cerebral artery.[11] Hemorrhagic transformation of the infarct is somewhat more common with large embolic strokes, presumably because lysis of the embolus and reperfusion of a large, severely ischemic region of brain allows blood to infuse the infarct. Using the more sensitive imaging technique of MRI, hemorrhagic transformation can be demonstrated in more than two-thirds of cardioembolic infarcts.[12]

Most hemorrhagic transformations are not associated with neurologic deterioration unless the patient is anticoagulated at the time of transformation. This observation is the basis for the recommendation of this author and others to avoid immediate anticoagulation of patients with stroke of cardioembolic source until a CT done 36 hours from stroke onset confirms the absence of hemorrhagic transformation. At this time, small- or medium-sized infarcts may be anticoagulated if the patient is considered a safe candidate for anticoagulation. Large infarcts are particularly prone to hemorrhagic transformation, and anticoagulation should be withheld if possible for 7 to 10 days. Of course, each case must be considered individually, weighing the estimated risk of recurrent embolus against the risk of intracerebral hemorrhage aggravated by full anticoagulation.

Uncertainty about the utility and risk of long-term warfarin therapy led to the design of five randomized clinical treatment trials of anticoagulation in individuals with AF.[13–20] All trials compared various intensities of anticoagulation to a non-anticoagulated control population. Two trials, AFASAK and SPAF I, included an aspirin-treated group.[15,16,18] Two of the trials, CAFA and SPINAF, were designed with a double-blind comparison of warfarin and placebo.[14,20] The remaining trials managed the warfarin-treated patients in an open-label design.[13,15,16–18]

The benefit of warfarin for prevention of stroke was proven consistently and conclusively by these randomized clinical trials. Warfarin-assigned AF patients had the risk of ischemic stroke or systemic embolus reduced by about two-thirds in each of the trials. On average, the annual rate of stroke was reduced from 4.5% to 1.5% (Figure 6.1). The true efficacy of warfarin is undoubtedly greater when the outcomes in these trials are viewed with an on-treatment analysis. Most patients suffering an ischemic stroke had no or inadequate anticoagulation at the time of the stroke.[21,22] Patients willing and able to continue warfarin treatment experienced an 80% or greater reduction in stroke risk.

The prospective randomized treatment trials of patients with AF have defined a number of coexistent conditions that influence the risk of stroke. Multivariate analyses have consistently shown that hypertension, prior TIA or stroke, and left ventricular systolic dysfunction are independently predictive of stroke in AF patients.[21,23–26] In other studies, additional risks were coronary artery disease, diabetes, and age.[21,24,26]

The condition of greatest predictive value for risk of stroke in patients with AF is a prior stroke or TIA. This fact was well established by the European Atrial Fibrillation Trial (EAFT).[27] In this trial, 669 patients with AF and a recent TIA

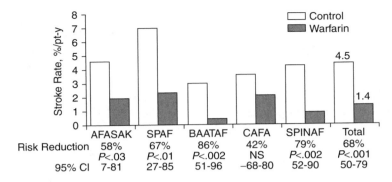

FIGURE 6.1. Stroke rate (percent per patient-year [pt-y]. in patients randomized to warfarin and in control subjects (intention-to-treat analysis). Strokes represent all strokes, regardless of suspected cause. Transient ischemic attacks, systemic emboli, and intracranial hemorrhages are not included. Control subjects received placebo in all studies except BAATAF. (In BAATAF, 46% of the control patients took aspirin and 54% received "no treatment".) P values by chi square analysis. Reprinted by permission.[22]

or minor stroke considered candidates for anticoagulation were randomized to open anticoagulation or double-blind treatment with either 300 mg. aspirin per day or placebo. An additional 338 patients considered not candidates for anticoagulation were randomized to either aspirin or placebo. After a mean follow-up of 2.3 years, the risk of stroke in the placebo-treated group was 12% per year, compared to 4% per year in the anticoagulated group (Figure 6.2). Major bleeds occurred in 2.8% of the anticoagulated patients each year, compared to 0.9% per year in the aspirin-treated patients.

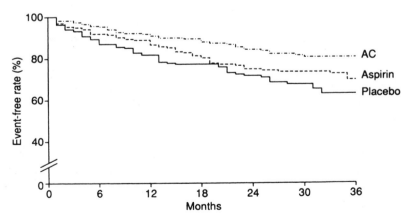

FIGURE 6.2. Survival analysis for primary outcome event: group 1. Vascular death, nonfatal stroke, nonfatal myocardial infarction, or nonfatal systemic embolism, whichever came first: anticoagulation (AC), aspirin, and placebo. Reprinted by permission.[27]

The practical clinical management decision is often whether a patient with AF has a stroke risk that justifies the bleeding risk and inconvenience of warfarin anticoagulation or can be managed with aspirin alone or some simpler treatment regimen. The SPAF III study was designed to determine whether patients with increased stroke risk could be treated with a low fixed dose of warfarin (1–3 mg) and aspirin effectively and safely. This study was stopped early when, after a mean follow-up of only 1.1 years, the rate of ischemic stroke and systemic embolus was 7.9% per year in the patients on the low-dose combination therapy and only 1.9% per year in the patients treated with warfarin adjusted to an INR of 2.0-3.0 (Figure 6.3).[28]

The predictors of stroke risk in patients treated only with aspirin was addressed in the SPAF I–III studies. More than 2000 participants were treated with aspirin or the above-noted low-dose warfarin combination with aspirin. A multivariate logistic regression analysis of predictors yielded a number of significant factors.[29] The predictors were age with a relative risk (RR) of 1.8 per decade, a history of hypertension (RR = 2.0), female gender (RR = 1.6), systolic blood pressure >160 torr (RR = 2.3), and prior stroke or TIA (RR = 2.9). These predictors were significant at the p = <0.001 level. Consumption of ≥14 alcohol drinks per week reduced stroke risk (RR = 0.4, p = 0.04). Estrogen hormone replacement in women in the SPAF studies was associated with an increased risk of stroke (RR = 3.2, p = 0.007).

Echocardiography is a commonly applied diagnostic tool in the assessment of patients for a potential cardiac source of embolus, including patients with AF.

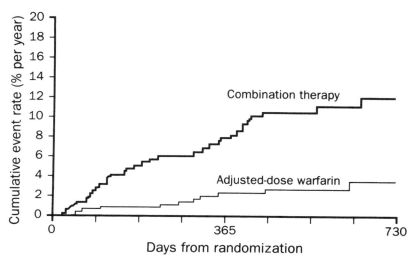

FIGURE 6.3. Cumulative rate of ischemic stroke or systemic embolism (primary events. in adjusted-dose warfarin group (n = 523) and combination therapy group (n = 521). The relative risk reduction by adjusted-dose warfarin was 74% (95% CI 50,87, p < 0.0001).[28]

Transthoracic echocardiography (TTE) fails to adequately visualize the left atrium. The ability of transesophageal echocardiography (TEE) to outline the atrial anatomy and contents has made it the favored technique for evaluation of the heart in patients with AF. TEE is consistently superior to TTE in detecting left atrial thrombi. In the SPAF cohort of patients undergoing TEE, 13% had left atrial thrombi detected.[30] Nineteen percent had dense spontaneous echo contrast, a finding predictive of thrombus formation and stroke. A reduced flow velocity (<20 cm/sec.) in the left atrium also predicted the presence of thrombus. Spontaneous echo contrast is presumed to be a consequence of reduced flow of blood, allowing the clumping together of red blood cells that slowly swirl and reflect the echocardiographic signals to yield a smoke-like illusion. The SPAF TEE studies also found that complex aortic atherosclerotic plaque was more common in patients with prior stroke.

The optimal intensity of anticoagulation has been evaluated directly and indirectly by a number of investigators. SPAF III demonstrated that low doses of warfarin, even with aspirin, were ineffective in preventing thromboembolism in high-risk AF patients. Other investigators have addressed the optimal range of international normalized ratio (INR) to prevent stroke and minimize the risk for major bleeding, especially intracerebral bleed. An analysis of the 214 patients who received anticoagulant therapy in the European Atrial Fibrillation Trial calculated incidence rates for both ischemic and major hemorrhagic events as they related to the patients' INR. The optimal intensity of anticoagulation was found to lie between an INR of 2.0 and 3.9. No treatment effect was apparent with anticoagulation below an INR of 2.0. The rate of thromboembolic events was lowest at INRs from 2.0 to 3.9, and most major bleeding complications occurred with treatment at INRs of 5.0 and above.[31]

TABLE 6.1. Primary Prevention of Ischemic Stroke: Source of Potential Cardiogenic Emboli

NONVALVULAR ATRIAL FIBRILLATION	RECOMMENDED TREATMENT AND COMMENTS
High risk (stroke rate 8%/year) Prior TIA or stroke Age >75 years Left ventricle dysfunction SBP >160 mm Hg	Warfarin, target INR 2.5 (2.0–3.0) Alternative therapy for patients with contraindication to warfarin: aspirin
Moderate risk (stroke rate 4%/year) History of hypertension Age 65–75 years	Aspirin *or* warfarin, target INR 2.5 (2.0–3.0), depending on individual patient preferences and bleeding risks
Low risk (stroke rate 1%/year) <65 years No high-risk factors	Aspirin
"Lone" atrial fibrillation	Primary prevention not recommended

Another case control study concluded that the optimal INR range was 2.0–3.0, although some effect in prevention of thromboembolism was noted with INRs below 2.0.[26] Given the difficulties in maintaining a consistent INR level over time, it seems most prudent to target an INR of 2.5 (range 2.0–3.0). Randomized trials have observed that about 20% of INR levels over an extended period of time will fall below the target range. Thus, the practice of targeting a low INR in an attempt to avoid bleeding complications may cause periods of inadequate anticoagulation, placing the patient at risk for stroke. The major predictor of intracerebral hemorrhage seems to be advanced age. Poorly controlled hypertension is also considered to increase the risk of intracerebral bleed. Based on the available information about the predictors of stroke risk, the value of warfarin and aspirin therapy, and the bleeding risks of warfarin therapy, a recommendation can be made for the management of these patients as outlined in Table 6.1 and Figure 6.4.

The potential for stroke prevention in patients with AF is great. The number of individuals with this common arrhythmia is increasing as a consequence of an aging population. The evidence is overwhelming as to the risk of thromboembolism without treatment and the risks reduction with appropriate therapy. Information is available to allow identification of patients at highest risk for stroke and to reduce their stroke risk by a remarkable 65%–80%. The greatest challenge is to identify these patients at risk and to manage them with the appropriate therapy, thereby preventing the devastating consequences of unheralded stroke.

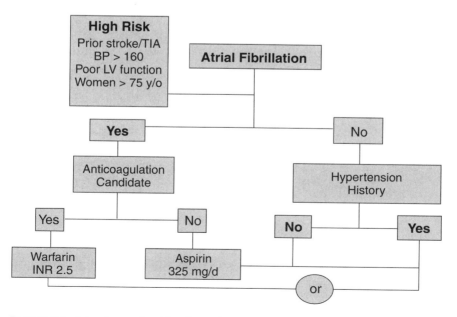

FIGURE 6.4. A treatment algorithm for patients with atrial fibrillation.

REFERENCES

1. Wolf PA, Abbott RD, Kannel WB. Atrial fibrillation: a major contributor to stroke in the elderly—The Framingham Study. *Arch Intern Med* 1987;147:1561–1564.
2. Sherman DG, Goldman L, Whiting RB, Jurgensen K, Kaste M, Easton JD. Thromboembolism in patients with atrial fibrillation. *Arch Neurol* 1984;41:708–710.
3. Wolf PA, Kannel WB, McGee DL, Meeks SL, Bharucha NE, McNamara PM. Duration of atrial fibrillation and imminence of stroke: The Framingham study. *Stroke* 1983;14:664–667.
4. Wolf PA, Dawber TR, Thomas HE, Jr., Kannel WB. Epidemiologic assessment of chronic atrial fibrillation and risk of stroke: Fhe Framingham study. *Neurology* 1978; 28:973–977.
5. Censori B, Camerlingo M, Casto L, Ferraro B, Gazzaniga GC, Cesana B, Mamoli A. Prognostic factors in first-ever stroke in the carotid artery territory seen within 6 hours after onset. *Stroke* 1993;24:532–535.
6. Lin HJ, Wolf PA, Kelly-Hayes M, Beiser AS, Kase CS, Benjamin EJ, D'Agostino RB. Stroke severity in atrial fibrillation. The Framingham Study. *Stroke* 1996;27(10): 1760–1764.
7. Sandercock P, Bamford J, Dennis M, Burn J, Slattery J, Jones L, Boonyakarnkul S, Warlow C. Atrial fibrillation and stroke: Prevalence in different types of stroke and influence on early and long term prognosis (Oxfordshire Community Stroke Project). *BMJ* 1992;305:1460–1465.
8. Caplan LR, Hier DB, D'Cruz I. Cerebral embolism in the Michael Reese Stroke Registry. *Stroke* 1983;14:530–536.
9. Bogousslavsky J, Hachinski VC, Boughner DR, Fox AJ, Vi:nuela F, Barnett HJ. Clinical predictors of cardiac and arterial lesions in carotid transient ischemic attacks. *Arch Neurol* 1986;43:229–233.
10. Bogousslavsky J, Cachin C, Regli F, Despland PA, Van Melle G, Kappenberger L. Cardiac sources of embolism and cerebral infarction—clinical consequences and vascular concomitants: The Lausanne Stroke Registry. *Neurology* 1991;41:855–859.
11. Tomsick TA, Brott TG, Chambers AA, Fox AJ, Gaskill MFLR, Pleatman CW, Wiot JG, Bourekas E. Hyperdense middle cerebral artery sign on CT: Efficacy in detecting middle cerebral artery thrombosis. *Am J Neuroradiol* 1990;11(3):473–477.
12. Hornig CR, Dorndorf W, Agnoli AL. Hemorrhagic cerebral infarction—a prospective study. *Stroke* 1986;17:179–185.
13. The Boston Area Anticoagulation Trial for Atrila Fibrillation Investigators. The effect of low-dose warfarin on the risk of stroke in patients with nonrheumatic atrial fibrillation. *N Engl J Med* 1990;323:1505–1511.
14. Ezekowitz MD, Bridgerws SL, James KE, Carliner NH, Colling CL, Gornick CC, Krause-Steinrouf H, Kurtzke JK, Nazarian SM, Radford MJ, et al. Warfarin in the prevention of stroke associated with nonrheumatic atrial fibrillation. *N Engl J Med* 1992;327:1406–1412.
15. Petersen P, Boysen G, Godtfredsen J, Andersen ED, Andersen B. Placebo-controlled, randomised trial of warfarin and aspirin for prevention of thromboembolic complications in chronic atrial fibrillation. The Copenhagen AFASAK Study. *Lancet* 1989;1: 175–179.
16. Petersen P, Kastrup J, Helweg-Larsen S, Boysen G, Godtfredsen J. Risk factors for thromboembolic complications in chronic atrial fibrillation. The Copenhagen AFASAK Study. *Arch Intern Med* 1990;150:819–821.

17. Stroke Prevention in Atrial Fibrillation Investigators. Preliminary report of the Stroke Prevention in Atrial Fibrillation Study. *N Engl J Med* 1990;322:863–868.
18. Stroke Prevention in Atrial Fibrillation Investigators. Stroke Prevention in Atrial Fibrillation Study: Final results. *Circulation* 1991;84:527–539.
19. Stroke Prevention in Atrial Fibrillation Investigators. Warfarin versus aspirin for prevention of thromboembolism in atrial fibrillation: Stroke Prevention in Atrial Fibrillation II Study. *Lancet* 1994;343:687–691.
20. Connolly SJ, Laupacis A, Gent M, Roberts RS, Cairns JA, Joyner C. Canadian Atrial Fibrillation Anticoagulation (CAFA. Study. *J Am Coll Cardiol* 1991;18:349–355.
21. Atrial Fibrillation Investigators. Risk factors for stroke and efficacy of antithrombotic therapy in atrial fibrillation: Analysis of pooled data from five randomized controlled trials. *Arch Intern Med* 1994;154:1449–1457.
22. Albers GW. Choice of antithrombotic therapy for stroke prevention in atrial fibrillation: warfarin, aspirin, or both? *Arch Intern Med* 1998;158(14):1487–1491.
23. Atrial Fibrillation Investigators. Echocardiographic predictors of stroke in patients with atrial fibrillation: A prospective study of 1066 patients from 3 clinical trials. *Arch Intern Med* 1998;158(12):1316–1320.
24. The Stroke Prevention in Atrial Fibrillatin Investigators. Predictors of thromboembolism in atrial fibrillation: I. Clinical features of patients at risk. *Ann Intern Med* 1992;116:1–5.
25. The Stroke Prevention in Atrial Fibrillation Investigators. Predictors of thromboembolism in atrial fibrillation: II. Echocardiographic features of patients at risk. *Ann Intern Med* 1992;116:6–12.
26. Hylek EM, Skates SJ, Sheehan MA, Singer DE. An analysis of the lowest effective intensity of prophylactic anticoagulation for patients with nonrheumatic atrial fibrillation. *N Engl J Med* 1996;335:540–546.
27. European Atrial Fibrillation Trial Study Group. Secondary prevention in nonrheumatic atrial fibrillation after transient ischaemic attack or minor stroke. EAFT (European Atrial Fibrillation Trial. Study Group. *Lancet* 1993;342(8882):1255–1262.
28. Stroke Prevention in Atrial Fibrillation Investigators. Adjusted-dose warfarin versus low-intensity, fixed-dose warfarin plus aspirin for high-risk patients with atrial fibrillation: Stroke Prevention in Atrial Fibrillation III randomised clinical trial. *Lancet* 1996;348(9028):633–638.
29. Hart RG, Pearce LA, McBride R, Roghbart RM, Asinger RW, for the Stroke Prevention in Atrial Fibrillation Investigators. Factors associated with ischemic stroke during aspirin therapy in atrial fibrillation: Analysis of 2012 participants in the SPAF I-III clinical trials. *Stroke* 1999;30:1223–1229.
30. The Stroke Prevention in Atrial Fibrillation Investigators Committee on Echocardiography. Transesophageal echocardiographic correlates of thromboembolism in high-risk patients with nonvalvular atrial fibrillation. The Stroke Prevention in Atrial Fibrillation Investigators Committee on Echocardiography. *Ann Intern Med* 1998;128(8):639–647.
31. European Atrial Fibrillation Trial Study Group. Optimal oral anticoagulant therapy in patients with nonrheumatic atrial fibrillation and recent cerebral ischemia. *N Engl J Med* 1995;333(1):5–10.

7

PREVENTION AND SCREENING PROGRAMS

Philip B. Gorelick

Stroke is well-suited for prevention because it has a high prevalence, burden of illness and economic cost, and effective preventive measures.[1–3] Although stroke is preventable, recent surveys suggest that there is a lack of awareness of stroke warning signs and risk factors by the public and underutilization or possible mis-application of stroke prevention methods by physicians.[5,6] This should not come as a surprise, because implementation rates of clinical prevention services lag far behind the dissemination of prevention service goals.[7,8] A major barrier to the delivery of preventive services may be a perceived lack of time to implement such measures in the ambulatory office setting.

With rising prosperity one sees increasing interest in future health, healthy living, and a healthy environment.[9] Ironically, physicians are trained to care for the sick, but preventive training may not receive appropriate emphasis in medical school and postgraduate training programs. Furthermore, as resources for health care remain limited, politics and money increasingly determine health policy. The humanitarian argument that favors preventive medicine[9] may not be the highest priority of health planners, who must juggle limited financial resources.

SCREENING: CONCEPTS, DIAGNOSTIC TECHNOLOGY, AND VALUES

Screening is a public health strategy designed to separate persons with higher from persons with lower probabilities of disease. Those who screen "positive" are then referred to medical attention for definitive diagnosis.[11] For screening to do more good than harm, the following guidelines must be considered.[11]

1. Is the program effective judged on the basis of a randomized trial?
2. If an effectiveness trial has not been carried out, (a) are there efficacious treatments for the primary disorder or prevention measures for its sequelae? and (b) does the burden of disease warrant screening?
3. Is there a good screening test?
4. Does the program serve those who need it?
5. Can the health system accommodate the screening program?
6. Will those screened comply with advice and treatment plans?

To better understand screening in the context of prevention, one must appreciate the stages of chronic disease.[12] Chronic disease usually has a long latent period before clinical symptoms are manifested. Risk factors or exposures are thought to cause pathophysiologic changes that may eventually lead to clinically active disease. In the natural history of chronic disease, the earliest period is the susceptibility stage, in which one is susceptible to pathogenetic tissue change when exposed to risk factors. If the risk factor can be prevented from developing, disease may be thwarted or postponed. At this stage prevention may be possible through health promotion and intervention.

The second period is the presymptomatic stage, when pathogenetic damage has occurred but clinical symptoms have not yet appeared. Early detection, diagnosis, and treatment of modifiable risk factors may be the key to prevention at this stage. In the last two stages, clinical disease and disability or recovery, clinical disease is manifest and intervention is aimed at limiting disability and prevention of recurrent disease. Some have likened the first two stages to being 'upstream' and the latter two stages to being 'downstream'.[1] The upstream/downstream analogy refers, in the former case, to the point in time before disease becomes overt but may be prevented, and in the latter case to the point of manifest disease and its sequelae. Ideally, one strives to prevent risk factor development, and thus, intervene at the earliest possible stage (i.e., the upstream stage).

Public health dogma advocates screening and early intervention for modifiable risk factors. Risk factor modification is most effective when the factor is prevalent in the population; when there is a strong association between the favorable effects of treating the risk factor and the target disease; and when there are valid, safe, and cost-effective screening procedures and treatments. Thus, screening plays an important role in the public health model of disease prevention.

Effective screening depends on diagnostic technology. The purpose of diagnostic technology is to heighten the quality of health care.[13,14] Many technologies, however, have entered the market without adequate assessment of their effects on the quality of health care. Diagnostic tests directly affect those who are being screened. Those being screened value *safety* and *efficacy* as the most important characteristics of a technology. Thus, can a screening test be performed with minimal inconvenience and discomfort? Do side effects outweigh diagnostic benefits? With regard to efficacy of the technology one must consider the following:[13]

1. *Technical capability*—Does the diagnostic test meet the accepted standards of showing what it is expected to?
2. *Diagnostic accuracy*—What is the true positive rate (sensitivity), or the ability of the test to detect disease correctly when present? What is the true negative rate (specificity), or the test's ability to exclude disease when not present? Accuracy reflects both sensitivity and specificity (true positive plus true negative results divided by the total number of tests administered). A "gold-standard" is used to determine the "true" state of the screened.
3. *Diagnostic and therapeutic impact*—Does the technology change the diagnosis, add significant information, or change patient management?

Key factors to be considered when evaluating a medical diagnostic test are listed in Table 7.1.[15]

The complexity of a diagnostic screening instrument may vary considerably. For example, consider the differences in complexity of the following screening techniques: manual pulse rate estimation, blood pressure cuff, biochemical assay, and magnetic resonance spectroscopy system. Furthermore, in the current medical environment of cost-containment, flawed or unnecessary screening tests can lead to inappropriate referral for treatment, false reassurance, or even disability. To assist in the evaluation of a screening instrument, a technology assessment is employed to identify reliable, useful, and positive impact tests.[13]

To better understand the usefulness of a screening test, some basic terms and measures (e.g., validity, sensitivity, specificity) are listed and defined in Table 7.2.[13,15,16] Sox et al.[13] and Rocca[17] provide an in-depth review of these and other concepts that relate to the interpretation and assessment of screening tests.

TABLE 7.1. Factors to be Considered When Evaluating a Medical Diagnostic Test[15]

1. Is there a gold standard to define the disease?
2. Has an abnormal test result been clearly and prospectively defined?
3. Has the test assessment been done in a blind manner?
4. Has the technology been tested in a wide spectrum of disease, among those without the disease, and in the practice setting in which it is intended to be used?
5. Has test validity been specified?
6. How do other types of tests compare?

TABLE 7.2. Commonly Used Definitions and Measures for Screening Tests[13,15,16]

TERM	DEFINITION
Validity	The extent by which a test measures what it is intended to measure (lack of validity is referred to as bias or systematic error).
Precision	Reproducibility of a study. Lack of precision refers to random error. Studies with too few subjects allow for random error. Low precision corresponds to wide confidence intervals.
Sensitivity (true-positive rate)	The likelihood of a positive test in a diseased person: $$\frac{\#\text{diseased with }(+)\text{ test}}{\#\text{ diseased}}$$
Specificity (true-negative rate)	The likelihood of a negative test in a person without disease: $$\frac{\#\text{ nondiseased with }(-)\text{ test}}{\#\text{ nondiseased}}$$
Positive Predictive Value (PPV)	Probability of disease if the test is positive, or how likely it is that the person has the disease if the test is abnormal. A high PPV rules in disease.
Negative Predictive Value (NPV)	Probability of the absence of disease if a test is negative, or how likely is it that the person is disease-free if the test is normal. A high NPV rules out disease.
False Positive Rate	Likelihood of a $(+)$ test in a patient without disease: $$\frac{\#\text{ nondiseased with }(+)\text{ test}}{\#\text{ nondiseased}}$$
False Negative Rate	Likelihood of $(-)$ test in a patient with disease: $$\frac{\#\text{ diseased with }(-)\text{ test}}{\#\text{ diseased}}$$

"Truth table" to calculate sensitivity (Sen), specificity (Sp), PPV, and NPV:

	DISEASE	NO DISEASE
Test(+)	TP	FP
Result(−)	FN	TN

TP = true positive, FP = false positive, FN = false negative, TN = true negative. Sen = TP/TP+FN, Sp = TN/TN+FP, PPV = TP/TP+FP, NPV = TN/TN+FN.

Studies of diagnostic (screening) tests are evaluated according to evidence-based rules. One such system that has been used by the American Academy of Neurology[18] rates quality of evidence by class designation and strength of the recommendation (Table 7.3). Such rating systems are important because they emphasize the rigor by which a test was assessed in the context of a recommendation for use based on safety and efficacy.

TABLE 7.3. Quality of Evidence and Strength of Recommendation Ratings for Diagnostic Tests[18]

QUALITY OF EVIDENCE RATINGS	
Class I:	1 or more well-designed studies of a diverse population, blind assessment, gold standard comparison
Class II:	Restricted population, blinded, reference test
Class III:	Expert opinion, nonrandomized, historical controls, or case series
STRENGTH OF RECOMMENDATIONS	
Type A:	Class I or overwhelming Class II
Type B:	Class II
Type C:	Strong consensus of Class III
Type D:	Negative recommendation, inconclusive, or conflicting Class II
Type E:	Strongly negative, based on Class I or II

APPROACHES TO PREVENTION

Two basic public health strategies have been advocated for prevention of chronic disease, the mass approach and the high-risk approach.[9,19] The mass approach is advanced through health education, legislation, and economic measures that discourage exposure to risk factors or the development of risk factors. Lifestyle modification is used to achieve modest reductions in the levels of a risk factor in the community. It is believed that prevention of disease among the many persons in the community with mild or moderate levels of risk will yield large absolute benefit from a public health standpoint.

The high-risk approach is typically used by practicing physicians to identify individuals with high levels of a risk factor. Medication is usually prescribed to achieve substantial reductions in the risk factor. The high-risk approach can result in a substantial and expensive case-finding procedure if applied on a large scale and may fail to prevent a high percentage of disease among those in the community with lower levels of a risk factor.

The relation of hypertension and stroke may serve as an example of the latter paradox. Although there may be a large relative benefit for stroke prevention by identification and treatment of persons with severe hypertension, the bulk of strokes occur in those with less severe hypertension,[20] who may not be identified and treated by the high-risk approach. One must also keep in mind, however, that measures that may bring large absolute benefit to the general community through modest reductions in risk factor levels for all may offer little in the way of advantage for some individuals in the community (i.e., those with highest levels of the risk factor and highest risk of disease).[9] The high-risk and mass prevention approaches should be considered complementary strategies.[1–3]

SCREENING FOR STROKE RISK: EVIDENCE-BASED EXAMPLES

This section explores several evidence-based examples of screening for stroke risk. These examples have been chosen because they include risk-benefit or cost-effectiveness.[21]

Asymptomatic Carotid Stenosis

Several recent clinical trials suggest that carotid endarterectomy is efficacious to reduce risk of cerebral ischemia in patients with asymptomatic carotid stenosis.[22,23] Asymptomatic carotid stenosis is common, and community physicians may be uncertain if it is appropriate to obtain diagnostic studies, such as noninvasive carotid blood flow, or offer treatment, such as carotid endarterectomy, to patients with carotid bruit.[24–26]

One must first decide if noninvasive carotid artery tests are an adequate predictor of stenosis. Blakeley et al.[27] carried out a meta-analytic review of noninvasive carotid tests when carotid angiography was the reference standard. Sensitivity, specificity, receiver operator curves (ROC), and summary measures of effectiveness for each test were determined. Carotid duplex ultrasound, carotid doppler ultrasound, and magnetic resonance angiography had sensitivities between 0.82 and 0.86, with specificities of 0.98 and test effectiveness measures at or exceeding 3.0 for predicting 100% occlusion. For carotid stenosis $\geq 70\%$, there were sensitivities at 0.83 to 0.86, specificities at 0.89 to 0.94, test effectiveness approaching 3.0, and composite ROC at 0.91 to 0.92. These latter analyses included supraorbital doppler ultrasonography. The authors concluded that the noninvasive procedures were similarly successful at predicting carotid occlusion and 70% stenosis. Feinberg has cautioned however, about the tendency for noninvasive tests to overestimate carotid stenosis and their inability to discriminate total occlusion from very high-grade stenosis in some cases.[28]

Models have been developed to assess the cost-effectiveness and efficacy of noninvasive screening for patients with asymptomatic carotid stenosis, or neck bruits. These models are based on various assumptions that may or may not be valid in a particular practice setting or for an individual case. Lee et al.[29] based their model on the screening of 65-year-old men and simulated the Asymptomatic Carotid Atherosclerosis Study (ACAS) experience.[23] Markov modeling was used to estimate annual transitions by different health states. The authors concluded that if $\geq 60\%$ carotid stenosis was detected by ultrasonography and confirmed by cerebral angiography, carotid endarterectomy offered a modest absolute reduction in the rate of stroke, but at a cost greater than is usually considered acceptable. Obuchowski et al.[30] developed a model based on literature estimates of the prevalence and incidence of carotid artery stenosis and associated morbidity and mortality and used a Markov cohort simulation to estimate mean quality-adjusted life years and monetary costs. They concluded that asymptomatic patients with carotid bruits may benefit from screening if the prevalence rate is ≥20%, the benefits and associated risks of surgery are similar to those of ACAS,[23] and the quality of life with stroke was substantially lower than that without stroke.

The Canadian Stroke Consortium does not recommend screening asymptomatic patients for carotid endarterectomy or, in general, performing carotid endarterectomy for asymptomatic carotid stenosis.[31] This recommendation is based on the belief that widespread screening would detect relatively few patients who were suitable for surgery, and a large number of noninvasive and potentially dangerous invasive diagnostic procedures would be necessary and the modest benefit of carotid endarterectomy could be nullified by limited generalizeability of the procedure based on ACAS.[23] Furthermore, serial carotid ultrasound studies may be of limited usefulness in predicting cerebrovascular events and death in persons with asymptomatic carotid stenosis.[32] From the standpoint of population-based medicine, screening for asymptomatic carotid stenosis does not appear to be useful.[33] For some high-risk individuals in the population with asymptomatic carotid stenosis, however, carotid endarterectomy may be indicated[34] and may be diagnosed by high-quality, noninvasive studies only, as some have advocated.[35]

Major Cardiovascular Risk Factors

Prevention guidelines and consensus statements for stroke invariably target cardiovascular risk factors and promotion of a healthy lifestyle.[36,37] Substantial clinical trial or observational epidemiologic evidence suggests that treatment of hypertension, hypercholesterolemia in coronary heart disease patients, atrial fibrillation with antithrombotic agents, and cessation of cigarette smoking or heavy alcohol consumption will reduce the risk of a first stroke.[1-3] Furthermore, cardiovascular risk factor screening instruments, such as the one developed by the Framingham Study investigators,[38,39] that assess stroke risk based on age, blood pressure, antihypertensive therapy use, medical history of diabetes mellitus, cigarette smoking, cardiovascular disease, atrial fibrillation, and left ventricular hypertrophy are available and have been applied in populations at risk for stroke.[40] Although treatment or modification of the aforementioned cardiovascular risk factors may reduce the risk of stroke, there is generally a paucity of information concerning the cost-effectiveness of mass screening for stroke prevention. As noted above, mass screening may be expensive and may fail to prevent a high percentage of strokes.[9,19] The mass approach to prevention, however, may have special merit as attempts are made to shift a community's risk factor profile or likelihood of developing a risk factor(s) downward,[1] yet formal mass screening may not be needed.

Atrial Fibrillation and Echocardiography

Two other evidenced-based examples of the application of screening technology in stroke merit mention. The first relates to screening and treatment for atrial fibrillation. The National Stroke Association has recently launched a campaign for self-detection of atrial fibrillation.[41] Should this method turn out to be useful, community members will be taught a screening method for atrial fibrillation by simply taking their own pulse. Once atrial fibrillation is confirmed by a physician, the screenee can be referred for evaluation of antithrombotic therapy. Several studies suggest that warfarin therapy is cost-effective for stroke prophylaxis in nonvalvular atrial fibrillation, provided that the risk of major adverse events is low or there are risk factors for stroke.[42,43]

A second example relates to the application and cost-effectiveness of echocardiography after stroke. McNamara et al.[44] developed a Markov model decision analysis for hypothetical patients with first stroke in normal sinus rhythm in a simulated practice in the United States. The authors concluded that transesophageal echocardiography alone was a cost-effective option for cardiac imaging after stroke. Assumptions necessary for the model include no obvious clinical cause of stroke, lack of antithrombotic medication use at the time of the stroke, ischemic stroke subtype independent of the underlying condition, transesophageal echocardiography did not cause discomfort or diminish quality of life, risk of recurrent stroke was independent of history of cardiac disease, the first major complication after stroke was considered in the analysis, and new onset or recurrent strokes had similar relative effects on quality of life and on risk of death.

SCREENING AND COST-EFFECTIVENESS

The examples cited above suggest that screening for stroke risk may not be cost-effective when taking into account diagnostic technology and treatment options. In some cases, however, screening may prove to be cost-effective for those at high risk, as has been demonstrated for prevention of coronary heart disease in the primary care setting.[45]

This may not translate to cost-effectiveness in the community at large, where case-finding may be an expensive proposition. No doubt, the aggregate cost of stroke in the United States is expensive—more than $30 billion, with an average cost of approximately $50,000 per case.[46] When societal concerns are weighed, which include resource constraint, mass screening for stroke has not been proven to be cost-effective as of yet and is difficult to sell to those with financial incentives in the real world. In the United States, the bulk of screening activities for stroke risk occur in the physician's office or local health clinic, with emphasis on identification of persons at high risk for cardiovascular disease.

PREVENTION PROGRAMS

It has been lamented that preventive action lags behind the state of public health science, and that under-investment in prevention remains a major drawback to effective public health action.[47] It is estimated that less that 5% of health care expenditures are spent on health promotion and disease prevention. Local health department expenditures for essential public health services average a dime per day per person in the United States.[48] It has been argued that preventive action fails to gain momentum unless three important components are in place: the knowledge base, political support, and a social strategy to accomplish change.[49] Whereas policy approaches to disease prevention have greater impact than individually oriented approaches, policy-imposed barriers need to be removed to reap the benefit.[50] Furthermore, decision makers need to be informed about the effectiveness of a proposed public health prevention strategy, costs, risks to those who will not benefit, and how the strategy compares with alternative strategies.[51]

Gains in life expectancy from preventive interventions in those at average risk have been reported to range from <1 month to slightly more that 1 year per person, with gains as high as 5 years or more for those at especially high risk of chronic disease.[52] The mean gain in life expectancy may be small for most members of the population (especially if the disease is rare) but is much larger for those at higher risk. Such gains, however, may be followed by sobering realizations when one considers that the largest gains may occur shortly after administration of the intervention or when cost is taken into account.[53]

Those with favorable cardiovascular risk profiles may have lower average annual Medicare charges in older age.[54] While this is good news, the cost-effectiveness of preventions for those in middle-life may yield 100-fold differences in life years depending on the target at-risk group.[55] Such results beg for the identification of more cost-effective interventions or identification of new risk factors that can be modified in a more cost-effective manner.

Community-based cardiovascular disease prevention programs have focused on reduced risk factors, maintenance of reduction of risk factors, and surveillance of cardiovascular morbidity and mortality. Key cardiovascular endpoints have included coronary heart disease (CHD) and stroke. In community studies, modest program effects have been blamed primarily on contamination of the control communities with the educational message aimed at the intervention communities.[56] In addition, insufficient sample size or inconsistent and insensitive outcome measures could contribute to insignificant effects.[57] Changes in secular trends in national cardiovascular health awareness, knowledge, and behavior may be largely attributed to national mass media campaigns.[58]

Stanford Five-City Project

This program, an outgrowth of a three-community study, is a community-based intervention trial designed to test whether a comprehensive program of community organization and health education resulted in favorable changes in cardiovascular risk factors, morbidity, and mortality in two treatment versus three control cities in northern California.[59] The education intervention began in 1980 and lasted six years. The intervention used mass media and interpersonal education programs for the public and health care professionals. The education arm was based on social learning and persuasion theories, social marketing theories, and community change theories. Community organization strategies were developed to create institutional and societal support for educational goals, with the plan to establish a self-sustaining health promotion structure within the communities that would continue to function after the conclusion of the project. Differences in risk factor change were assessed for women and men 25–74 years of age. A survey was again conducted in 1989–1990, three years after the intervention was completed.

After 30 to 64 months of education, significant net reductions in community averages that favored treatment occurred for plasma cholesterol level (2%), blood pressure (4%), resting pulse rate (3%), and smoking rate (13%).[60] Composite reductions occurred in total mortality risk scores (15%) and CHD risk scores (16%). Analysis of control cities over time showed improvements in respondents general cardiovascular disease risk factor knowledge and behaviors which was marked for cholesterol.[61]

When long-term effects were assessed, (1) blood pressure improvements were maintained in treatment but not control cities; (2) cholesterol levels continued to decline in treatment and control cities; (3) smoking rates leveled off or increased slightly in treatment cities but declined in control cities (net differences not significant); and (4) CHD and all-caused mortality risk scores were maintained or continued to improve with treatment, whereas they leveled off or rebounded in control cities. Overall, sustained, but only modest program effects were noted.[59]

Minnesota Heart Health Program (MHHP)

The MHHP, a research and demonstration project, was conducted from 1980 to 1990 for the primary prevention of CHD and stroke.[62–64] The intervention program included three communities in Minnesota and North Dakota. Of the three pairs of communities that were studied, each had one education and one comparison site. Communities were matched on size, type, and distance from Minneapolis-St. Paul. A 5-6 year intervention program was initiated in November 1981 in Mankato (small rural area), and 22 and 28 months later in Fargo-Moorhead (urban area) and Bloomington (large suburban area), respectively. Risk factors and health behaviors were measured over time. Morbidity and mortality endpoints were also collected and analyzed.

The intervention program emphasized hypertension prevention and control, healthy eating habits to lower cholesterol and blood pressure, cessation of smoking, and regular physical activity. The intervention was carried out at the individual, group, and community levels. Social learning theory, persuasive communication theory, and models for involvement of community leaders and institutions were used.

Overall, in the 30- to 74-year-old men and women enrollees, there were only modest program effects that were generally within chance levels, given a background of secular trends for health promotion and declining risk factors.[64] In the education communities, there were 2394 cases of CHD and 818 cases of stroke, versus 2526 and 739 cases, respectively, in the comparison communities.[63] The CHD event rate decreased by 1.8% per year in men ($p = .03$) and by 3.6% per year in women ($p = .007$). There were no significant trends for stroke. In addition, there were minimal effects of sustained intervention on risk factor levels, and no significant intervention effect on CHD or stroke morbidity or mortality.

Pawtucket Heart Health Program (PHHP)

Similar to the Stanford Five-City Project and the MHHP, the PHHP was designed to test the hypothesis that population risk factor intensity or prevalence and projected cardiovascular disease risk would decrease more in Pawtucket, the intervention city, than in a comparison city.[65] The theoretical base of the education program featured social learning theory. The program targeted risk factors, behavior change, and community activation.

There were small, insignificant differences in blood cholesterol and blood pressure that favored Pawtucket. A downward trend in smoking was slightly greater in the control city. In cross-sectional surveys, but not in the cohort surveys, body mass index increased significantly in the control city. Projected cardiovascular disease rates were 16% less in Pawtucket during the intervention program, but this declined to 8% post-education. Overall, cardiovascular risk reduction was feasible, but maintenance of statistically significant differences between the intervention and control cities was not.

North Karelia Project (NKP)

The NKP was launched in 1972 in Finland in response to high CHD rates and levels of cardiovascular disease risk factors. Given the status of secular trends for cardiovascular disease by decade, the NKP was carried out in a community with very high cardiovascular disease rates in comparison to, for example, the MHHP, where rates stayed within the medium range.[63] The aim of NKP[66-70] was to carry out a systematic and comprehensive intervention to reduce mortality and morbidity rates of CHD and related cardiovascular diseases in the entire population, and particularly middle-aged men. Reduction of risk factors, such as smoking, high serum cholesterol, and hypertension, were the main targets. There was a comprehensive educational and service-oriented program to modify risk factors based on local community action and service structure. Practical skills, social support for change, and environmental modifications were provided. The program was notable for the high motivation for participation and support by the local population, local health services, and local and national administrations. The program community was compared to other communities in Finland.

The study showed that a community-wide intervention was feasible and could lead to risk factor changes.[70] Cardiovascular mortality decreased more in North Karelia than in the rest of Finland.[69] Based on potential sources of bias and theoretical issues regarding causal inference, it may be difficult to conclude what excess proportion of the mortality decline was attributable to the program.[70]

Hypertension Control Program in Rural Northeastern Japan

Hypertension is the most important modifiable risk factor for stroke.[1-3] In Japan, stroke rates have been traditionally high, and hypertension has been a prevalent risk factor. In the early 1960s a community-based hypertension control program was begun in two rural communities in northeastern Japan.[71] In one of the communities, the municipal government began to charge participants for blood pressure screenings after 1968 and failed to replace the public health nurse after she retired in 1973. In the other community, the program had continuous support. In the full intervention, community residents ≥30 years of age were offered blood pressure screenings. High risk individuals were referred to local clinics for antihypertensive medication and were rescreened annually. The remainder of the community was rescreened at four-year intervals. Treatment of hypertension was carried out by local physicians, who used thiazide diuretics and, secondarily, beta-adrenergic blocking agents. Calcium channel blockers and angiotensin-converting enzyme inhibitors were used infrequently before the mid-1980s. Health education for hypertensives was carried out at screening sites and also included adult classes, nurse home visits, volunteers for health education ("healthy diet" volunteers), and community-wide media to encourage participation in blood pressure screening and reduced salt intake.[72] Because the traditional Japanese diet was high in salt (20g/day), education on how to reduce salt intake was a major focus of the program.

In the minimal intervention community, blood pressure rescreening occurred at two-year intervals. Program components were similar to the full educational intervention but did not include adult classes or community-wide media education. About 75% of the referred hypertensives attended a clinic outside the community.

Six-year stroke incidence rates, adjusted for sex and age, did not differ between the two groups in the period 1964 to 1969. Subsequently, stroke incidence declined in men, more so in the full intervention than the minimal intervention group (42% decrease vs. 5% increase for 1970 to 1975; 53% vs. 19% decrease for 1976 to 1981; and 75% vs. 29% decrease for 1982 to 1987). For women, however, there was no difference in stroke rates in the three later periods. Stroke prevalence declined in the full intervention group for men in periods subsequent to 1972. In women, stroke prevalence declined in both intervention groups and was reduced in the full intervention group as compared to the minimal intervention group only in 1982.

For men and women aged 40 to 69 years, age-adjusted blood pressures, prevalence of hypertension, and hypertensive end-organ defects were nearly identical in the study communities. For men, the full intervention group showed a 3–4 mm Hg lower mean systolic blood pressure in the early 1970s and 1980s. This was not maintained in the mid-1980s. For women, a difference in systolic blood pressure was found only in the early 1980s. Unexpectedly, among those with hypertension, the proportion previously undetected was greater and the proportion treated and controlled was lower in the full intervention group. For the most part, there were no major differences in the prevalence of diabetes mellitus or atrial fibrillation in either community.

The investigators concluded that active use of existing health resources, high participation in blood pressure screenings and follow-up exams, and community-wide health education for hypertension control augmented the decline in stroke incidence and prevalence among men. Control of hypertension in the community has been shown to yield benefits for cardiovascular disease prevention in other studies,[73,74] but in one study it had little impact on stroke risk.[75] Many hypertensive persons in the community, however, have blood pressures that are not well-controlled, and there is a trend for falling awareness, treatment, and control of hypertension in the United States.[76,77]

Community Intervention Trial for Smoking Cessation (COMMIT)

Cigarette smoking is a well-documented risk factor for stroke.[1–3] Furthermore, the risk of stroke reverses substantially within two to five years after smoking cessation. COMMIT was a community-level, multichannel, four-year intervention designed to increase quit rates.[78,79] The trial included two matched pairs of community, one randomly assigned to intervention and the other as a control. The intervention focused on public education through media and community-wide events, work-sites and other organizations, health care providers and other organizations, and cessation resources. Mandated activities were carried out primarily by community volunteers, local staff, or agencies and were implemented by community task forces. The target smoking group was between 25 and 64 years old and included heavy smokers (≥25 cigarettes per day) and light to moderate smokers.

There was a modest impact of the intervention on light to moderate smokers, but the quit rate of heavy smokers did not increase.[78] Smoking prevalence was not affected significantly beyond existent favorable secular trends.[79] It has been estimated that preventive interventions for smoking cessation may be extremely cost-effective.[80]

Work-site health promotion has been advocated as part of community intervention programs because a large percentage of the community may be employed, more than a third of one's waking hours are spent at work, and the potential public health benefits of work-site health promotion may be substantial.[81] Work-site interventions may address multiple risk factors or single risk factors. Work-site interventions may be aimed at organizational and environmental change or individual change (e.g., screening, educational, behavioral counseling, and incentives). Behavioral counseling may be an effective strategy for reduction of some cardiovascular disease risk factors.[81,82]

COMMUNITY PREVENTION PROGRAMS IN PERSPECTIVE

Secular trends for improvements in cardiovascular risk factor profiles have been substantial and are believed largely to account for the generally insignificant differences between intervention and comparison communities. These secular trends became prominent from the 1960s through the 1980s. With the recent realization that stroke rates may be on the rise[83] and that high stroke rates exist in some areas of the world where cardiovascular risk factor frequency is high and presumably adequate treatment is lacking,[84] there is concern that stroke rates may be moving backward in the direction of past decades, when stroke rates were high.[85] This has led to a battle cry to redouble efforts to control cardiovascular risk factors in the community and to identify new risk factors and treatments. Thus, there is a need to continue to advocate for public health policy for mass and high-risk approaches to community prevention.

FUTURE TARGETS OF SCREENING AND PREVENTION

Since atherosclerosis seems to begin in childhood and cardiovascular risk factors or their precursors may manifest in this time period, interest has been increasing in cardiovascular screening and prevention of children, adolescents, and young adults.[86–97] Risk factor variables such as ponderal index; systolic blood pressure and total cholesterol;[96] triglycerides, insulin, and blood pressure[92] may cluster in children or young adults and predict susceptibility to cardiovascular disease later in life. Evidence from tracking studies suggests, for example, that young adult men in the top quintile of blood pressure distribution are likely to remain in the top quintile.[97] Thus, a number of risk factors or precursors of risk factors may manifest early in life that could be modified by lifestyle changes (e.g., weight loss, exercise, diet). These windows of opportunity need to be investigated to determine if stroke and other cardiovascular diseases can be prevented or postponed by early-life modification of these factors.[3] Low-cost, high-yield population strategies may be the most cost-effective options.[98] Sensitivity analyses must be taken into account and consideration given to the duration of the intervention's expected effect, society's willingness to pay for additional quality-adjusted years of life, the cost and risk associated with the development of the intervention, and the size of the target population expected to comply with the intervention recommendations.

Beyond biological aging, much illness and disability in the elderly is related to risk factors that are present in midlife.[99] If the foundation for subclinical disease is being established in childhood and young adulthood, our public health policy for screening and prevention should begin to explore health promotion for leading causes of chronic illness of the elderly during this early time period.

REFERENCES

1. Gorelick PB. Stroke prevention. An opportunity for efficient utilization of health care resources during the coming decade. *Stroke* 1994;25:220–224.
2. Gorelick PB. Stroke prevention. *Arch Neurol* 1995;52:347–355.
3. Gorelick PB. Stroke prevention: Windows of opportunity and failed expectations? A discussion of modifiable cardiovascular risk factors and a prevention proposal. *Neuroepidemiology* 1997;16:163–173.
4. Pancioli AM, Broderick J, Kothari R, Brott T, Tuchfarber A, Miller R, Khoury J, Jauch E. Public perception of stroke warning signs and knowledge of potential risk factors. *JAMA* 1998;279:1288–1292.
5. Brass LM, Krumholz HM, Scinto JM, Radford M. Warfarin use among patients with atrial fibrillation. *Stroke* 1997;28:2328–2389.
6. Goldstein LB, Bonito AJ, Matchar DB, Duncan PW, Samsa GP. National survey of physician practices for secondary and tertiary prevention of ischemic stroke: Medical therapy in patients with carotid artery stenosis. *Stroke* 1996;27:1473–1478.
7. Kottke TE, Brekke ML, Solberg LI. Making "time" for preventive services. *Mayo Clin Proc* 1993;68:785–791.
8. Kottke TE, Solberg LI, Brekke ML, Cabrera A, Marquez MA. Delivery rates for preventive services in 44 Midwestern clinics. *Mayo Clin Proc* 1997;72:515–523.
9. Rose G. *The Strategy of Preventive Medicine.* New York: Oxford University Press, 1994:1–138.
10. Fletcher SW. Evidence-based screening: What kind of evidence is needed? *ACP J Club* May/June 1998:A12–A14.
11. Sackett DL, Haynes RB, Tugwell P. *Clinical Epidemiology. A Basic Science for Clinical Medicine.* Boston: Little Brown, 1985:139, 302–310.
12. Mausner JS, Kramer S. *Mausner and Bahn Epidemiology—An Introductory Text.* Philadelphia: WB Saunders, 1985;1–42.
13. Sox H, Stern S, Owens D, Abrams HL. *Assessment of Diagnostic Technology in Health Care. Rationale, Methods, Problems and Directions.* Washington, DC: Institute of Medicine, National Academy Press, 1989:8–54.
14. Silverman WA. Doing more good than harm. In: Warren KS, Mosteller F, (eds). *Doing More Good than Harm: The Evaluation of Health Care Interventions.* New York: Annals of the New York Academy of Sciences, vol 703, 1993:5–11.
15. Nuwer M. On the process for evaluating proposed new diagnostic EEG tests. *Brain Topogr* 1992;4(4):243–247.

16. Ahlbom A, Norell S. *Introduction to Modern Epidemiology.* Chestnut Hills, MA: Epidemiology Resources, 1990:24–27, 57–60.
17. Rocca WA. Clinical trials in neurology: Reliability and validity of rating scales. In: Gorelick PB, Alter MA, eds. *Handbook of Neuroepidemiology.* New York: Marcell Dekker, 1994:63–74.
18. American Academy of Neurology, Therapeutics and Technology Assessment Subcommittee. *Assessment Workbook.* 1997.
19. Dunbabin DW, Sandercock PAG. Preventing stroke by modification of risk factors. *Stroke* 1990;21(suppl IV):IV-36–IV-39.
20. Joseph LN, Kase CS, Beiser AS, Wolf PA. Mild blood pressure elevation and stroke: The Framingham Study. 23rd International Conference on Stroke and Cerebral Circulation, Orlando, Florida, February 5–7, 1998 (abstract).
21. Ringel SP, Hughes HL. Evidence-based medicine, critical pathways, practice guidelines, and managed care: Reflections on the prevention and care of stroke. *Arch Neurol* 1996;53:867–871.
22. Hobson RW, Weiss DG, Fields WS, Goldstone J, Moore WS, Towne JB, Wright CB, Veterans Affairs Cooperative Study Group. Efficacy of carotid endarterectomy for asymptomatic carotid stenosis. *N Engl J Med* 1993;328:221–227.
23. Executive Committee for the Asymptomatic Carotid Atherosclerosis Study. Endarterectomy for asymptomatic carotid artery stenosis. *JAMA* 1995;273:1421–1428.
24. Feussner JR, Matchar D. When and how to study the carotid arteries. *Ann Intern Med* 1988;109:805–818.
25. Health and Public Policy Committee, American College of Physicians. Diagnostic evaluation of the carotid arteries. *Ann Intern Med* 1988;109:835–837.
26. Sauve J-S, Laupacis A, Ostbye T, Feagan B, Sackett DL. Does the patient have a clinically important carotid bruit? *JAMA* 1993; 270: 2843–2845.
27. Blakeley DD, Oddone EZ, Hasselbad V, Simel DL, Matcher DB. Noninvasive carotid artery testing: A meta-analytic review. *Ann Intern Med* 1995;122:360–367.
28. Feinberg AW. Commentary. *ACP J Club* July/August 1995:17.
29. Lee TT, Solomon NA, Heidenreich PA, Oehlert J, Garber AM. Cost-effectiveness of screening for carotid stenosis in asymptomatic patients. *Ann Intern Med* 1997;126: 337–346.
30. Obuchowski NA, Modic MT, Magdenic M, Masaryk TJ. Assessment of the efficacy of noninvasive screening for patients with asymptomatic neck bruits. *Stroke* 1997;28: 1330–1339.
31. Perry JR, Szalai JP, Norris JW, for the Canadian Stroke Consortium. Consensus against both endarterectomy and routine screening for asymptomatic carotid artery stenosis. *Arch Neurol* 1997;54:25–28.
32. Lewis RF, Abrahamowicz M, Cote R, Battista RN. Predictive power of duplex ultrasound in asymptomatic carotid disease. *Ann Intern Med* 1997;127:13–20.
33. Lanska DJ, Kryscio RJ. Endarterectomy for asymptomatic internal carotid artery stenosis. *Neurology* 1997;48:1481–1490.
34. Sarasin FP, Bounameaux H, Bogousslavsky J. Asymptomatic severe carotid stenosis: Immediate surgery or watchful waiting? A decision analysis. *Neurology* 1995;45: 2147–2153.
35. Strandess DE. Angiography before carotid endarterectomy-no. *Arch Neurol* 1995; 52:832–833.
36. Organizing Committees (Program, Advisory and Local): Asia Pacific Consensus Forum on Stroke Management. *Stroke* 1998;29:1730–1736.

37. National Stroke Association Prevention Advisory Board. National Stroke Association stroke prevention guidelines. *Journal of Stroke and Cerebrovascular Diseases* 1998;7: 162–164.

38. Wolf PA, D'Agostino RB, Belanger AJ, Kannel WB. Probability of stroke: A risk profile from the Framingham Study. *Stroke* 1991;22:312–318.

39. D'Agostino RB, Wolf PA, Belanger AJ, Kannel WB. Stroke risk profile: Adjustment for antihypertensive medication. The Framingham Study. *Stroke* 1994;25:40–43.

40. Sitzer M, Skutta M, Siebler M, Sitzer G, Siegrist J, Steinmetz H. Modifiable stroke risk factors in volunteers willing to participate in a prevention program. *Neuroepidemiology* 1998;17:179–187.

41. National Stroke Association. *Check Your Pulse America*! 1998.

42. Gustafsson C, Asplund K, Britten M, Norrving B, Olsson B, Marke L-A. Cost-effectiveness of primary stroke prevention in atrial fibrillation: Swedish national perspective. *BMJ* 1992;305:1457–1460.

43. Gage BF, Cardinalli AB, Albers GW, Owens DK. Cost-effectiveness of warfarin and aspirin for prophylaxis of stroke in patients with nonvalvular atrial fibrillation. *JAMA* 1995;274:1839–1845.

44. McNamara RL, Lima JAC, Whelton PK, Powe NR. Echocardiographic identification of cardiovascular sources of emboli to guide clinical management of stroke: A cost-effectiveness analysis. *Ann Intern Med* 1997;127:775–787.

45. Field K, Thorogood M, Silagy C, Normand C, O'Neill C, Muir J. Strategies for reducing coronary risk factors in primary care: Which is most cost effective? *BMJ* 1995;310:1109–1112.

46. Matchar DB. The value of stroke prevention and treatment. *Neurology* 1998;51(Suppl 3):S31–S35.

47. Atwood K, Colditz GA, Kawachi I. From public health science to prevention policy: Placing science in its social and political contexts. *Am J Public Health* 1997;87:1603–1606.

48. Gordon RL, Gerzoff RB, Richards TB. Determinants of US local health department expenditures, 1992 through 1993. *Am J Public Health* 1997;87:91–95.

49. Richmond JB, Kotelchuck M. Co-ordinating and development of strategies and policy for public health promotion in the United States. In: Holland WW, Detels L, Knox G, eds. *Oxford Textbook of Public Health*. Oxford: Oxford Medical Publications, 1991.

50. Brownson RC, Newschaffer CJ, Ali-Abarghoui F. Policy research for disease prevention: Challenges and practical recommendations. *Am J Public Health* 1997;87: 735–739.

51. Russell LB. The knowledge base for public health strategies (annotation). *Am J Public Health* 1997;87:1597–1588.

52. Wright JC, Weinstein MC. Gains in life expectancy from medical interventions—standardizing data on outcome. *N Engl J Med* 1998;339:380–386.

53. Detsky AS, Redelmeier DA. Measuring health outcomes—putting gains into perspective. *N Engl J Med* 1998;339:402–404.

54. Daviglus ML, Greenland P, Dyer AR, Garside DB, Manheim L, Lowe LP, Rodin MB, Lubitz J, Stamler J. Benefit of a favorable cardiovascular risk-factor profile in middle age with respect to medicare costs. *N Engl J Med* 1998;339:1122–1129.

55. Russell LB. Prevention and Medicare costs. *N Engl J Med* 1998;339:1158–1160.

56. Feinlieb M. New directions for community intervention studies (editorial). *Am J Public Health* 1996;86:1696–1698.

57. Fishbein M. Great expectations, or do we ask too much from community-level interventions (editorial)? *Am J Public Health* 1996;86:1075–1076.
58. Niknian M, Lefebvre C, Carleton RA. Are people more health conscious? A longitudinal study of one community. *Am J Public Health* 1991;81:203–205.
59. Winkleby MA, Taylor LB, Jatulis D, Fortmann SP. The long-term effects of a cardiovascular disease prevention trial: The Stanford Five City Project. *Am J Public Health* 1996;86:1773–1779.
60. Farquhar JW, Fortmann SP, Flora JA, Taylor CB, Haskell WL, Williams PT, Maccoby N, Wood PD. Effects of community wide education on cardiovascular disease risk factors: The Stanford Five City Project. *JAMA* 1990;264:359–365.
61. Frank E, Winkleby M, Fortmann SP, Farquhar JW. Cardiovascular disease risk factors: Improvements in knowledge and behavior in the 1980s. *Am J Public Health* 1993;83:590–593.
62. Murray DM. Design and analysis of community trials: Lessons from the Minnesota Heart Health Program. *Am J Epidemiol* 1995;142:569–575.
63. Luepker RV, Rastam L, Hannam PJ, Murray DM, Gray C, Baker WL, Crow R, Jacobs AR, Pirie PL, Mascioli SR, Mittlemark MB, Blackburn H. Community education for cardiovascular disease prevention: Morbidity and Mortality results from the Minnesota Heart Health Program. *Am J Epidemiol* 1996;144:351–362.
64. Luepker RV, Murray DM, Jacobs DR, Mittelmark MB, Bracht N, Carlaw R, et al. Community education for cardiovascular disease prevention: Risk factor changes in the Minnesota Heart Health Program. *Am J Public Health* 1994;84:1383–1393.
65. Carleton RA, Lasator TM, Assaf AR, Feldman HA, McKinlay S, and the Pawtucket Heart Health Program Writing Group. The Pawtucket Heart Health Program: Community changes in cardiovascular risk factors and projected disease risk. *Am J Public Health* 1995;85:772–785.
66. Salonen JT, Puska P. Kotte TE, Tuomilheto J. Changes in smoking, serum cholesterol and blood pressure levels during a community-based cardiovascular disease prevention program: The North Karelia Project. *Am J Epidemiol* 1981;114:81–94.
67. Paska P, Toumilehto J, Nissinen A, Salonen JT, Vartiainen E, Pietinen P, Koskela K, Korhonen HJ. The North Karelia Project: 15 years of community-based prevention of coronary heart disease. *Ann Med* 1989;21:169–173.
68. Salonen JT, Puska P, Mustaniemi H. Change in morbidity and mortality during comprehensive community program to control cardiovascular diseases during 1972–7 in North Karelia. *BMJ* 1979;2:1178–1183.
69. Tuomilehto J, Geboeas J, Salonen JT, Nissinen A, Kuulasmaa K, Puska P. Decline in cardiovascular mortality in North Karelia and other parts of Finland. *BMJ* 1986;293: 1068–1071.
70. Salonen JT. Did the North Karelia project reduce coronary mortality (letter). *Lancet* 1987;2:269.
71. Shimamoto T, Komachi Y, Inada H, Doi M, Iso H, Sato S, et al. Trends for coronary heart disease and stroke and their risk factors in Japan. *Circulation* 1989;79:503–515.
72. Iso H, Shimamoto T, Naito Y, Sato S, Kitamura A, Iida M, et al. Effects of a long-term hypertension control program on stroke incidence and prevalence in a rural community in Northeastern Japan. *Stroke* 1998;29:1510–1518.
73. Krishan I, Davis CS, Nobrega FT, Smoldt RK. The Mayo Three-Community Hypertension Control Program, IV: Five-year outcomes of intervention in entire communities. *Mayo Clin Proc* 1981;56:3–10.
74. Kotchen JM, McKean HE, Jackson-Thayer S, Moore RW, Straus R, Kotchen TA. Im-

pact of a rural high blood pressure control program on hypertension control and cardiovascular disease mortality. *JAMA* 1986;255:2177–2182.

75. Whisnant JP. Effectiveness versus efficacy of treatment of hypertension for stroke prevention. *Neurology* 1996:46:301–307.

76. Berlowitz DR, Ash AS, Hickey EC, Friedman RH, Clickman M, Kader B, Moskowitz MA. Inadequate management of blood pressure in a hypertensive population. *N Engl J Med* 1998;339:1957–1963.

77. The Sixth Report of the Joint National Committee on Prevention, Detection, Evaluation, and treatment of High Blood Pressure. NIH Publication No. 98-4080, November 1997:3.

78. The COMMIT Research Group: Community Intervention Trial for Smoking Cessation: I. Cohort results from a four-year community intervention. *Am J Public Health* 1995;85:183–192.

79. The COMMIT Research Group: Community Intervention Trial for Smoking Cessation (COMMIT): II. Changes in Adult cigarette smoking prevalence. *Am J Public Health* 1995;85:193–200.

80. Cromwell J, Bartosch WJ, Fiore MC, Hasselblad J, Baker T. Cost-effectiveness of the clinical practice recommendations in the AHCPR guideline for smoking cessation. *JAMA* 1997;278:1759–1766.

81. Gomel M, Oldenburg B, Simpson JM, Owen N. Work-site cardiovascular risk reduction: A randomized trial of health risk assessment, education, counseling, and incentives. *Am J Public Health* 1993;83:1231–1238.

82. Gomel MK, Oldenburg B, Simpson JM, Chilvers M, Owen N. Composite cardiovascular risk outcomes of a work-site trial. *Am J Public Health* 1997;87:673–676.

83. Brown RD, Whisnant JP, Sicks JD, O'Fallon WM, Wiebers DO. Stroke incidence, prevalence and survival: Secular trends in Rochester, Minnesota, through 1989. *Stroke* 1996;27:373–380.

84. Feigin VL, Wiebers DO, Nikitin YP, O'Fallon WM, Whisnant JP. Stroke epidemiology in Novosibirsk, Russia: A population-based study. *Mayo Clin Proc* 1995;70:847–852.

85. Gillum RF. Secular trends in stroke mortality in African Americans: The role of urbanization, diabetes and obesity. *Neuroepidemiology* 1997;16:180–184.

86. Hurbert HB, Faker ED, Garrison RJ. Life styles correlates of risk factor change in young adults: An eight-year study of coronary heart disease risk factors in the Framingham offspring. *Am J Epidemiol* 1987;125:812–831.

87. Hovell MF, Slymen DJ, Jones JA, Hofstetter CR, Burkham-Kreitner S, Conway TL, Rubin B, Noel D. An adolescent tobacco-use prevention trial in orthodontic offices. *Am J Public Health* 1996;86:1760–1766.

88. Blum RW, Beuhring T, Wunderlich M, Resnick MD. Don't ask, they won't tell: The quality of adolescent health screenings in five practice settings. *Am J Public Health* 1996;86:1767–1772.

89. Barnett HL. Preventive screening for health risks among adolescents (annotation). *Am J Public Health* 1996;86:1701.

90. Khoury MJ and the Genetics Working Group. From genes to public health: The applications of genetic technology in disease prevention. *Am J Public Health* 1996;86:1717–1722.

91. Raitakari OT, Leino M, Raikkonen K, Porkka KVK, Taimela S, Rasanen L, Vikari JSA. Clustering of risk habits in young adults: The Cardiovascular Risk in Young Finns Study. *Am J Epidemiol* 1995;142:36–44.

92. Guillaume M, Lapidus L, Beckers F, Lamberta A, Bjorntorp P. Cardiovascular risk factors in children from the Belgian province of Luxembourg: The Belgian Luxembourg Child Study. *Am J Epidemiol* 1996;144:867–880.
93. Twisk JWR, Kemper HCG, van Mechelen KW, Post GB. Tracking of risk factors for coronary heart disease over a 14–year period: A comparison between lifestyle and biologic risk factors with data from the Amsterdam Growth and Health Study. *Am J Epidemiol* 1997;145:888–898.
94. Lewis CE, Smith DE, Wallace DD, Williams OD, Bild DE, Jacobs DR. Seven-year trends in body weight and associations with lifestyle and behavioral characteristics in black and white young adults: The CARDIA Study. *Am J Public Health* 1997;87:635–642.
95. Vartiainen E, Paavola M, McAlister A, Puska P. Fifteen-year follow-up of smoking prevention effects in the North Karelia Youth Project. *Am J Public Health* 1998;88:81–85.
96. Meyers L, Coughlin SS, Webber LS, Srinivasan SR, Berenson GS. Prediction of adult cardiovascular multfactorial risk status from childhood risk factor levels: The Bogalusa Heart Study. *Am J Epidemiol* 1995;142:918–924.
97. Tate RB, Manfreda J, Krahn AD, Cuddy TE. Tracking of blood pressure over a 40–year period in the University of Manitoba Follow-Up Study, 1948–1988. *Am J Epidemiol* 1995;142:946–954.
98. Hornberger J. A cost-benefit analysis of a cardiovascular disease prevention trial, using folate supplementation as an example. *Am J Public Health* 1998;88:61–67.
99. Reed DW, Foley DJ, White LR, Heimovitz H, Burchfiel CM, Masak K. Predictors of healthy aging in men with high life expectancies. *Am J Public Health* 1998;88:1463–1468.

8

HORMONES AND STROKE PREVENTION

Diana B. Petitti

The belief that use of estrogenic hormones by postmenopausal women prevents coronary artery disease is widespread. It is often assumed that if hormone replacement therapy prevents coronary disease, it will prevent stroke.

Sex differences in stroke incidence and mortality, studies of estrogen and experimental stroke in animals, and studies of the effects of exogenous hormones on the mediators of stroke provide information pertinent to this issue. Data on these topics, as well as data from randomized trials and observational epidemiology, are reviewed in this chapter. Although epidemiologic studies show that use of combined estrogen/progestin oral contraceptives does not prevent stroke and probably increases the risk of ischemic and hemorrhagic stroke in some women, the chapter also reviews recent information on this topic.

STROKE INCIDENCE AND MORTALITY IN MEN AND WOMEN

The incidence of stroke is higher in men than in women.[1–2] Figure 8.1, which summarizes data on stroke incidence from the WHO MONICA study,[1] shows that this is true throughout the world. Table 8.1 shows that stroke mortality is also higher in men than in women, at least up to age 85. While the data in this table are from the United States, they are consistent with data from other settings.

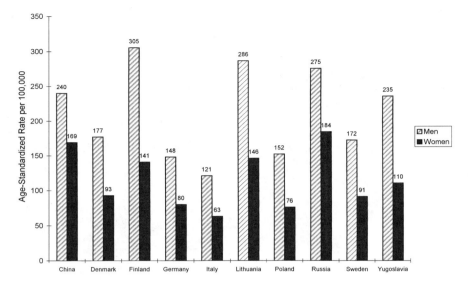

FIGURE 8.1. Age-standardized stroke incidence rates in men and women by country, WHO Monica Project. *Source*: Thorvaldsen et al. Stroke incidence, case fatality, and mortality in the WHO Monica Project. *Stroke* 1995;26:361–367. Rates from multiple sites in one country were averaged

Higher rates of cigarette smoking or diabetes, more poorly controlled blood pressure, or other lifestyle factors could explain the difference in stroke incidence and mortality between men and women. However, the fact that the relationship between male sex and a higher stroke risk (or female sex and a lower stroke risk) holds in so many different geographic settings suggests that sex differences in endogenous hormones may be responsible for at least some of the difference.

TABLE 8.1. Stroke Mortality Rate/100,000 for Men and Women in the United States by Race and Age

	WHITE		BLACK	
AGE	**Men**	**Women**	**Men**	**Women**
0–34	0.9	0.8	2.0	2.4
35–44	5.1	4.4	25.1	17.0
45–54	15.0	13.3	67.3	44.6
55–64	47.9	35.8	136.5	100.2
65–74	153.4	118.6	303.6	249.7
75–84	558.3	482.9	720.1	705.5
85+	1578.0	1705.7	1343.2	1428.1

Source: *Stroke 1980–1989*. National Center for Chronic Disease Prevention and Health Promotion, Centers for Disease Control and Prevention, Atlanta, Georgia, 1994.

ANIMAL STUDIES OF ESTROGEN AND STROKE OUTCOME

Young adult female rats and gerbils have lower mortality and less cerebral ischemia than males after experimental occlusion of the cerebral arteries that produces stroke.[3,4] The protection against experimental ischemic brain injury disappears after reproductive senescence in middle-aged female rats.[5] Ovariectomy in young female rats increases infarct size after experimental cerebral occlusion,[6] and administration of exogenous estradiol decreases ischemic injury in both old and young animals,[5–7] with a therapeutic window of three hours.[7] The mechanism of protection from injury was found to be independent of blood flow in two different experiments.[5,7] This line of research raises the tantalizing possibility that exogenous estrogen might prevent death and disability after stroke, even if estrogen does not decrease the incidence of stroke.

EFFECTS OF EXOGENOUS ESTROGEN AND ESTROGEN/PROGESTIN COMBINATIONS ON THE MEDIATORS OF STROKE

The mechanisms of stroke are not completely understood. Glucose metabolism, blood pressure, coagulation and fibrinolysis, the interaction of platelets and the endothelium, and the renin-angiotensin-aldosterone system all may play a role in the development of stroke. Some of these factors may also modify the extent of damage following stroke. Lipid levels may affect stroke risk directly or indirectly through their effects on coagulability and platelet function.

For both stroke and coronary disease, the distinctions between atherogenesis and thrombosis are being replaced by integrated models of vascular function. The complexity of the mechanisms of stroke and the incompleteness of our understanding of stroke pathogenesis complicate the interpretation of information on the effect of exogenous hormones on factors that mediate stroke.

Estrogen and Estrogen/Progestin Combinations in Postmenopausal Women

The literature on the effect of exogenous estrogen and estrogen/progestin combinations on potential mediators of stroke in postmenopausal women is vast. Table 8.2 summarizes five recent particularly well-conducted studies of this topic.[8–12]

Postmenopausal estrogen and estrogen/progestin combinations decrease fasting serum glucose and insulin levels and do not affect blood pressure. Studies are consistent in showing a favorable effect of the combined estrogen/progestin therapies currently in widespread use on levels of total cholesterol and high-density and low-density lipoprotein cholesterol levels, but they increase triglycerides. The effect of combined therapy on lipids is generally less than that of estrogen alone. That is, the combination therapies are generally more "lipid neutral" than estrogen alone.

TABLE 8.2. Effects of Postmenopausal Estrogen and Estrogen/Progestin Combinations on Proven and Possible Mediators of Stroke Risk

MEDIATOR	ESTROGEN ALONE	ESTROGEN PLUS MPA[1]	REFERENCE(S)
Insulin[2]	↓	↓	8–10
Glucose[2]	↓	↓	8–9
Blood pressure	No effect	No effect	8–9
Triglyceride	↑	↑	8–10
LDL-cholesterol	↓	↓	8–11
HDL-cholesterol	↑	No effect	8–11
Lp(a)	↓	↓	9–10
Fibrinogen	↓	↓	8–9,11
Fibrinopeptide A	↑	?	12
F_{1+2}[3]	↑	?	12
D-dimer	↑ (?)	No effect	10
Plasminogen activator inhibitor-1	↓	↓	10
Factor VII, % activity	↑	No effect	9,11
Factor VIII, %	No effect	No effect	9
Antithrombin III	↓	No effect	9,12
Protein C	↑	No effect	9,12
Protein S	↓	?	12

Note: Unless otherwise indicated, effect is on level of the mediator.
[1]MPA = medroxyprogesterone acetate.
[2]Fasting.
[3]Marker of factor Xa action on prothrombin.

The effects of postmenopausal estrogen and estrogen/progestin combinations on factors that affect coagulation and measures of fibrinolysis are complex. Summarizing the data, estrogens, and probably also postmenopausal estrogen/progestin combinations, enhance both coagulability and fibrinolysis.

Considering these effects, postmenopausal estrogen and estrogen/progestin combinations might be predicted to increase, decrease, or have no effect on the occurrence of stroke. The net effect of estrogens and estrogen/progestin combinations might be different for ischemic than for hemorrhagic stroke. That is, the data on the effects of postmenopausal hormones on mediators of stroke are compatible with any observed effect on stroke incidence, and they are compatible with effects on the incidence of hemorrhagic stroke that are different from those on ischemic stroke.

Estrogen/Progestin Combinations as Oral Contraceptives

The literature on the effects of oral contraceptives on potential mediators of stroke risk in postmenopausal women is also vast. Table 8.3 summarizes the conclu-

TABLE 8.3. Effects of Combined Low Estrogen Dose (<50 Micrograms) Oral
Contraceptives on Proven and Possible Mediators of Stroke Risk and Whether the Type
of Progestin Modifies the Effect (adapted from refs. 13–15)

MEDIATOR	OVERALL	PROGESTIN MODIFIES
Insulin[1]	No effect	Yes
Glucose[1]	No effect	Yes
Insulin resistance	↑	Yes
Blood pressure	↑	Yes
Triglyceride	↑	Yes
LDL-cholesterol	No effect	Yes
HDL-cholesterol	↓, No effect, ↑	Yes, large differences
Lp(a)	No effect	No
Fibrinogen	No effect	No
Plasminogen activator inhibitor-1	↓	No
Factor VII, % activity	↑	?
Factor VIII, %	↑	No

Note: Unless otherwise indicated, effect is on level of the mediator.
[1]Fasting.

sions of three recent reviews of the effects of low-dose (less than 50 micrograms
of ethinyl estradiol) combined estrogen/progestin and progestin-only oral contraceptives on various mediators of stroke risk.[13–15] As with postmenopausal hormone replacement therapy, these data are compatible with any observed effect of
combined estrogen/progestin oral contraceptives on stroke incidence and with effects on the incidence of hemorrhagic stroke that are different from those on ischemic stroke.

For oral contraceptives, much attention has been paid to their effects on factors that predispose to venous thromboembolic disease. These data are also difficult to interpret, although there is an emerging consensus that combined
estrogen/progestin oral contraceptives may cause thromboembolism in women
with resistance to activated protein C, a hereditary thrombophilia, and perhaps
in women with other inherited thrombophilias. Winkler[15] discusses in detail the
data on thrombophilia and oral contraceptives and the many theories about why
they increase the risk of venous thrombosis.

HORMONE REPLACEMENT AND CAROTID THICKNESS

The Cardiovascular Health Study[11] reported on the results of a cross-sectional
analysis of ultrasound assessment of carotid artery thickness and percent of stenosis in relation to postmenopausal hormone use. The study involved 2955 women
65 or more years of age at the time of the ultrasound assessment at entry to the
study. Of these women, 356 were current users of estrogen or estrogen/progestin

TABLE 8.4. Ultrasound Assessment of Carotid Intimal-Medial Thickness and Percent Carotid Stenosis in Estrogen Users and Nonusers in the Cardiovascular Health Study (ref 11)

| | ESTROGEN USE | | |
	CURRENT	PAST	NEVER
Common carotid thickness, mm	0.94	0.97	0.98[1]
Internal carotid thickness, mm	1.25	1.41	1.42[1]
Percentage with carotid stenosis ≥50%	1.8	4.5	5.8[1]

Source: Manolio, Furberg, Shenanski, et al. Associations of postmenopausal estrogen use with cardiovascular disease and its risk factors in older women. *Circulation*, 1993:88:2163–2171.
[1]$p < 0.05$ comparing current users with never plus past users.

and an additional 784 had used postmenopausal hormones prior to examination. The near and far wall maximal intimal-medial thickness of the carotid arteries and the percent of carotid stenosis were assessed using duplex ultrasonography.

Table 8.4 summarizes the results of this cross-sectional analysis. Common and internal carotid thicknesses were both statistically significantly less in current hormone users than in noncurrent users. The percentage of current hormone users with 50% or more stenosis of the carotid artery (1.8%) was significantly less than in noncurrent users (5.6%). The association of current estrogen use with a thinner common carotid wall persisted after adjustment for age, hysterectomy, race, income, smoking, fasting glucose, factor VII, and use of lipid-lowering medication. The association of current estrogen use with a thinner carotid artery wall was attenuated by further adjustment for high-density and low-density lipoprotein cholesterol levels. The authors interpreted this as evidence that the benefits of hormone replacement act through their effects on lipid levels.

RANDOMIZED TRIALS OF POSTMENOPAUSAL HORMONE REPLACEMENT THERAPY

The Hormone Estrogen/Progestin Replacement Study (HERS) was a randomized, blinded, placebo-controlled study that involved 2763 postmenopausal women with coronary disease that was specifically designed to assess the effect of hormone replacement therapy on cardiovascular disease endpoints.[16] Women were assigned to placebo or to 0.625 milligrams of conjugated equine estrogen plus 2.5 milligrams of medroxyprogesterone acetate as a continuous combined regimen. After an average of 4.1 years of follow-up, 108 of the 1380 women assigned to estrogen/progestin therapy and 96 of the 1383 women assigned to placebo had a stroke or transient ischemic attack (TIA). The relative risk of ischemic stroke plus TIA in women assigned to hormone use was 1.13 (95% CI 0.85–1.48).

Hemminki and McPherson[17] extracted data on cardiovascular disease from 22 published randomized trials of postmenopausal estrogen replacement therapy that were conducted to assess outcomes other than cardiovascular disease and did a meta-analysis of these data. The 22 trials identified for the meta-analysis involved more than 4000 women who had been assigned to hormone replacement or to placebo and to no treatment or vitamins and minerals. The odds ratio for all cardiovascular disease in women assigned to hormone therapy was 1.39 (95% CI 0.48–3.95). The meta-analysis did not present data on the rate or risk of stroke in hormone users.

Hemminki and McPherson's meta-analysis excluded a large randomized trial (1265 subjects) reported by Speroff et al.[18] that compared estradiol alone, estradiol plus norethindrone acetate as continuous combined therapy, or placebo alone. No data on stroke were presented in the only publication from this study.

The Women's Health Initiative is an on-going randomized trial that was also designed specifically to address the effect of postmenopausal estrogen only and estrogen/progestin therapy on cardiovascular endpoints.[19] Data on stroke incidence and mortality are not yet available.

OBSERVATIONAL STUDIES OF HORMONE REPLACEMENT THERAPY

A number of observational epidemiologic studies have been performed specifically to assess the effect of postmenopausal hormone replacement therapy and the risk of stroke. Other studies provide data on the risk of stroke but were not done specifically to address this topic. Table 8.5 describes the overall designs of the studies that provide data on postmenopausal hormone replacement therapy and the risk of stroke.[20–44]

The observational studies that provide data on hormone replacement therapy and stroke varied in the degree to which they used rigorous definitions of stroke and included review to confirm cases. Some prospective studies ascertained hormone use only at entry to the study, and the results thus pertain to ever having used of hormone replacement therapy, an exposure variable that is difficult to interpret. Some cohort studies included women with a past history of stroke at entry. Some studies did not control for potential confounders, the most important being hypertension, diabetes, and cigarette smoking, which are known to differ between hormone users and nonusers and are also strong risk factors for stroke. Some studies can be inferred to pertain only to use of estrogen alone because of the era in which they were conducted, and some present estimates of the risk of stroke separately in users of estrogen and estrogen/progestin combination. However, for many studies, the exact hormone regimen used by women in the study cannot be determined. The data in the next tables should be interpreted recognizing these limitations.

TABLE 8.5. Summary of Studies that Provide Estimates of the Relative Risk of Stroke in Users of Postmenopausal Hormone Replacement Therapy

STUDY POPULATION	DESIGN	YEARS OF CASE ASCERTAINMENT	CASE REVIEW	FIRST-EVER	CONTROL FOR HBP, SMOKING DIABETES	REFERENCE(S)
Leisure World I	Case control	1964–1973	Yes	Yes	Yes	20
Kaiser Permanente Northern California						
Case Control Study I	Case control	1972–1974	Yes	Yes[1]	Yes	21
England/Wales	Case control	1978	No	No	No	22
Framingham	Case control	1972–1980	Yes	Yes	Yes	23
Lipid Research Clinics	Cohort	1972–1984 (?)[1]	Yes	?	No	24
Walnut Creek Contraceptive Drug Study	Cohort	1969–1976 nonfatal; 1969–1977 fatal	Yes/no[2]	Yes/no[3]	Yes	25, 26
Copenhagen City Heart Study	Cohort	1976–1988	Yes	Yes	Yes	27, 28
British Menopause Clinics	Cohort	1978–1988	No	No	No	29, 30
Leisure World II	Case control	1981–1987 all fatal; 1981–1989 (?)[4] ischemic	No	No	No	31, 32
National Health and Nutrition Examination Survey	Cohort	1971–1987	No	Yes	Yes	33, 34
King County, Washington	Case control	1987–1989	Yes	Yes	Yes	35
Iowa Women's Health Study	Cohort	1986–1991	No	No	Yes	36
Nurses' Health Study	Cohort	1976–1994 fatal; 1976–1992 nonfatal	Yes/no[1]	Yes	Yes	37, 38
Danish Patient Register	Case control	1990–1992	Yes	Yes	Yes	39
Kaiser Permanente Northern California						
Case Control Study II	Case control	1991–1994	Yes	Yes	Yes	40
Turku Mammography Cohort	Cohort	1987–1995	No	No	Yes	41
Rancho Bernardo Study	Cohort	1984–1996	No	Yes	Yes	42
Uppsala	Cohort	1977–1995	No	Yes	Yes	43, 44

[1]Study recruitment 1972 to 1976; analysis from visit 2; 8.5 years of average follow-up. [2]Case review for nonfatal events. [3]First-ever for nonfatal events. [4]Cannot determine closing date for analysis for ischemic stroke.

Table 8.6 shows the results of the eight studies that provided an estimate of risk for all fatal and nonfatal stroke in users of hormone replacement therapy. Three studies provided an estimate of the risk of stroke separately in current and past hormone users. All three studies were rigorous, had clear case definitions, and controlled for hypertension, diabetes, and smoking. The relative risk estimates from these studies were all very close to 1.0 in current hormone users. The studies showed that an effect of hormone use, if there is an effect, does not persist after cessation of use.

Table 8.7 shows the results of the nine studies that provided an estimate of the risk of ischemic stroke only in users of hormone replacement therapy. Six studies provided an estimate of the risk of ischemic stroke separately in current hormone users and three provided an estimate in past users. All six studies that provided risk estimates in current users had clear case definitions and case review, were limited to first-ever stroke, and controlled for hypertension, diabetes, and smoking. In four of the six studies, the relative risk of ischemic stroke was higher in current users of hormone replacement therapy than in nonusers. The four largest studies included more than 1500 women with ischemic stroke. All four studies reported relative risk estimates for ischemic stroke that were greater than 1.0, although the 95% CIs included 1.0 in all studies except the Nurses' Health Study. The estimated relative risks of ischemic stroke in past users of hormone replacement therapy were close to 1.0 in all three studies that estimated risk in past hormone users.

Table 8.8 shows the results of the seven studies that provided an estimate of the risk of hemorrhagic stroke only in users of hormone replacement therapy. Four studies were limited to subarachnoid hemorrhage. Five studies provided an estimate of the risk of hemorrhagic stroke separately in current hormone users and two provided an estimate in past users. The results of these studies were extremely heterogenous. Risk estimates for hemorrhagic stroke in current users of replacement hormone therapy ranged from 0.33 to 1.6. Even the three largest studies, all well-conducted, were contradictory, with risk estimates for hemorrhagic stroke in current users of hormone replacement therapy of 0.38, 0.90, and 1.00. No conclusion about the effect of current use of hormone replacement therapy on the risk of hemorrhagic stroke can be drawn.

Table 8.9 shows the results of the nine studies that provided an estimate of the risk of fatal stroke in users of hormone replacement therapy. Data on fatal stroke are of particular interest because of the findings in animal studies. Four studies provided an estimate of the risk of fatal stroke separately in current hormone users and three provided an estimate in past users. Unfortunately, these studies often did not include clear definitions of what qualified as a fatal stroke and did not include case review. The results were heterogenous. The estimated relative risks of fatal stroke in current users of hormone replacement therapy ranged from 0.16 to 0.95. On the other hand, the risk estimates for current use were all less

TABLE 8.6. All Stroke: Estimated Relative Risk in Users of Postmenopausal Hormone Replacement Therapy

POPULATION	NUMBER	CURRENT USE	EVER USE	PAST USE	REFERENCE
Leisure World I	210	—	1.12 (0.79–1.57)	—	20
Framingham	45	—	2.27 (1.22–4.23)	—	23
Copenhagen City Heart Study	97[1]	—	1.0 (0.5–1.9)	—	27
National Health and Nutrition Examination Survey	250	—	0.82 (0.46–1.47)[1]	—	34
Nurses' Health Study	552	1.03 (0.82–1.31)	1.01 (0.86–1.18)[3]	0.99 (0.80–1.22)	37
Turku Mammography Cohort	111	0.86 (0.42–1.75)[4]	0.97 (0.59–1.59)[3]	1.08 (0.55–2.10)	41
Rancho Bernardo	57	—	1.39 (0.59–3.26)[5]	—	42
Uppsala	289	0.88 (0.65–1.19)[6]	0.91 (0.71–1.17)	0.93 (0.71–1.22)	44

[1]Excludes subarachnoid hemorrhage.

[2]Self-report.

[3]Summary estimate was calculated as variance weighted average of current and past use.

[4]Summary estimate was calculated as variance weighted average of estrogen replacement therapy and combined estrogen/progestin replacement therapy.

[5]Summary estimate was calculated as variance weighted average of fatal and nonfatal.

[6]"Recent" use.

[7]Includes TIA.

TABLE 8.7. Ischemic Stroke: Estimated Relative Risk in Users of Postmenopausal Hormone Replacement Therapy

POPULATION	NUMBER	CURRENT USE	EVER USE	PAST USE	REFERENCE
Leisure World I	158	—	1.0 (N.R.)	—	20
Kaiser Permanente Northern California	198	1.32 (0.84–2.09)	—	—	22
Case Control Study I					
Framingham	21	—	2.60 (N.R.)	—	23
Walnut Creek Contraceptive Drug Study	23	0.9 (0.4–1.8)	—	—	25
Leisure World II	92	—	0.63 (0.40–0.97)[1]	—	32
Nurses' Health Study	281	1.40 (1.02–1.92)	1.19 (0.95–1.48)[2]	1.01 (0.74–1.36)	37
Danish Patient Register	846	1.17 (0.97–1.41)[3]	1.13 (0.98–1.31)[2]	1.08 (0.86–1.35)	39
Kaiser Permanente Northern California	374	1.03 (0.65–1.65)	0.93 (0.67–1.27)[2]	0.84 (0.54–1.32)	40
Case Control Study II					
Uppsala	198	0.79 (0.54–1.16)[4]	0.94 (0.69–1.27)	—	44

N.R. = not reported, cannot be calculated

[1]Fatal only.

[2]Summary estimate was calculated as variance-weighted coverage of current and past use.

[3]Summary estimate was calculated as variance-weighted average of estrogen replacement therapy and combined estrogen/progestin.

[4]"Recent use."

TABLE 8.8. Hemorrhagic Stroke: Estimated Relative Risk in Users of Postmenopausal Hormone Replacement Therapy

POPULATION	NUMBER	CURRENT USE	EVER USE	PAST USE	REFERENCE
Medical Research Council	23[1]	—	0.64 (0.06–6.52)[2]	—	22
Walnut Creek Contraceptive Drug Study	11[1]	1.6 (0.7–3.8)	—	—	25
King County, Washington	103[1]	0.38 (0.17–0.84)	0.47 (0.26–0.86)	—	35
Nurses' Health Study	155[1]	0.90 (0.57–1.41)[3]	0.85 (0.62–1.17)[4]	0.81 (0.52–1.25)	37
Danish Patient Register	160[1]	1.01 (0.69–1.48)[3]	0.93 (0.69–1.26)[4]	0.81 (0.49–1.33)	39
	95[5]	0.99 (0.55–1.76)[3]	0.97 (0.63–1.49)[4]	0.95 (0.51–1.76)	39
	255[6]	1.00 (0.73–1.38)[3]	0.94 (0.74–1.21)[4]	0.86 (0.58–1.28)	39
Kaiser Permanent Northern California Case Control Study II	83[6]	0.33 (0.12–0.96)	—	—	40
Uppsala	45[6]	—	0.79 (0.69–1.27)	—	44

[1]Subarachnoid hemorrhage only.
[2]Confidence interval was calculated from data in publication.
[3]Summary estimate was calculated as variance-weighted average of estrogen replacement therapy and combined estrogen/progestin replacement therapy.
[4]Summary estimate was calculated as variance-weighted average of current and past use of hormone replacement therapy.
[5]Intracerebral hemorrhage.
[6]All hemorrhagic stroke.

TABLE 8.9. Fatal Stroke: Estimated Relative Risk in Users of Postmenopausal Hormone Replacement Therapy

POPULATION	NUMBER	CURRENT USE	EVER USE	PAST USE	REFERENCE
Lipid Research Clinics	8	—	0.40 (0.01–3.07)	—	24
Walnut Creek Contraceptive Drug Study	9	0.6 (0.2–2.2)	—	—	26
British Menopause Clinics	23	—	0.54 (0.24–0.84)	—	30
Leisure World II	63[1]	—	0.53 (0.31–0.91)[1]	—	31
National Health and Nutrition Examination Survey	64	—	0.86 (0.28–2.66)[2]	—	34
Iowa Women's Health Study	90	0.95 (0.37–2.43)	0.90 (0.54–1.50)	0.88 (0.48–1.61)	36
Nurses' Health Study	167	0.68 (0.39–1.16)	0.89 (0.63–1.27)[3]	1.07 (0.68–1.69)	38
Turku Mammography Study	51	0.16 (0.2–1.18)	0.76 (0.32–1.80)[3]	1.05 (0.41–2.68)	41
Rancho Bernardo	37	—	0.92 (0.34–2.49)	—	42

[1]All fatal stroke.

[2]Self-reported hormone use.

[3]Summary estimate was calculated as variance-weighted average of current and past use.

than 1.0, and the data do not rule out the possibility of an effect of estrogen in limiting ischemic damage following stroke.

RANDOMIZED TRIALS OF EXOGENOUS ESTROGEN AND STROKE IN MEN

The Coronary Drug Project was a large, randomized trial of lipid-lowering drugs in men with coronary disease that included two estrogen treatment arms, conjugated equine estrogen, at two doses, 2.5 and 5.0 milligrams. Data on the incidence of fatal stroke were presented in the publication about the results from the 2.5 milligram treatment arm.[45] Data on estrogen and fatal stroke also were presented in a publication about the results of randomized trials of the Veterans Administration (VA) Cooperative Prostate Cancer Treatment trial.[46]

Table 8.10 shows that in the Coronary Drug Project the rate of fatal stroke was slightly lower in men treated with 2.5 milligrams of estrogen. In contrast, in the VA Cooperative Study, the rate of fatal stroke in men treated with 5.0 milligrams of diethylstilbestrol was elevated substantially. The number of fatal strokes was small in both studies. The dose of estrogen used in the VA trial was very large. The studies do not provide evidence that estrogen prevents fatal stroke, but they do not out rule out this possibility.

COMBINED ESTROGEN/PROGESTIN ORAL CONTRACEPTIVES AND STROKE

Since oral contraceptives were first marketed in the early 1960's, the dose of both estrogen and progestin has decreased markedly. Early studies of stroke and oral contraceptive use are consistent in finding an increased risk of ischemic stroke in current oral contraceptive users, but these studies are not relevant to oral contraceptive formulations now in widespread use.

Early studies on the relationship between oral contraceptives and hemorrhagic stroke are inconsistent. The unavailability and infrequency of use of radiologic tests (CT and MRI scans) that would distinguish between ischemic and hemorrhagic stroke makes these early studies difficult to interpret, and elevations in the risk of hemorrhagic stroke might be due to misclassification of ischemic stroke as hemorrhagic because of presentation with headache.

Table 8.11 summarizes the results of four recent large studies of stroke and oral contraceptive use in which a high percentage of cases had CT or MRI scan to define the type of stroke.[47–51] Importantly, these studies also assessed smoking and hypertension as possible confounders and effect modifiers.

The two studies done in the United States[47,48] found no overall increase in the risk of ischemic stroke in current oral contraceptive users. Both the WHO study[49,50]

TABLE 8.10. Effect of Estrogen on Fatal Stroke in Randomized Trials in Men

STUDY AND REFERENCE	SUBJECTS	ESTROGEN	ESTROGEN NO. OF STROKES AND RATE/100		PLACEBO NO. OF STROKES AND RATE/100		RELATIVE RISK IN ESTROGEN USERS
Coronary Drug Project[45]	Men with coronary artery disease	2.5 mg Premarin	4	1.8	11	2.1	0.86
VA Cooperative Urologic Research Group[46]	Men with prostate cancer	5 mg diethylstilbestrol	37	3.6	14	1.4	2.6

TABLE 8.11. Summary of Four Studies of Stroke Risk in Current Users of Combination Oral Contraceptives

| | ISCHEMIC STROKE | | HEMORRHAGIC STROKE | |
STUDY AND REFERENCE	NUMBER	RR (95% C.I.)	NUMBER	RR (95% C.I.)
Kaiser Permanente[47]	144	1.2 (0.5–2.6)	151	1.1 (0.6–2.2)
Washington State[48]	60	1.4 (0.5–3.8)	102	1.4 (0.7–3.0)
WHO[49,50]				
Developing countries	556	2.9 (2.2–4.0)	821	1.8 (1.3–2.3)
Europe	141	3.0 (1.7–5.4)	247	1.4 (0.8–2.3)
Transnational[51]	220	3.6 (2.4–5.4)	—	—

and the Transnational Study[51] reported a three- to four-fold increase in the risk of ischemic stroke in current oral contraceptive users.

The U.S. studies found either no increase in the risk of hemorrhagic stroke in current oral contraceptive users or only a small increase.[47,48] The WHO study reported a relative risk of hemorrhagic stroke in current oral contraceptive users of 1.8 (95% CI 1.3–2.3) in developing countries and 1.4 (95% CI 0.8–2.3) in European countries.[50]

The WHO study had a sufficiently large number of subjects to assess in detail the degree to which hypertension, smoking, age, and estrogen dose modified the effect of current oral contraceptive use for stroke. Table 8.12 shows estimates of the relative risk of ischemic and hemorrhagic stroke in current oral contraceptive users according to hypertension, smoking, age, and estrogen dose from the WHO study. The relative risks of both ischemic and hemorrhagic stroke were dramatically higher in current oral contraceptive users with hypertension than in current oral contraceptives without hypertension. The relative risks of both ischemic and hemorrhagic stroke were also higher in current oral contraceptive users who smoked than in current users who did not smoke, but the magnitude of the difference in the risk of stroke between the current users who smoked and did not smoke was less than for women with and without hypertension.

In the European centers of the WHO study, higher estrogen dose oral contraceptives were associated with a higher risk of ischemic, but not hemorrhagic, stroke. The relative risks of hemorrhagic stroke in current oral contraceptive users who did not have hypertension, in non-smokers, and in women less than 35 years of age all were 1.1–1.4. In the European centers, the relative risk of ischemic stroke in current users of low-estrogen oral contraceptives was 1.36. The latter risks from the WHO study are about the same as the overall relative risks of hemorrhagic stroke and ischemic stroke in current oral contraceptive users in the two U.S. studies. In both U.S. studies, current use of oral contraceptives in women with hypertension and in women more than 35 years of age was rare, and the

TABLE 8.12. Estimated Relative Risk of Stroke in Current Oral Contraceptives Users by Presence or Absence of Hypertension, Smoking, Age >35, and Estrogen Dose: WHO Collaborative Study

	ISCHEMIC STROKE		HEMORRHAGIC STROKE	
	DEVELOPING COUNTRIES	EUROPE	DEVELOPING COUNTRIES	EUROPE
RISK FACTOR	RR (95% C.I.)	RR (95% C.I.)	RR (95% C.I.)	RR (95% C.I.)
No hypertension	2.73 (1.97–3.77)	2.71 (1.47–4.99)	1.43 (1.06–1.93)	1.05 (0.61–1.80)
Hypertension	14.5 (5.36–39.0)	10.7 (2.04–56.6)	14.3 (6.72–30.4)	10.3 (3.27–32.3)
Nonsmoker	2.64 (1.85–3.77)	2.09 (1.03– 4.5)	1.49 (1.05–2.10)	1.19 (0.58–2.44)
Smoker	4.83 (2.76–8.43)	7.20 (3.23–16.1)	3.73 (2.43–5.71)	3.10 (1.65–5.83)
Age <35	NR[1]	—	1.11 (0.75–1.66)	0.85 (0.43–1.68)
Age ≥35	NR[1]	—	2.46 (1.67–3.62)	2.17 (1.08–4.36)
Estrogen <50mg	3.39 (2.24–5.13)	1.36 (0.60–3.07)	1.66 (1.16–2.37)	1.27 (0.70–2.32)
Estrogen ≥50mg	2.95 (1.69–5.14)	5.56 (2.43–12.7)	1.65 (1.11–2.47)	1.42 (0.67–2.97)

[1]NR = not reported.

Source: WHO Collaborative Study of Cardiovascular Disease and Steroid Hormone Contraception: Ischaemic stroke and combined oral contraceptives: Results of an international, multicentre, case-control study. *Lancet* 1996;348:498–505; and WHO Collaborative Study of Cardiovascular Disease and Steroid Hormone Contraception: Haemorrhagic stroke, overall stroke risk, and combined oral contraceptives: Results of an international, multicentre, case-control study. *Lancet* 1996;348:505–510.

prevalence of smoking was low. In the U.S. studies, virtually all women used low estrogen formulations. Taken as a whole, recent studies show that current low-estrogen oral contraceptive use does not increase the risk of ischemic or hemorrhagic stroke in young women without hypertension who do not smoke. Combined estrogen/progestin oral contraceptives, and probably even low-estrogen oral contraceptives, greatly increase the risk of both hemorrhagic and ischemic stroke in women with hypertension.

SUMMARY AND CONCLUSIONS

Stroke incidence and mortality are higher in men than women, suggesting that hormonal factors may influence the development of stroke or its outcome. Studies in rats show that endogenous and exogenous estrogen affect the extent of ischemic injury after experimental occlusive stroke, suggesting a possible effect of estrogen in preventing death and disability following stroke.

Exogenous estrogen and estrogen/progestin combinations affect a number of factors that may mediate the occurrence of stroke in postmenopausal women. The net effect of the complex changes on stroke risk in the whole animal cannot be predicted. The possibility that the net effect might be to decrease the risk of stroke cannot be ruled out.

The only randomized trial that has provided data on the effect of postmenopausal hormones on the risk of stroke in women showed no effect of combined estrogen/progestin therapy on the risk of a combined endpoint of ischemic stroke plus TIA. Observational studies of postmenopausal hormones and stroke, taken as a whole, show no decrease in the risk of ischemic stroke in current users. Observational studies on the effect of hormone replacement therapy on hemorrhagic stroke are inconsistent, and no firm conclusion can be drawn from them. Epidemiologic studies confined to fatal stroke do not rule out the possibility that estrogen might decrease the risk of death following stroke, as suggested by animal studies.

The body of evidence on low-estrogen and combined estrogen/progestin oral contraceptives and stroke shows that current oral contraceptive use does not increase the risk of stroke in young women who do not have hypertension and do not smoke.

REFERENCES

1. Thorvaldsen P, Asplund K, Kuulasmaa K, et al. Stroke incidence, case fatality, and mortality in the WHO MONICA project. *Stroke* 1995;26:361–367.
2. Alter M, Shang ZX, Sobel E, et al. Standardized incidence ratios of stroke: A worldwide review. *Neuroepidemiology* 1986;5:148–158.
3. Alkayed NH, Harukuni I, Kimes AS, et al. Gender-linked brain injury in experimental stroke. *Stroke* 1998;29:159–165.

4. Hurn PD, Alkayed NJ, Tong TJK. Female vs. male: Injury in experimental stroke. In: Crieglstein J, ed. *Pharmacology of Cerebral Ischemia*. Stuttgart, Germany: Medpharm Scientific Publishers, 1998.

5. Alkayed NJ, Murphy SJ, Traystman RJ, et al. Neuroprotective effects of female gonadal steroids in reproductively senescent female rats. *Stroke* 2000;31:161–168.

6. Fukuda K, Yao H, Ibayashi S, et al. Ovariectomy exacerbates and estrogen replacement attenuates photothrombotic focal ischemic brain injury in rats. *Stroke* 2000;31: 155–160.

7. Yang SH, Shi J, Day AL, et al. Estradiol exerts neuroprotective effects when administered after ischemic insult. *Stroke* 2000;31:745–749.

8. The Writing Group for the PEPI Trial. Effects of estrogen or estrogen/progestin regimens on heart disease risk factors in postmenopausal women. The Postmenopausal Estrogen/Progestin Interventions (PEPI) Trial. *JAMA* 1995;273:199–208.

9. Nabulsi AA, Folsom AR, White A, et al. Association of hormone-replacement therapy with various cardiovascular risk factors in postmenopausal women. *N Engl J Med* 1993;328:1069–1075.

10. Koh KK, Mincemoyer R, Bui MN, et al. Effects of hormone-replacement therapy on fibrinolysis in postmenopausal women. *N Engl J Med* 1997;336:683–690.

11. Manolio TA, Furberg CD, Shemanski L, et al. Associations of postmenopausal estrogen use with cardiovascular disease and its risk factors in older women. *Circulation* 1993;88:2163–2171.

12. Caine YG, Bauer KA, Barzegar S, et al. Coagulation activation following estrogen administration to postmenopausal women. *Thromb Haemost* 1992;68:392–395.

13. Crook D, Godsland I. Safety evaluation of modern oral contraceptives. Effects on lipoprotein and carbohydrate metabolism. *Contraception* 1998;57:189–201.

14. Winkler U. Blood coagulation and oral contraceptives. *Contraception* 1998;57:203–209.

15. WHO Scientific Group. Cardiovascular disease and steroid hormone contraception: Report of a WHO scientific group. WHO technical report series 877. Geneva, Switzerland, 1997.

16. Hulley S, Grady D, Bush T, et al. Randomized trial of estrogen plus progestin for secondary prevention of coronary heart disease in postmenopausal women. *JAMA* 1998; 280:605–613.

17. Hemminki E, McPherson K. Impact of postmenopausal hormone therapy on cardiovascular events and cancer: Pooled data from clinical trials. BMJ 1997;315:149–153.

18. Speroff L, Rowan J, Symons J, et al. The comparative effect on bone density, endometrium, and lipids of continuous hormones as replacement therapy (CHART Study). *JAMA* 1996;276:1397–1403.

19. The Women's Health Initiative Study Group. Design of the Women's Health Initiative clinical trial and observational study. *Controlled Clin Trials* 1998;19:61–109.

20. Pfeffer RI, Van Den Noort S. Estrogen use and stroke risk in postmenopausal women. *Am J Epidemiol* 1976;103:445–456.

21. Rosenberg SH, Fausone V, Clark R. The role of estrogens as a risk factor for stroke in postmenopausal women. *West J Med* 1980;133:292–296.

22. Adam S, Williams V, Vessey MP. Cardiovascular disease and hormone replacement treatment: A pilot case-control study. *BMJ* 1981;282:1277–1278.

23. Wilson PW, Garrison RJ, Castelli WP. Postmenopausal estrogen use, cigarette smoking, and cardiovascular morbidity in women over 50: The Framingham Study. *N Engl J Med* 1985;313:1038–1043.

24. Bush TL, Barrett-Connor E, Cowan LD, et al. Cardiovascular mortality and noncontraceptive use of estrogen in women: Results from the Lipid Research Clinics Program Follow-up Study. *Circulation* 1987;75:1102–1109.
25. Petitti DB, Wingerd J, Pellegrin F, et al. Risk of vascular disease in women: Smoking, oral contraceptives, noncontraceptive estrogens, and other factors. *JAMA* 1979; 242:1150–1154.
26. Petitti DB, Perlman JA, Sidney S. Noncontraceptive estrogens and mortality: Long-term follow-up of women in the Walnut Creek Study. *Obstet Gynecol* 1987;70:289–293.
27. Boysen G, Nyboe J, Appleyard M, et al. Stroke incidence and risk factors for stroke in Copenhagen, Denmark. *Stroke* 1988;19:1345–1353.
28. Lindenstrom E, Boysen G, Nyboe J. Lifestyle factors and risk of cerebrovascular disease in women: The Copenhagen City Heart Study. *Stroke* 1993;24:1468–1472.
29. Hunt K, Vessey M, McPherson K, et al. Long-term surveillance of mortality and cancer incidence in women receiving hormone replacement therapy. *Br J Obstet Gynaecol* 1987;94:620–635.
30. Hunt K, Vessey M, McPherson K. Mortality in a cohort of long-term users of hormone replacement therapy: An updated analysis. *Br J Obstet Gynaecol* 1990;97:1080–1086.
31. Paganini-Hill A, Ross RK, Henderson BE. Postmenopausal oestrogen treatment and stroke: A prospective study. *BMJ* 1988;297:519–522.
32. Henderson BE, Paganini-Hill A, Ross RK. Decreased mortality in users of estrogen replacement therapy. *Arch Intern Med* 1991;151:75–78.
33. Wolf PH, Madans JH, Finucane FF, et al. Reduction of cardiovascular disease-related mortality among postmenopausal women who use hormones: Evidence from a national cohort. *Am J Obstet Gynecol* 1991;164:489–494.
34. Finucane FF, Madans JH, Bush TL, et al. Decreased risk of stroke among postmenopausal hormone users: Results from a national cohort. *Arch Intern Med* 1993; 153:73–79.
35. Longstreth WT, Nelson LM, Koepsell TD, et al. Subarachnoid hemorrhage and hormonal factors in women: A population-based case-control study. *Ann Intern Med* 1994;121:168–173.
36. Folsom AR, Mink PJ, Sellers TA, et al. Hormonal replacement therapy and morbidity and mortality in a prospective study of postmenopausal women. *Am J Public Health* 1995;85:1128–1132.
37. Grodstein F, Stampfer MJ, Manson JE, et al. Postmenopausal estrogen and progestin use and the risk of cardiovascular disease. *N Engl J Med* 1996;335:453–461.
38. Grodstein F, Stampfer MJ, Colditz GA, et al. Postmenopausal hormone therapy and mortality. *Engl J Med* 1997;336:1769–1775.
39. Pedersen AT, Lidegaard O, Kreiner S, et al. Hormone replacement therapy and risk of non-fatal stroke. *Lancet* 1997;350:1277–1283.
40. Petitti DB, Sidney S, Quesenberry CP Jr, et al. Ischemic stroke and use of estrogen and estrogen/progestogen as hormone replacement therapy. *Stroke* 1998;29:23–28.
41. Sourander L, Rajala T, Raiha I, et al. Cardiovascular and cancer morbidity and mortality and sudden cardiac death in postmenopausal women on oestrogen replacement therapy (ERT). *Lancet* 1998;352:1965–1969.
42. Fung MM, Barrett-Connor E, Bettencourt RR. Hormone replacement therapy and stroke risk in older women. *J Womens Health* 1999;8:359–364.
43. Falkeborn M, Persson I, Terent A, et al. Hormone replacement therapy and the risk

of stroke: Follow-up of a population-based cohort in Sweden. *Arch Intern Med* 1993;153:1201–1209.

44. Grodstein F, Stampfer MJ, Falkeborn M, et al. Postmenopausal hormone therapy and risk of cardiovascular disease and hip fracture in a cohort of Swedish women. *Epidemiology* 1999;10:476–480.

45. The Coronary Drug Project Research Group. The Coronary Drug Project: Findings leading to discontinuation of the 2.5–mg day estrogen group. *JAMA* 1973;226:652–657.

46. The Veterans Administration Co-operative Urological Research Group. Treatment and survival of patients with cancer of the prostate. *Surg Gynecol Obstet* 1967;124:1011–1017.

47. Petitti DB, Sidney S, Bernstein A, et al. Stroke in users of low-dose oral contraceptives. *N Engl J Med* 1996;335:8–15.

48. Schwartz SM, Siscovick DS, Longstreth WT Jr., et al. Use of low-dose oral contraceptives and stroke in young women. *Ann Intern Med* 1997;127:596–603.

49. WHO Collaborative Study of Cardiovascular Disease and Steroid Hormone Contraception. Ischaemic stroke and combined oral contraceptives: Results of an international, multicentre, case-control study. *Lancet* 1996;348:498–505.

50. WHO Collaborative Study of Cardiovascular Disease and Steroid Hormone Contraception. Haemorrhagic stroke, overall stroke risk, and combined oral contraceptives: Results of an international, multicentre, case-control study. *Lancet* 1996;348:505–510.

51. Heinemann LAJ, Lewis MA, Thorogood M, et al. Oral contraceptives and risk of thromboembolic stroke: Results for the Transnational Study on Oral Contraceptives and the Health of Young Women. *BMJ* 1997;315:1502–1504.

II

SECONDARY PREVENTION

9

CARDIAC ANOMALIES

G. Devuyst and J. Bogousslavsky

The aims in treating stroke are three-fold: (1) to reopen an occluded cerebral artery (thrombolysis), (2) to provide protection against the metabolic cascade caused by ischemic injury leading to neuronal death (neuroprotection), and (3) to prevent recurrent stroke (secondary prevention). Secondary prevention of stroke is the most important of these three since neither thrombolysis nor neuroprotection are currently practical in the majority of patients. In studies performed before the 1980s, the stroke recurrence rate varied from 2%–13% in the first month, irrespective of treatment, and from 2%–22% in untreated patients.[1]

No difference has been found in the early recurrence rate among patients with vascular causes compared to those with presumed cardioembolic stroke (CES).[2,3] In strokes with cardiac causes, 13%–21% will experience a recurrence within two weeks, which worsens the prognosis.[4–7] The Cerebral Embolism Study[8] found the risk of recurrence was slightly higher during the first 6 days, and Yasaka et al.[7] noted that recurrence was especially frequent 2–14 days after the initial stroke.

Little information exists about the recurrence rates of stroke for the various types of cardioembolic sources, except for rheumatic heart disease, in which recurrence rates differ among subgroups of patients with the same cardioembolic source, e.g. atrial fibrillation. Therapeutic strategies include anticoagulants, antiplatelet agents, and surgical procedures (e.g., closure of patent foramen ovale).

Three levels of credibility of clinical diagnosis for stroke of cardiac origin have been suggested—possible, probable or definite depending on the source, and treatment is specific to each of these.[9] This chapter provides an overview of the recurrent stroke risk and the risk–benefit ratio for secondary preventive therapies in patients with stroke of cardiac origin.

ATRIAL FIBRILLATION (AF)

Approximately 16% (11%–29%) of all ischemic strokes are associated with non-valvular AF,[10] and among patients over 70 years old with ischemic stroke, more than one-third suffer AF.[11,12] AF increases the relative risk of ischemic stroke about five-fold, roughly 1%–5% per year for elderly people.[10] Wolf et al.[12,13] reported a five-fold increase in stroke incidence in patients with nonrheumatic atrial fibrillation compared with a normal age matched population. The stroke risk associated with AF was 0.2 per 1,000 in the 30–39 year age group, and 39 per 1,000 in the 80–89 year age group. The risk of very early stroke recurrence among patients with AF (the most common cause of cardiogenic embolism) is estimated at 0.1%–1.3% per day during the first two weeks.[2,3,14–24] Moreover, AF patients with prior ischemic stroke or transient ischemic attack (TIA) have a high risk for recurrence of 12% per year for the subsequent two to three years.[25,26] Those with more remote stroke or TIA have a similar high risk.[27] These variations of recurrence rates are due to the retrospective design of most studies and also to the inclusion of AF patients irrespective of a coexistent cardiac disorder.

Nine recent randomised clinical trials—AFASAK, SPAF I, BAATAF, CAFA, SPINAF, SPAF II, EAFT, ESPS II, SPAF III—have convincingly demonstrated the efficacy of anticoagulants and aspirin in stroke prevention in nonvalvular AF,[28,29] but only two—EAFT[25] and ESPS II[26]—dealt specifically with secondary prevention.

Five trials of primary prevention—AFASAK, SPAF I, BAATAF, CAFA, SPINAF—comparing warfarin vs. placebo found a relative risk reduction of 33%–86% per year for ischemic stroke and 2.5%–4.7% per year for absolute rate reduction.[10,30] The Atrial Fibrillation investigators,[30] analyzing pooled data from the first five primary prevention trials, found an annual stroke rate of 4.5% in controls vs. 1.4% in the warfarin group (risk reduction = 68%). The death rate and combined outcome rate (stroke, death, systemic embolism) were also significantly reduced in the treatment group.

The efficacy of aspirin for stroke prevention in AF patients has been studied in only two of the original five primary prevention trials (AFASAK and SPAF I) and in one secondary prevention trial (EAFT), yielding a pooled risk reduction of 20%, a modest reduction compared to placebo.[10] In the SPAF II trial of primary prevention, warfarin [international normalized ration (INR 2.0–4.5)] produced a 50% risk reduction compared to aspirin at 325 mg/day.[31] Evaluation of the combined results of AFASAK, SPAF I, BAATAF, CAFA, SPINAF, and EAFT, indicates that warfarin reduces ischemic stroke by nearly 70%, compared to placebo.[10]

The stroke prevention benefit of warfarin carried no serious risk of major bleeding in most of these trials: 1.0% for placebo, 1.0% for aspirin, and 1.3% for warfarin.[10,30] Also, the incremental increase in severe haemorrhage among elderly, anticoagulated AF patients in these trials was only 0.3%–2.0% per year with INR 1.5–4.0,[10] although trial patients have a lower bleeding risk than those in clinical settings. The risk of major hemorrhage in AF patients receiving warfarin was related to the intensity of anticoagulation, patient age, and fluctuation in INRs.[10] "High-risk" AF patients, defined as those with prior TIA or stroke, a history of hypertension, or a substantially impaired left ventricular systolic function, had a higher risk of stroke (>7% per year) that was significantly reduced by warfarin.[10]

In the SPAF III study,[29] 892 patients with AF who were at low risk of stroke and taking 325 mg aspirin per day were followed for a mean of 2.0 years. The rate of primary events (ischemic stroke and systemic embolism) was 2.2% per year, while for all ischemic stroke it was 2.0% per year and for disabling ischemic stroke it was 0.8% per year. Those with hypertension had a significantly higher rate of primary events (3.6% per year vs. 1.1% per year), while the rate of disabling stroke was low. This study illustrates that AF patients with a low risk of ischemic stroke benefited less with anticoagulation than with aspirin.

Risk Stratification for Patients with AF Based on Primary Prevention Studies

The risk of stroke from AF depends on various factors, including age,[13] duration of fibrillation,[32] coexisting heart failure and hypertension.[33] One evaluation of pooled data from five randomized primary stroke prevention trials found that the major risk factors were prior stroke or TIA, diabetes, hypertension, and age, while angina, previous myocardial infarction, and congestive heart failure were also significant.[34] Mitral stenosis and thyrotoxicosis were also associated with increased stroke risk in retrospective series.[34]

The annual rate of ischemic stroke in AF is about 5%, varying between 0.5% and 12% depending upon the subgroup at risk.[28] Patients with paroxysmal AF tend to be younger and have less cardiovascular disease, so that their risk of stroke is less.[28]

In the SPAF III study,[29] patients were divided into high-risk and low-risk groups depending upon four prespecified risk factors: (1) left ventricular function associated with congestive heart failure or reduced extraction fraction on echocardiography; (2) systolic blood pressure >160 mm Hg; (3) prior ischemic stroke, TIA, or systemic embolism; and (4) female and older than 75 years. The results of this trial indicated 3 levels of risk: (1) low (about 1.0% per year) for those without thromboembolic risk factors or hypertension, (2) moderate (about 3.5 % per year) for those with hypertension but no risk factors, and (3) high (about 8% per year) for those with all the risk factors.

Based on these findings, Hart et al.[9,10] recommended aspirin at 325 mg/day for low-risk patients, aspirin or warfarin for moderate risk patients, and warfarin, INR 2.0–3.0, for patients ≤75 years, and 1.6–2.5 for patients >75 years and for high-risk patients.[28]

Echocardiography helps gauge the risk stratification, but it is unclear at present if left ventricular dysfunction, left atrial size, and mitral annular calcification diagnosed by transthoracic echocardiography (TTE) represent consistent additional stroke risk factors in AF patients. A pooled analysis of three studies, BAATAF, SPINAF, and SPAF I, showed that moderate to severe left ventricular dysfunction diagnosed by TTE was an independent predictor of stroke, but not left atrial size.[35,36] Similarly, Shively et al.[37] noted increased stroke risk associated with decreased left atrial flow velocity (<15 cm/sec), left ventricular dilatation, and decreased left atrial ejection fraction in patients with AF and left atrial enlargement. In another study, spontaneous echo contrast was significantly associated with AF-related stroke, possibly by changing blood coagulability consecutive to atrial stasis.[38]

Transesophageal echocardiography (TEE) in the SPAF III study[39] showed that the presence of complex aortic plaques (≥4 mm or mobile) carried an annual stroke risk of 16%, compared with 4% in high-risk patients without such plaques. Unlike TEE, TTE is very insensitive for atrial thrombi detection.[40]

The decision to use anticoagulant or aspirin therapy depends upon risk stratification of patients with AF. Aspirin carries a lower bleeding risk and requires less medical monitoring than do anticoagulants, and at 325 mg/day reduces the stroke risk in these patients from 6.3% per year in the placebo group to 3.6% per year in the aspirin group, a risk reduction of 42%.[36] This therapeutic effect was higher in noncardiac sources of stroke than in those from arterial causes. In AF patients with a low stroke risk (1% per year) on aspirin, only small reductions in ischemic stroke could be expected from anticoagulation, but this causes a higher risk of intracranial bleeding. In those with a high risk of stroke (6%–12% per year) on aspirin, a much greater reduction can be expected with warfarin.

Secondary Prevention Strategies

The only large placebo-controlled trial of secondary prevention of stroke in AF, the European Atrial Fibrillation Trial (EAFT),[25,41] enrolled AF patients with prior TIAs or minor ischemic strokes and was divided into three groups: warfarin alone, aspirin 300 mg/day alone, and warfarin vs. aspirin. The rate of recurrent stroke, 12% per year in the placebo group, was reduced by 17% in the aspirin group (n.s.) and 66% in the warfarin group ($p = 0.001$).

In this trial, the INRs varied between 2.5 and 4.0, but values of 2.0 to 2.9 reduced the stroke risk (including hemorrhagic events) by 80%, compared to INRs of less than 2.0. INRs between 3.0 and 3.9 reduced the rate by 40 %. Only INRs higher than 3.9 increased the complication rate, principally because of hemorrhagic complications.

In the ESPS II trial,[26] in which dipyridamole with aspirin reduced recurrent stroke, this therapeutic effect was not seen in the subgroup of patients with AF.[26,42] In a similar secondary prevention study, Studio Italiano Fibrillazione Atriale,[43] using indobufen (100 mg–200 mg twice a day) or warfarin (INR, 2.0–3.5) no superiority of one treatment over the other was detected, and bleeding complications were low. Hence, indobufen is an acceptable alternative therapy to anticoagulation in AF patients.

Some questions remain unanswered, such as the efficacy of ticlopidine and anti-glycoprotein IIb/IIIa inhibitors in preventing recurrent stroke in AF patients, especially in elderly or hypertensive patients in whom anticoagulation is more risky, as well as the efficacy of thrombolytic agents. Finally, there is no convincing evidence that restoring sinus rhythm by cardioversion reduces cerebral embolic potential (Table 9.1).

ATRIAL FLUTTER AND ATRIAL FIBRILLATION-FLUTTER

Data concerning this uncommon cardiac disorder are scant, and the exact risk of stroke associated with atrial flutter is unknown. Nevertheless, in a recent small retrospective study in patients without history of brain ischemia, the annual risk of stroke was only 1.6%.[44] Available data suggest that the risk of embolism from atrial flutter is less than AF following cardioversion. Atrial fibrillation-flutter carries the same risk of stroke as AF and so requires the same management

SICK SINUS SYNDROME (SSS)

In a recent prospective study of sick sinus syndrome, previous cerebral ischemic events, an age >65 years, left atrial spontaneous echocardiographic contrast and depressed atrial ejection force were independent risk factors for stroke.[45] Those with AF showed a thromboembolic rate of 5% per year, compared to 3.5% per year in those without AF,[10] though a more recent study reported a stroke rate of 10% per year.[45] Dual-chamber cardiac pacemakers reduced both the occurrence of AF as well as thromboembolism in comparison to ventricular pacing.

For secondary prevention in patients with well established SSS, anticoagulation should be considered, irrespective of the presence or absence of AF.[10] The value of antiplatelets, the optimal intensity of anticoagulation, and the safety of chronic anticoagulation in elderly patients remains uncertain.

TABLE 9.1. Prevention of Stroke in Atrial Fibrillation Patients: Recommendations

	PRIMARY PREVENTION			SECONDARY PREVENTION	
Studies	**Risk stratification**	**Risk of stroke***	**Therapy**	**Studies**	**Therapy**
AFASAK	AFI criteria	without therapy	≤75 y.	EAFT	warfarin
SPAF 1	*high risk*	±6% / year	warfarin INR 2.5	ESPS II	INR 3.0
BAATAF	hypertension history		(20-30=	SIFA	(2.5–4.0)
CAFA	diabetes		>75 y.		aspirin if warfarin is contraindicated
SPINAF	prior stroke or TIA		warfarin INR 2.0		indobufen if aspirin is
SPAF II	coronary disease		(1.6–2.5)		contraindicated
SPAF III	congestive heart failure				aspirin with dipyridamole but needs
	moderate risk	±2% / year	aspirin or warfarin		confirmation
	age ≥65 years				
	no high risks				
	low risk	±1%	aspirin 325 mg/d		
	age <65 years				
	no high risks				
	SPAF III criteria	under aspirin			
	high risk	±8%			
	systolic BP >160 m Hg				
	left ventricular dysfunction				
	prior stroke or TIA				
	women >75 years				
	moderate risk	±3.5%/year			
	history of hypertension				
	no high risks				
	low risk	±1%/year			
	no high risks				
	no history of hypertension				

*In unselected AF patients: 5 %/year on aspirin.

PATENT FORAMEN OVALE

During the last decade, there has been an increasing emphasis on the role of patent foramen ovale (PFO) in the genesis of ischemic stroke, particularly in the young. Several case control studies[46–54] have shown that PFO was significantly associated with stroke in patients younger than 60 years of age. Cerebral paradoxical embolism is usually a presumed diagnosis, because direct evidence, such as a thrombus lodged in the PFO shown on transesophageal echocardiography or the discovery of a deep venous thrombosis, is commonly lacking.[46,49–56] Despite these ongoing controversies, it is reasonable to incriminate a cerebral paradoxical embolism in young patients with no other identified cause of stroke than PFO.

The optimal treatment of these patients remains a matter of debate, mainly because of a lack of controlled clinical trials. There are four therapeutic options: antiplatelets drugs, anticoagulants, closure of PFO by transcatheterization or closure of PTO by surgery. The only two studies[57–58] of secondary prevention of stroke in patients with PFO show that the risk of recurrent stroke is relatively low, about 1% per year, in patients treated with aspirin or short-term anticoagulation.[10] In the Lausanne Study[57] and the French Study Group,[58] the annual rate of TIA was 3.8% and 3.4%, and of stroke alone, 1.9% and 1.2%, respectively.

At present, there is little information on the risk of stroke recurrence in those with PFO associated with an atrial septal aneurysm (ASA) compared to PFO alone, and some have suggested that PFO with an ASA, or large PFOs with right-to-left shunting, have more stroke risk.[59–62] On these grounds, Nendaz et al.[63] created a decision analysis model for the clinician. This model indicates that for a stroke risk recurrence of 0.8%–to 7% per year, there was more benefit from surgical closure of the PFO than from any other treatment. When the risk exceeds 0.8%–1.4% per year, anticoagulants and antiaggregants are better than placebo, while when it is <0.8% per year, neither medical nor surgical treatment is indicated. Further studies are planned to determine the stroke risk in subgroups of PFO patients using transcranial Doppler ultrasound with the microbubble technique, which may be more accurate than TEE.[64] At present, treatment is limited to the application of empirical clinical criteria.

Surgical closure of PFO without recurrence of stroke has been reported,[65–67] but others have not been so fortunate.[68] An alternate procedure consists of transcatheter closure of the PFO, which was effective in 82% of cases, but recurrence occurred in 4 of 34 patients on follow-up.[69] Considerably more information is needed concerning the efficiency, safety, and long-term complications of the transcatheter technique before it can replace surgery.

The use of anticoagulants is risky in young patients with a long life expectancy because of the major bleeding risk, estimated at 1.5%–11% per year.[67] The authors recommend anticoagulants when a deep venous thrombosis (DVT) is demonstrated by ultrasound investigation or by venography, and before closing the PFO surgically in those with a presumed higher risk of stroke recurrence. In practice, and until results of future studies focusing on risk stratification are reported, the authors apply the following criteria to decide secondary prevention therapy in patients with stroke and PFO: (1) more than one cerebrovascular event clinically or on MRI scan, (2) a history of Valsalva's manoeuvre just before the clinical event, (3) significant right-to-left shunting through the PFO documented by TEE or Doppler, and (4) PFO associated with ASA. In these patients we recommend aspirin of 300 mg/day, or closure of the PFO by surgery or catheter, depending upon the criteria listed above (Table 9.2).

PROSTHETIC HEART VALVES (PHV)

Thromboembolic events occur at a rate of 1–5% per year in patients with prosthetic heart valves, despite oral anticoagulation, and 85% of these are cerebral.[68] Stroke may occur from either inadequate anticoagulation or because thrombogenic factors are inadequately suppressed despite adequate anticoagulation therapy. The precise pathophysiology of thromboembolism in patients with PHV remains uncertain. Increased shear rates at the valve surfaces may activate platelets, generating platelet-derived microparticles, which could have potent procoagulant activity.[71] Also, the presence of microemboli, frequently encountered in these patients, may result from harmless gaseous bubbles (cavitation) rather than from actual particulate elements.[70,71] High-intensity transient signals (HITS) detected by the Doppler technique are seen overwhelmingly with mechanical heart valves compared to biological prostheses, and these may produce a cognitive alteration.[72] Even with the combination of anticoagulation and antiplatelets, the annual incidence rate of thromboembolism in patients with PHV remained at 2% to 3%.[70]

As yet, no prospective randomized studies have been done in patients with mechanical valves to assess the efficacy of antithrombotic therapy. In a meta-analysis comprising more than 53,000 patient-years, the major embolism rate without antithrombotic therapy was 4.0% per year, reduced to 2.2% per year with antiplatelets and to 1.0% per year with anticoagulants.[73] The embolic rate with a combination of anticoagulants and antiplatelets was higher, at 1.7% per year, than for anticoagulants alone, and much higher with dipyridamole, at 5.4% per year than with aspirin alone, at 1.4% per year. Major embolism is more frequent with mitral valves, with mitral plus aortic valves, and with caged ball prostheses.

The exact level of anticoagulation needed to prevent thromboembolism in patients with mechanical valves remains uncertain. In the past, high-intensity anticoagulation was used, and a recent meta-analysis based on 12 studies found an INR of 2.5–3.6 was best, resulting in an American College of Chest Physicians

TABLE 9.2. Secondary Prevention in Patients with Patent Foramen Ovale–Associated Stroke: Recommendations (Risk of stroke on aspirin: ±1%/year [0–4% / year])

PRESUMED RISK STRATIFICATION	HIGH RISK	MODERATE RISK	LOW RISK
Absolute criterion			
No other potential cause of stroke than PFO	Required	Required	Required
Relative criteria			
Valsalva strain before stroke	>2 criteria	2 criteria	1 criterion
Interatrial septal aneurysm			
Massive right-to-left shunting (>50 bubbles)			
Multiple clinical cerebrovascular events and/or multiple ischemic lesions at brain MRI			
Recommended therapy:	Surgical closure of PFO	Transcatheter closure of PFO	Aspirin at 325 mg/day

recommendation of 2.5–3.5.[74] A similar study involving St. Jude valves confirmed this level of anticoagulation.[75] Another study showed that higher levels of anti-coagulation, with INRs of 3.0–4.0, were needed, but this may reflect a type of valve with a particularly high embolic rate.[76] The presence of other risk factors, such as AF, left ventricular dysfunction, spontaneous echocardiographic contrast (SEC) in the left atrium and increasing age increase the chance of embolism.[77] A meta-analysis of five controlled trials that combined antiplatelets and anti-agulants noted a 67% reduction in embolism risk, but a 65% increased risk of hemorrhage and a 250% increase of major gastrointestinal bleeding. These trials used high doses of aspirin (>400 mg/day).[78] Low doses of aspirin (100 mg/day) are safe in combination with an INR of 2.5–3.5, but it is uncertain if the com-bined therapy is significantly more effective than anticoagulation alone with a target INR of 2.5–3.5.

ACUTE MYOCARDIAL INFARCTION (AMI)

About 1% to 5% of patients with AMI have an ischemic stroke, most of them cardioembolic, occurring within two to four weeks. Stroke occurred especially in those with anterior AMI, in whom the risk of ischemic stroke was 12%,[10] and in patients with large anterior infarcts.[79,80] In the first month after AMI, incidence rates were 1%–3.2%, and AF and ST segment elevation were significant risk factors.[81]

Left ventricular thrombi (LVT), in older patients with large infarcts, especially those with congestive heart failure, have an increased risk of stroke. TTE is needed to diagnose ventricular thrombi, but it should be performed at least 24 hours af-ter AMI, because since these develop 1–10 days after AMI. Approximately 15% of AMI patients with recognised LVT will suffer stroke, while β-adrenergic block-ing drugs may favor the development of LVT.[10]

No randomised trials have been carried out comparing aspirin to anticoagu-lants to prevent stroke following AMI, though anticoagulants alone were shown effective in preventing recurrent AMI (INR 2.8–4.8) and stroke in the Anticoag-ulants in Secondary Prevention of Events in Coronary Thrombosis (ASPECT) trial. No comparison with aspirin was made.[82] Early randomised trials showed that heparin followed by low-intensity oral anticoagulation (INR 1.6–2.5) reduced stroke by about 70% in the weeks following AMI (mean rate 2.9%–1.2%).[10] Be-cause the stroke rate three months after AMI is so low, long-term anticoagula-tion beyond three months is not justified unless other major cardiac embolic risk factors, such as mural thrombosis, are present.

A risk stratification approach may be useful. Early treatment with low-dose hep-arin and aspirin for those with uncomplicated AMI is recommended, but full dose anticoagulation is needed for patients with LVT detected by echocardiography.

TIMING OF ANTICOAGULANT TREATMENT

Prevention of recurrent stroke by anticoagulantion in patients with cardioembolic stroke remains controversial, and the stroke risk must be balanced against the risk of hemorrhagic transformation of the cerebral infarct. The timing of anticoagulation is uncertain. In the International Stroke Trial[83] and other studies, neither heparin nor heparinoid were efficacious because the benefit of reducing recurrent ischemic strokes was offset by an increase in hemorrhagic strokes. Until adequate data are available from randomized trials, the therapeutic decisions for these patients will remain arbitrary.

REFERENCES

1. Koudstaal PJ. Prevention of early recurrences in acute stroke. In: J. Bogousslavsky, ed. *Acute Stroke Treatment*. London: Martin Dunitz, 1997:285–296.
2. Sandercock P, Bamford J, Dennis M, et al. Atrial fibrillation and stroke: Prevalence in different types of stroke and influence on early and long term prognosis. *BMJ* 1992; 305:1460–1465.
3. Broderick JP, Phillips SJ, O'Fallon WM, Frye RL, Whisnant JP. Relationship of cardiac disease to stroke occurrence, recurrence, and mortality. *Stroke* 1992;23:1250–1256.
4. Leonard AD, Newburg S. Cardioembolic stroke. *J Neurosci Nurs* 1992;24:69–76.
5. Takano K, Yamaguchi T, Kato H, Omae T. Activation of coagulqtion in acute cardioembolic stroke. *Stroke* 1991;22:12–16.
6. Yasaka M, Yamaguchi T. Immediate anticoagulation for intracardiac thrombus in acute cardioembolic stroke. *Angiology* 1992;(Nov):886–891.
7. Yasaka M, Yamaguchi T, Oita J, Sawada T, Shichiri M, Omae T. Clinical features of recurrent embolization in acute cardioembolic stroke. *Stroke* 1993;24:1681–1685.
8. Devuyst G, Bogousslavsky J. Which cardiac diagnosis tests apply in the acute phase of stroke and when are they useful? In: J. Bogousslavsky, ed.: *Acute Stroke Treatment*. London: Martin Dumitz, 1997:65–78.
9. Hart RG. Cardiogenic embolism to the brain. *Lancet* 1992;339:589–594.
10. Hart RG, Albers GW, Koudstaal PJ. Cardioembolic stroke. In: Ginsberg MD, Bogousslavsky J, eds. *Cerebrovascular Disease*, Malden, Mass.: Blackwell, 1998:vol 2, 1392–1429.
11. Asplund K, Carlberg B, Sundstrom G. Stroke in the elderly. *Cerebrovasc Dis* 1992;2: 152–157.
12. Wolf PA, Abbott RD, Kannel WB. Atrial fibrillation: A major contributor to stroke in the elderly. *Arch Intern Med* 1987;147:1561–1564.
13. Wolf PA, Dawber TR, Thomas HE, Kannel WB. Epidemiologic assessment of chronic atrial fibrillation and risk of stroke: The Framingham Study. Neurology 1978;28: 973–977.
14. Bogousslavsky J, van Melle G, Regli F, Kappenberger L. Pathogenesis of anterior circulation stroke in patients with nonvalvular atrial fibrillation: The Lausanne Stroke Registry. *Neurology* 1990;40:1046–4050.
15. Anonymous. Cariogenic brain embolism: The second report of the Cerebral Embolism Task Force. *Arch Neurol* 1989;46:727–743.

16. Hornig CR, Dorndorf W. Early outcome and recurrences after cardiogenic brain embolism. *Acta Neurol Scand* 1993;88:23–31.
17. Gustafsson C, Britton M. Pathogenetic mechanism of stroke in non-valvular atrial fibrillation: Follow-up of stroke patients with and without atrial fibrillation. *J Intern Med* 1991;230:11–16.
18. Bogousslavsky J, Adnet-Bonte C, Regli F, van Melle G; Kappenberger L. Lone atrial fibrillation and stroke. *Acta Neurol Scand* 1990;82:143–146.
19. Yamanouchi H, Shimada H, Tomonaga M, Matsushita S. Recurrence of embolic stroke in non-valvular atrial fibrillation (NVAF): An autopsy study. *Acta Neurol Scand* 1989; 80:123–129.
20. Kelley RE, Berger JR, Alter M, Kovacs AG. Cerebral ischemia and atrial fibrillation: Prospective study. *Neurology* 1984;34:1285–1291.
21. Wolf PA, Kannel WB, McGee DL, Meeks SL, Bharucha NE, McNamara PM. Duration of atrial fibrillation and imminence of stroke: The Framingham study. *Stroke* 1983;14:664–667.
22. Sage JI, Van Uitert RL. Risk of recurrent stroke in patients with atrial fibrillation and non-valvular heart disease. *Stroke* 1983;14:537–540.
23. Hart RG, Coull BM, Hart D. Early recurrent embolism associated with nonvalvular atrial fibrillation: A retrospective study. Stroke 1983;14:688–693.
24. Sherman DG, Goldman L, Whiting RB, Jurgensen K, Kaste M, Easton JD. Thromboembolism in patients with atrial fibrillation. *Arch Neurol* 1984;41:708–710.
25. European Atrial Fibrillation Trial Study Group. Secondary prevention of vascular events in patients with nonrheumatic atrial fibrillation and recent transient ischemic attack or minor ischemic stroke. *Lancet* 1993;342:1255–1262.
26. Diener HC, Forbes C, Riekkinin PJ, Sivenius J, Smets P, Lowenthal A. European stroke Prevention Study II: Efficacy and safety data. *J Neurol Sci* 1997;151:S13–S17.
27. Stroke Prevention in Atrial Fibrillation Investigators. Adjusted-dose warfarin versus low-intensity, fixed-dose warfarin plus aspirin for high-risk patients with atrial fibrillation: The Stroke Prevention in Atrial Fibrillation III randomized clinical trial. *Lancet* 1996;348:633–638.
28. Hart RG, Sherman DG, Easton JD, Cairns JA. Prevention of stroke in patients with nonvalvular atrial fibrillation: Views and reviews. *Neurology* 1998;51:674–681.
29. The SPAFF III Writing Committee for the Stroke Prevention in Atrial Fibrillation Investigators. Patients with nonvalvular atrial fibrillation at low risk of stroke during treatment with aspirin. *JAMA* 1998;279:1273–1277.
30. Atrial Fibrillation Investigators. Risk factors for stroke and efficacy of anti-thrombotics therapy in atrial fibrillation: An analysis of pooled data from five randomized control trials. *Arch Intern Med* 1994;154:1449–1457.
31. Stroke Prevention in Atrial Fibrillation Investigators. Warfarin versus aspirin for prevention of thromboembolism in atrial fibrillation: Stroke Prevention in Atrial Fibrillation II Study. *Lancet* 1994;343:687–691.
32. Wolf PA, Abbott RD, Kannel WB. Atrial fibrillation: A major contributor to stroke in the elderly. *Arch Intern Med* 1987;147:1561–1564.
33. Petersen P. Thromboembolic complications in atrial fibrillation. *Stroke* 1990;21:4–13.
34. Woolfenden AR, Albers GW. Cardioembolic stroke. In: Fisher M, Bogousslavsky J, eds. *Current Review of Cerebrovascular Disease.* Philadelphia: Current Medicine, 1999:93–105.
35. The stroke Prevention in Atrial Fibrillation Investigators Committee on Echocardiography. Transesophageal echocardiographic correlates of thromboembolism in high-risk patients with nonvalvular atrial fibrillation. *Ann Intern Med* 1998;128:639–647.

36. Souvik S, Oppenheimer SM. Cardiac disorders and stroke. *Curr Opin Neurol* 1998;11: 51–56.

37. Shively BK, Gelgland EA, Crawford MH. Regional left atrial stasis during atrial fibrillation and flutter. *J Am Coll Cardiol* 1996;27:1722–1729.

38. Chimowitz MI, De Georgia MA, Poole RM, Hepner A, Armstrong WM. Left atrial spontaneous echo contrast highly associated with previous stroke in patients with atrial fibrillation or mitral stenosis. *Stroke* 1993;24:1015–1019.

39. The Stroke Prevention in Atrial Fibrillation Investigators Committee on Echocardiography. Transesophageal echocardiographic correlates of thromboembolism in high-risk patients with nonvalvular atrial fibrillation. *Ann Intern Med* 1998;128:639–647.

40. Mugge A, Kuhn H, Daniel WG. The role of transesophageal echocardiography in the detection of left atrial thrombi. *Echocardiography* 1993;10:405–417.

41. European Atrial Fibrillation Trial Study Group. Optimal oral anticoagulant therapy in patients with nonrheumatic atrial fibrillation and recent cerebral ischemia. *N Engl J Med* 1995;333:5–10.

42. Diener HC, Lowenthal A. Antiplatelet therapy to prevent stroke: Risk of brain hemorrhage and efficacy in atrial fibrillation. *J Neurol Sci* 1997;153:112.

43. Morocutti C, Amabile G, Fattapposta F, et al. for the SIFA (Studio Italiano Fibrillazione Atriale) Investigators: Indobufen versus warfarin in the secondary prevention of major vascular events in nonrheumatic atrial fibrillation. *Stroke* 1997;28:1015–1021.

44. Wood KA, Eisenberg SI, Kalman JM, et al. Risk of thromboembolism in chronic atrial flutter. *Am J Cardiol* 1997;79:1043–1047.

45. Mattioli AV, Castellani ET, Fusco C, Mattioli G. Stroke in paced patients with sick sinus syndrome: Relevance of atrial mechanical function, pacing mode and clinical characteristics. *Cardiology* 1997;88:264–270.

46. Harvey JR, Teague SM, Anderson JL, Voyles WF, Thadani U. Clinically silent atrial septal defects with evidence for cerebral embolization. *Ann Intern Med* 1986;105: 695–697.

47. Lechat PH, Mas JL, Lascault G, et al. Prevalence of patent foramen ovale in patients with stroke. *N Engl J Med* 1988;318:1148–1152.

48. Webster MWI, Chancellor AM, Smith HJ, et al. Patent foramen ovale in young stroke patients. *Lancet* 1988;2:11–12.

49. Biller J, Adams HP Jr, Johnson MR, Kerber RE, Toffol GJ. Paradoxical cerebral embolism: Eight cases. *Neurology* 1986;36:1356–1360.

50. Jeanrenaud X, Bogousslavsky J, Stauffer JC, Payot M, Regli F, Kappenberger L. Foramen ovale perméable et infarctus cÈrÈbral du sujet jeune. *Schweiz Med Wochenschr* 1990;120:823–829.

51. Jeanrenaud X, Kappenberger L. Patent foramen ovale and stroke of unknown origin. *Cerebrovasc Dis* 1991;1:184–192.

52. Gautier JC, Dürr A, Koussa S, Lascault G, Grosgogeat Y. Paradoxical cerebral embolism with a patent foramen ovale. *Cerebrovasc Dis* 1991;1:193–202.

53. De Belder MA, Tourikis L, Leech G, Camm AJ. Risk of patent foramen ovale for thromboembolic events in all age groups. *Am J Cardiol* 1992;63:1316–1320.

54. Di Tullio M, Sacco RL, Gopal A, Mohr JP, Homma S. Patent foramen ovale as a risk factor for cryptogenic stroke. *Ann Intern Med* 1992;117:461–465.

55. Daniel WG. Transcatheter closure of patent foramen ovale: Therapeutic overkill or elegant management for selected patients at risk? *Circulation* 1992;86:2013–2015.

56. Ranoux D, Cohen A, Cabanes L, Amarenco P, Bousser MG, Mas JL. Patent foramen ovale: Is stroke due to paradoxical embolism? *Stroke* 1993;24:31–34.

57. Bogousslavsky J, Garazi S, Jeanrenaud X, Aebischer N, van Melle G. Stroke recurrence in patients with patent foramen ovale: The Lausanne Study, Lausanne Stroke with Paradoxal embolism Study Group. *Neurology* 1996;46:1301–1305.
58. Mas JL, Zuber M. Recurrent cerebrovascular events in patients with patent foramen ovale, atrial septal aneurysm or both and cryptogenic stroke or transient ischemic attack: French Study Group on Patent Foramen Ovale an Atrial Septal Aneurysm. *Am Heart J* 1995;130:1083–1088.
59. Homma S, Di Tullio MR, Sacco RL, Mihalatos D, Li Mandri G, Mohr JP. Characteristics of patent foramen ovale associated with cryptogenic stroke: A biplane transesophageal echocardiographic study. *Stroke* 1994;25:582–586.
60. Stone DA, Godard J, Coretti MC, Kittner SJ, Sample C, Price TR, Plotnick GD. Patent foramen ovale: Association between the degree of shunt by contrast transesophageal echocardiography and the risk of future ischemic neurologic events. *Am Heart J* 1996;131:158–161.
61. Hausmann D, Mügge A, Daniel WG. Identification of patent foramen ovale permitting paradoxic embolism. *J Am Coll Cardiol* 1995;26:1030–1038.
62. Steiner MM, Di Tullio MR, Rundek T, Gan R, Chen X, Liguori C, Brainin M, Homma S, Sacco RL. Patent foramen ovale size and embolic brain imaging findings among patients with ischemic stroke. *Stroke* 1998;29:944–948.
63. Nendaz MR, Sarasin FP, Junod AF, Bogousslavsky J. Preventing stroke recurrence in patients with patent oframen ovale: Antithrombotic therapy, foramen closure or therapeutic abstention? A decision analytic perspective. *Am Heart J* 1998;135:532–541.
64. Devuyst G, Despland PA, Bogousslavsky J, Regli F. Complementarity of contrast transcranial Doppler and contrast transesophageal echocardiography for the detection of patent foramen ovale in stroke patients. *Eur Neurol* 1997;38:21–25.
65. Harvey JR, Teague SM, Anderson JL, Voyles WF, Thadani U. Clinically silent atrial septal defects with evidence for cerebral embolization. *Ann Intern Med* 1986;105:695–697.
66. Homma S, Di Tullio MR, Sacco RL, et al. Surgical closure of patent foramen ovale in selected patients with cryptogenic stroke: A preliminary experience (abstract). *Stroke* 1995;26:172.
67. Devuyst G, Bogousslavsky J, Ruchat P, Jeanrenaud X, Despland PA, Regli F, Aebischer N, Karpuz HM, Castillo V, Guffi M, Sadeghi H. Prognosis after stroke followed by surgical closure of patent foramen ovale: A prospective follow-up study with brain MRI and simultaneous transesophageal and transcranial Doppler ultrasound. *Neurology* 1996;47:1162–1166.
68. Homma S, Di Tullio MR, Sacco RL, Sciacca RR, Smith C, Mohr JP. Surgical closure of patent foramen ovale in cryptogenic stroke patients. *Stroke* 1997;28(12):2376–2381.
69. Bridges ND, Hellenbrand W, Latson L, Filiano J, Newburger JW, Lock JE. Transcatheter closure of patent foramen ovale after presumed paradoxical embolism. *Circulation* 1992;86:1902–1908.
70. Geiser T, Sturzenegger M, Genewein U, Haeberli A, Beer JH. Mechanisms of cerebrovascular events as assessed by procoagulant activity, cerebral microemboli, and platelet microparticles inpatients with prosthetic heart valves. *Stroke* 1998;29:1770–1777.
71. Devuyst G. New trends in neurosonology. In: Fisher M, Bogousslavsky J. *Current Review of Cerebrovascular Disease*. Philadelphia: Current Medicine, 1999;65–76.
72. Deklunder G, Roussel M, Lecroart JL, Prat A, Gautier C. Microemboli in cerebral circulation and alteration of cognitive abilities in patients with mechanical prosthetic heart valves. *Stroke* 1998;29:1821–1826.

73. Cannegieter SC, Rosendaar FR, Briet E. Thromboembolic and bleeding complications in patients with mechanical heart valve prostheses. *Circulation* 1994;89:635–641.

74. Stein PD, Grandison D, Hua TA, et al. Therapeutic level of oral anticoagulation with warfarin in patients with mechanical heart valves: Review of literature and recommendations based on international normalzed ration. *Postgrad Med* 1994;70(suppl 1): S72–S83.

75. Horstkotte D, Schulte HD, Bircks W, Strauer BE. Lower intensity anticoagulation therapy results in lower complications rates with St. Jude medical prosthesis. *J Thorac Cardiovasc Surg* 1994;107:1136–1145.

76. Cannegieter SC, Rosendaal FR, Wintzen AR, et al. Optimal oral anticoagulant therapy in patients with mechanical heart valves. *N Engl J Med* 1995;333:11–17.

77. Vongpatanasin W, Hillis LD, Lange RA. Prosthetic heart valves. *N Engl J Med* 1996; 335:407–416.

78. Captell E, Fiore LD, Brophy MT, et al. Efficacy and safety of combined anticoagulant and antiplatelet therapy versus anticoagulant monotherapy after mechanical heart-valve replacement: A meta-analysis. *Am Heart J* 1995;130:547–552.

79. Sloan MA, Gore JM. Ischemic stroke and intracranial hemorrhage following thrombolytic therapy for acute myocardial infarction: A risk-benefit analysis. *Am J Cardiol* 1992;69:21A–38A.

80. Tanne D, Reicher-Reiss H, Boyko V, Behar S, for the SPRINT Study Group: Stroke risk after anterior wall acute myocardial infarction. *Am J Cardiol* 1995;76:825–826.

81. Mooe T, Eriksson P, Stegmayr B. Ischemic stroke after acute myocardial infarction: A population-based study. *Stroke* 1997;28:762–767.

82. Anticoagulants in the Secondary Prevention of Events in Coronary Thrombosis (ASPECT) Research Group. Effective long-term oral anticoagulant treatment on mortality and cardiovascular morbidity after myocardial infarction. *Lancet* 1994;343:499–503.

10

ACETYLSALICYLIC ACID (ASPIRIN)

Natan M. Bornstein

Aspirin is an old and widely-used drug. Its antithrombotic role is the base of its clinical use for prevention of stroke. The development of ASA as an active drug for stroke prevention underwent some important milestones over time. The salutary effects of willow bark (*saltix alba*) have been known to several cultures for centuries. Salicin, its active ingredient, is a bitter glycoside from which sodium salicylate was isolated in 1829 by Henri Leroux, who demonstrated its antipyretic effects. The pharmaceutical chemist Felix Hoffman found a way of acetylating the hydroxyl group on the benzene ring of salicylic acid to form acetylsalicylic acid, which was shown to have anti-inflammatory and analgesic effects.

Acetylsalicylic acid was introduced into clinical medicine at the turn of the nineteenth century under the name "aspirin," which was given to the new drug by Bayer's chief pharmacologist, Heinrich Dreser.[1] In 1953, Craven[2] suggested that aspirin may act as an anticoagulant and, in 1956, he suggested that it might prevent ischemic vascular disease.[3] In 1963, Blatrix[4] noted that aspirin increases bleeding time. The inhibitory effect of this compound on the action of blood platelets was not discovered until the late 1960s.[5] In 1968 O'Brien[6] described a specific inhibitory effect of aspirin on the aggregation response of blood. This property was then linked to the irreversible inhibition of the cyclooxygenase enzyme responsible for the synthesis of eicosanoids (prostacyclin and thromboxane) and involved in arachidonic acid metabolism,[7] which is responsible for the conversion of arachidonic acid to TxA_2 in platelets and for the conversion of arachidonic acid to prostacycline in the vascular wall.[8]

MECHANISM OF ACTION

Aspirin competes with arachidonic acid for binding to the hydroxyl group of single amino acid residue (serine 529) in the polypeptide chain of platelet prostaglandin G/H synthase 1. As a result, aspirin completely and irreversibly inhibits the action of the enzyme cyclooxygenase, thereby suppressing the production of thromboxane A_2 (TxA_2) in platelets, an affect that induces platelet aggregation and vasoconstriction. This irreversible effect persists for the life span of the platelet. On the other hand, aspirin reduces the production of prostacyclin (PGI_2) on the vessel wall, an effect that inhibits platelet aggregation and induces vasodilation and, therefore, might have some anti-thrombogenic effect . However, endothelial cells can rapidly recover the inhibitory effect of aspirin cyclooxygenase synthesis, in contrast to platelets.[9–10]

In addition to its anti-aggregate effect, aspirin has other actions that may potentially play a role in stroke prevention, namely; antiinflammatory and antioxidant activities. Aspirin is rapidly absorbed in the stomach and upper intestine: the peak plasma concentration occurs 15–20 minutes after ingestion and the anti-aggregate activity is evident within 1 hour after administration.[10] Thus, the inhibitory effect is rapid and lasts for the life-span of the platelet. Some mechanisms of aspirin on hemostasis are cyclooxygenase independent and should be taken into account. Aspirin may increase fibrinolytic activity for up to 4 hours after its administration,[11] and may lower vitamin K-dependent clotting factors II, VII, IX, and X.[12] However, the dose–response relationship, duration, occurrence in the clinical setting, and relevance to the antithrombotic effect of aspirin have not been established.

In summary, the two opposing actions of aspirin on blood platelets are blocking of the pro-aggregatory and vasoconstrictive effects of TxA_2 on the one hand and diminishing vasodilatation and anti-aggregate activity of prostacyclin on the other hand, which led to the coining of the term "aspirin dilemma".[13] The aspirin dilemma refers mainly to the debate concerning the use of higher vs. lower doses of aspirin in patients who are at high risk of cerebrovascular thrombosis.

ASPIRIN AND STROKE PREVENTION

Primary Prevention

Several trials aimed at investigating the use of aspirin for primary prevention of stroke yielded inconclusive results. The U.S. Physicians' Health Study[14] was a double-blind, placebo-controlled trial of 325 mg of aspirin taken every other day with or without beta carotene, conducted among 22,071 U.S. male physicians initially aged 40 to 84 years, with an average follow-up of 5 years. The study revealed a 44% reduction in the incidence of myocardial infarction, and that motivated the early termination of the study. Over the 5-year period, the incidence of cardiovascular death was similar in the aspirin and placebo groups, and a nonsignificantly increased risk of stroke of all types, particularly for the small subgroup of hemorrhagic strokes (23 vs. 12), was shown in the aspirin-treated group compared with placebo group. However, the number of events were too small to draw any firm conclusions.

The British Doctors' Trial[15] randomized 5139 male physicians initially aged 50 to 78 years in an open design between one group taking 500 mg of aspirin daily (two-thirds of the patients) and those advised to avoid aspirin (one-third of the patients). This trial was much smaller, unblinded, unbalanced, and less rigid than the U.S. Physicians' Health Study. After 6 years, no statistically significant difference was detected between the two groups, either for the combined outcome event "vascular death, stroke, or myocardial infarction," or for any of these events alone.[16] However, a slight increase in disabling strokes and a decrease in transient ischemic attacks (TIAs) among those allocated to aspirin. Only limited data were available on which of the strokes were hemorrhagic and which were thrombotic, but no excess of any particular type of stroke was shown with aspirin. Barnett[17] suggested that any future primary prevention studies designed to evaluate possible stroke reduction should be required to continue for 10 years longer or to involve a population of subjects 10 years older than the ones in these two studies, because stroke incidence peaks 10 years later in life than myocardial infarction.

An overview of these two trials of primary prevention[16,18] showed a 32% (SD ± 8%) reduction in the odds of suffering a nonfatal myocardial infarction, and a 13% (SD ± 6%) reduction of combined vascular events, but a nonsignificant increase for nonfatal stroke (18% SD ± 13%). The results of these two large studies led to the conclusion that the routine use of aspirin by healthy men should not be universally recommended when the side effects of aspirin are compared with the reduction in risk of nonfatal myocardial infarction.[16,19]

The Nurses' Health Study[20] included females taking from one to six aspirin per week or placebo was conducted in the United States. The analysis was based on 87,678 registered nurses aged 34 to 65 years and free of diagnosed coronary heart disease, stroke, and cancer at baseline. The study demonstrated that women who had taken aspirin had a reduced risk of a first myocardial infarction, but no alteration in the risk of stroke was observed. Cardiovascular death was slightly but nor significantly reduced.

Several points should be emphasized regarding these studies. They included individuals who were engaged in health services and could be considered as comprising an especially health-minded group. This also may explain the rate of vascular events being lower than expected in the general population. Kronmal et al.[21] have since reported the intriguing results that aspirin use was associated with increased risk for ischemic stroke in women and hemorrhagic stroke in both men and women in a cohort of elderly people. The authors mentioned the possibility of there having been some confounding of results stemming from aspirin use per se as opposed to cause and effect.

In another randomized study, the Hypertension Optimal Treatment (HOT) study,[22] in which 9391 hypertensive patients were assigned to receive 75 mg of daily aspirin and 9391 patients received placebo, there was a significant beneficial effect of aspirin on myocardial infarction reduced by 36% but there was no effect on stroke. In these studies, a small but definite chance of adverse events existed, with about 1 per 1000 cases of excessive bleeding due to aspirin.

A recent data analysis conducted by Hart et al.[23] concluded that aspirin is ineffective in primary prevention of stroke for individuals without clinically identified vascular disease. This is in contrast to its benefit in decreasing myocardial infarction and to its protective effect against stroke in patients with manifest vascular disease.

Efficacy of aspirin for stroke reduction in patients with asymptomatic carotid stenosis is doubtful. In a double-blind, placebo-controlled trial, Cote et al.[24] demonstrated that aspirin had no significant long-term protective effect in asymptomatic patients with high-grade (>50%) carotid stenosis. The median duration of follow-up was 2.3 years. The annual rate of all ischemic events and death from any cause was 12.3% for the placebo group and 11.0% for the aspirin group ($p = 0.61$). The annual rates for vascular events only were 11% for the placebo group and 10.7% for the aspirin group ($p = 0.99$).

The role of aspirin in preventing initial stroke in patients with nonvalvular atrial fibrillation remains unclear. Only two placebo-controlled, randomized, primary prevention trials in patients with atrial fibrillation have been performed, using warfarin and various doses of aspirin. They were terminated early as monitoring of the results showed significant differences.[25]

The Atrial Fibrillation, Aspirin, Anticoagulation (AFASAK) study from Copenhagen, Denmark,[26] and the Stroke Prevention in Atrial Fibrillation (SPAF) study from the United States[27] formally evaluated the use of aspirin as an alternative treatment. The AFASAK study used 75 mg of aspirin per day and the SPAF trial used 325 mg per day. Another study, Boston Area Anticoagulation Trial for Atrial Fibrillation (BAATAF),[28] which was not specifically designed to evaluate the role of aspirin, allowed patients in the placebo group to receive aspirin at a dose of 325 mg per day. The BAATAF and AFASAK trials were not blinded, and the SPAF study was blinded for ASA but not for warfarin therapy.

In the AFASAK,[26] 1007 patients were randomly allocated to receive warfarin, aspirin (75 mg/day), or placebo. At the end of 2 years, the incidence of stroke, TIA, and systemic embolism was significantly lower in the warfarin group (1.5%) than in the aspirin and placebo group (6% each). A reduction of about 20% in the risk of important vascular events occurred in the aspirin group, but because of very small numbers of events the results were inconclusive. The trial was reported as negative with respect to aspirin. However, its unblinded design and the fact that 38% of the patients assigned to the warfarin group withdrew from this study, together with the fact that the analysis was an efficacy analysis, necessitated confirmation of these findings by other trials.[25]

In the SPAF Study,[27] 588 patients with nonvalvular atrial fibrillation were randomly selected to receive warfarin, aspirin (325 mg/day), or placebo. In addition, 656 patients not eligible for treatment with warfarin received aspirin or placebo in a double-blind fashion. At the end of 1 year, the placebo arm of the study was terminated because active treatment (either warfarin or aspirin) reduced the risk of stroke and systemic embolism by an impressive 81%. The study also revealed that aspirin reduced the risk of stroke and embolism by 50% but was not effective in patients older than 75 years.

Various mechanisms of stroke may explain the lack of effectiveness of aspirin in the AFASAK study compared with that in the SPAF study. The AFASAK study entered older patients, who were probably at higher risk of stroke than those in the SPAF study. This difference may be related to a higher prevalence of left atrial or ventricular stasis-related thrombi, which are anticoagulant sensitive, in the older patients in the AFASAK study, as indicated by the threefold to fourfold higher incidence of heart failure and the twofold higher incidence of previous myocardial infarction in patients in that study. Aspirin reduced the occurrence of stroke categorized as noncardioembolic significantly ($p = 0.01$) more than it did those categorized as cardioembolic, an important finding of the SPAF investigation.[29] Another difference between the two studies was a lower (75 mg) dose of aspirin that was used in the AFASAK compared to 325 mg of aspirin in the SPAF. In addition, the Danish study included more females, and this also may be a confounder. Thus, ASA may have some stroke prevention benefit in patients with nonvalvular atrial fibrillation who tend to develop platelet rich in situ thrombi or emboli. In these patients, atrial fibrillation is probably only a marker of vascular disease rather than a cause of left arterial thromboembolism.[30]

In light of these findings, it emerges that there are presently no approved prescription indications for aspirin in the primary prevention of cerebrovascular and cerebrovascular disease, and that formal policy recommendations need to await the results of the randomized trials. In the meantime, the American Heart Association suggests that aspirin may outweigh the harm in men at high risk for coronary disease, but no guidelines have been issued for women.

Secondary Prevention

Since the late 1970s, many clinical trials have been conducted to determine the value of aspirin in the prevention of ischemic stroke. The first placebo-controlled randomized trial, which was done in Canada,[31] involved almost 600 patients (290 patients assigned to the two groups that included aspirin treatment were compared with 295 patients assigned to one of the two groups that did not take the drug) and showed that 1300 mg of aspirin per day reduced the incidence of stroke and death by 31%.

Another randomized controlled study conducted in France on 604 patients with previous TIA (16%) or completed stroke (84%) showed that 1000 mg of aspirin daily significantly reduced the risk of stroke (40%) in both sexes, but that the mortality rate was not reduced.[32] In this study, cotreatment with dipyridamole did not confer additional benefits. Since then, several other trials have been conducted with different doses of aspirin, ranging from 30 to 1000 mg per day. The results of three trials were published in 1991. One was the final report of the U.K. TIA aspirin trial,[33] in which 2435 patients with TIA or minor stroke were randomly allocated to receive "blind" treatment with aspirin at 1200 mg daily, aspirin at 300 mg daily, or placebo. Patients were followed for a mean of about 4 years. The outcomes (i.e., death, myocardial infarction, and stroke) were similar in the two groups that had been allocated aspirin—neither dose of aspirin was significantly better than placebo. It is noteworthy that the number of patients in each aspirin group was 815 and 806, which might be too small to rule out a type II error. In the final analysis, when both aspirin dose groups were combined, the investigators found a significant (15%) reduction in the risk of death, myocardial infarction, and stroke, but only a 7% reduction in disabling stroke and death, and 3% reduction in disabling stroke and vascular death. It is important to mention that the population of the U.K. TIA study was somewhat different from other stroke studies in that there was a relative low annual rate of stroke (3.2% in the placebo group, compared to 5.9%–7.3% reported in other studies.[31,34]

A randomized double-blind Dutch TIA trial[34] compared the effectiveness of 30 mg aspirin daily to 283 mg aspirin daily on the occurrence of nonfatal stroke, myocardial infarction, and vascular death in patients after TIA or minor stroke (there was no placebo group). A total of 3131 patients were included and followed for an average of 2.6 years. No significant difference was found in vascular events between the 30 mg daily group (14.7%) compared with the 283 mg daily group (15.2%).

The Swedish Aspirin Low-Dose Trial (SALT)[35] was a double-blind randomized trial that compared 75 mg of aspirin daily with placebo for the prevention of stroke and death following TIA or minor stroke. The 1360 study patients were followed for a mean of 32 months. A significant 18% reduction was found in the primary out come events (stroke or death).

The recently completed second European Stroke Prevention Study (ESPS-2) was a randomized, placebo-controlled, double-blind trial comparing the effect of low dose aspirin (50 mg daily), modified-release dipyridamole (DP, 400 mg daily), to the combination of both drugs with the effects of placebo in 6602 patients with a prior ischemic stroke or TIA.[36] The investigators reported that the combined therapy was more effective in preventing stroke (37% reduction) than aspirin alone (18.1% reduction) or DP alone (16.3% reduction). For the combination end-point of stroke death, the combination regimen was associated with a 24.4% risk reduction. The combination of aspirin and DP compared with aspirin alone was associated with a 12.9% (95% CI 0-25%; $p = 0.056$) relative risk reduction in primary outcome event of stroke and death, and 22% (95% CI:9–33%) relative event vascular death, nonfatal stroke, or nonfatal myocardial infarction.[37,38] None of the treatments significantly reduced the risk of death alone or of fatal stroke. Before the ESPS-2, the four studies that had compared the combination of aspirin and DP with aspirin alone in TIA/stroke patients had collectively shown that the combination of the two drugs was associated with only a 3% (95% CI: from −22 to 22%) reduction in the vascular events compared with aspirin alone.[10,31] These results are somewhat different from the result obtained by EPSP-2. A meta-analysis of all trials, including ESPS-2, indicates that among the 2473 patients with prior stroke or TIA who were assigned to the combination of aspirin and DP, 356 (14.6%) experienced vascular event compared with 419 (17.2%) of 2436 patients assigned to receive aspirin—a relative risk reduction of 15% ($p = 0.012$).[38] If the results of this meta-analysis are correct, the combination of aspirin and DP prevents twice as many vascular events as does aspirin alone. However, it is known that large randomized trials may contradict previous meta-analyses. In a recent review of all the DP, Wilterdink and Easton[39] concluded that. . . . "another randomized clinical trial showing a significant benefit of the combination of dipyridamole plus aspirin over aspirin alone may be needed before the addition of dipyridamole to aspirin is widely accepted for prevention of stroke."

The results of ESPS-2 were criticized on several issues:

1. There were ethical concerns regarding the use of a placebo arm when the efficacy of aspirin was proven.
2. There were concerns that emerged from one of the participating centers having been excluded from analysis after 438 fictitious patients were enrolled.
3. Among the 25% of patients who withdrew from the study, most were in the DP and the combination groups and compliance was higher among DP patients (97%) than in the aspirin groups (84%).
4. The low dose of aspirin (50 mg daily) was regarded by many as a placebo.
5. The predominant effect of the combination regimen was in reducing non-fatal stroke, with little effect on myocardial infarction and fatal stroke, which is different from the effect of other antiplatelet agents.

The Ticlopidine Aspirin Stroke Study (TASS)[40] was a "triple"-blind study comparing the effect of aspirin 1300 mg daily vs. ticlopidine 250 mg twice daily in

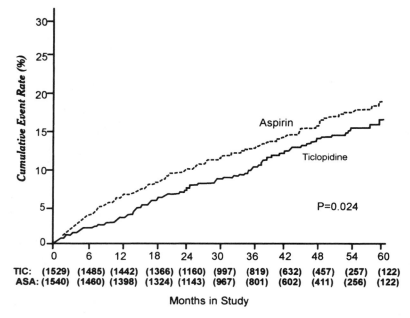

FIGURE 10.1. Cumulative event-rate curves for fatal and nonfatal stroke. Values in paren-theses indicate the number of patients in the ticlopidine (TIC) and aspirin (ASA) groups.

3069 patients with TIA (1300) and minor stroke who were followed for up to 5.8 years. The primary analysis was an "intention-to-treat" assessment of death from all causes or nonfatal stroke. Ticlopidine effected a 13% greater reduction than aspirin in the primary end-points and a reduction of 21% in the 3-year event rate for fatal or non-fatal stroke (Fig. 10.1). It was interesting to note that there was 42% relative risk reduction (RRR) for stroke and death in the first year and a 47% RRR for stroke and stroke death. This was largely maintained over the next 2 years, but the RRR declined to 21% after 3 years. The superiority of ticlo-pidine over aspirin in the reduction of stroke was seen in both males and females.

A large (19,185 patients) randomized blinded, international trial of clopido-grel vs. aspirin in patients at risk of ischemic events (CAPRIE) was conducted and reported in 1964.[41] CAPRIE was the largest clinical trial of a secondary pre-vention strategy to prevent various vascular end-points in a high-risk population. The trial was designed to assess the relative efficacy of clopidogrel 75 mg once daily and aspirin 325 mg daily in reducing the risk of a composite outcome clus-ter of ischemic stroke, myocardial infarction, or vascular death. Three groups of patients at significant risk of vascular events, those with recent ischemic stroke (6431), recent myocardial infarction (6302); or symptomatic peripheral arterial disease (6452), were followed for 1–3 years. The result of the outcome cluster showed a significant RRR of 8.7% in favor of clopidogrel (95% CI:0.3–16.5%; $p = 0.043$) and an absolute risk reduction of 0.51% (Fig. 10.2). There were no significant differences in adverse events between the two regimens: specifically, there was no increased risk of neutropenia in the clopidogrel group. In a post-hoc analysis, there were significant differences in the RRR for each of the three entry groups (stroke, myocardial infarction, and peripheral arterial disease), with the most striking effect appearing to be in patients with peripheral arterial disease (RRR 23.8%; CI 8.9–36.2). For stroke patients, there was nonsignificant benefit for clopidogrel over aspirin (RRR 7.3%; 95% CI 5.7–18.7). However, the trial was not powered to detect a realistic treatment effect in each of the three clinical subgroups. Moreover, an additional analysis of these patients in the ischemic stroke and peripheral arterial disease subgroups with a previous history of myocardial infarction demonstrated clear benefit for clopidogrel over aspirin. Hence, the conclusion of this study appears to strongly confirm and be consistent with the previous ticlopidine studies. When the absolute risk reduction of 0.5% is taken in consideration, it is calculated that 200 patients per year would need to be treated with clopidogrel rather than aspirin to save one end-point.

Thus, it seems probable that clopidogrel will replace ticlopidine but that it is less likely to replace aspirin as the first-line therapy for secondary stroke prevention, given its only modest superiority and presumed higher cost.

In 1994, the antiplatelet Trialists' Collaboration published the results of a meta-analysis[18] in which they analyzed 18 placebo-controlled clinical trials on 10,000

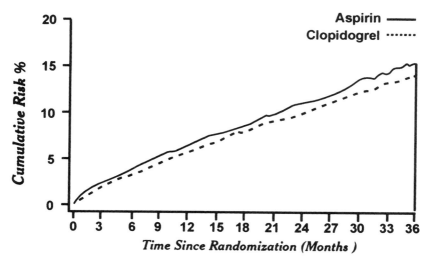

FIGURE 10.2. Cumulative risk of composite endpoint (ischemic stroke, myocardial infarction, and vascular death) in CAPRIE patients treated with aspirin or clopidogrel. Adapted from CAPRIE with permission.

patients with TIAs or minor stroke: allocation to a mean duration of 33 months of antiplatelet therapy produced a highly significant ($2p < 0.00001$) reduction of 37 per 1000 in risk of suffering another vascular events (i.e., myocardial infarction, stroke or vascular death) with a standard deviation (SD) of 8. The proportional reduction in important vascular events in these trial was 22% (SD 5%).

Algra and Van Gijn conducted a mini-meta analysis on data from 10 randomized trials of aspirin only vs. control treatment in 6171 patients after TIA or minor stroke.[42] They concluded that aspirin at any dose above 30 mg daily prevents 13% (95% CI; 4–12) of vascular event (i.e., vascular death, stroke, or myocardial infarction).

The data of meta-analyses are not free of criticism. If one wishes to compare the results of studies already published, one immediately is confronted with difficulties because of the strikingly different methodologies that were applied and diagnosis that was not always determined under the same conditions. One has to ask if the same therapy may be applied after TIA and after stroke. The criteria used to evaluate the efficiency of the therapy varied and very little information concerning the compliance of the patients to the criteria was given.

Comparisons can be direct or indirect, and the latter is not always acceptable. Dyken[43] warned that direct comparisons between clinical trials are difficult because of the types of patients entered, duration of treatment, quality of follow-ups, and because endpoint definitions often differ. He also warned that several variables other than the study drug could influence the sizes of risk reduction between trials. There are other problems with making comparisons between studies that test high doses of aspirin to those examining low doses. Many of the former studies were performed up to 15 years before the latter were carried out. The changes in medical treatment of hypertension of heart disease may have altered the impact of aspirin.

Adverse effects

Regular use of aspirin increases the risk of gastrointestinal (GI) side effects, such as epigastric pain, peptic ulcer, gastritis, and GI bleeding. Administration of enteric-coated aspirin, but not the buffered type, may lessen the damage to the gastric mucosa.[44–46] It is difficult to compare the incidence of these side effects among studies because the criteria and the definitions are not the same, nor are the auditing procedures. Therefore, comparison of bleeding complications between different groups within one study gives more valuable information.

In both the U.K. TIA[33] and the Dutch TIA trials, the bleeding complications were more frequent in the higher aspirin dose group. In the U.K. TIA trial, GI bleeding occurred in 1.6% of patients on placebo, 2.6% on 300 mg aspirin and per day, 4.7% on 1200 mg per day, and approximately half of the patients in each group required hospitalization. It is a widely held view that all-site bleeding with aspirin is not dose-related.[47] In the Dutch TIA, although major bleeding occurred only slightly less in the 30 mg group, minor bleeds were significantly less in that group.

Aspirin and risk of hemorrhagic stroke was recently evaluated using a meta-analysis of the data from 16 randomized controlled trials[48] involving 55,462 participants and 108 hemorrhagic strokes. The mean dosage of aspirin was 273 mg per day, and the mean duration of treatment was 37 months. Aspirin treatment was associated with an absolute risk increase in hemorrhagic stroke of 12 events per 10,000 persons (95% CI, 5–20, $p < 0.001$). However, the overall benefit of aspirin on myocardial infarction and ischemic stroke may outweigh its slight increase in the risk of hemorrhagic stroke.

Dose of Aspirin

The inhibition of platelet thromboxane (TxA_2) synthesis is presumed the major mediator of the clinical antithrombotic effect of aspirin. Therefore, an optimal aspirin dosage regimen must maximally suppress (TxA_2) production. It should be taken in consideration that the synthesis of the beneficial prostacyclin is also suppressed by aspirin. These opposite actions of aspirin were termed the "aspirin dilemma".[13]

Experimental Data

It was initially suggested that the higher doses of aspirin have a greater chance of platelet inhibition.[49] Weksler et al.[8] suggested that relatively large doses of aspirin (1000 mg–3000 per day) were necessary to inhibit the cyclooxygenase enzyme in both platelets and endothelial cells. The dose-dependent effect of aspirin on reduction of the stable metabolite TxA_2, thromboxane B_2 (TxB_2), was demonstrated by Thogi et al.[50] The serum (TxB_2)-generated ex-vivo incubation was reduced after 40 mg per day of aspirin (by 85%) and decreased further with increasing aspirin doses to 320 mg per day (by 96%) and 1280 mg per day (by 99%) aspirin doses. In another study,[51] serum TxB_2 synthesis was inhibited by more than 99% with 300 mg and 500 mg of aspirin 2 hours after the first administration.

Helgason et al.[52] had demonstrated that partial inhibition of platelet aggregation, named "aspirin resistance," occurred in the patients with or without acute stroke even when increasing doses of aspirin (325, 650, 975, and 1300 mg per day) were administered. Ackerman and Newman[53] noted that there was a progressive increase in the number of nonresponders as the dose of aspirin decreased below 975 mg per day. About 16% of those who received less than 65 per day were nonresponders, but all who were taking over 975 mg per day experienced a full effect.

Hormes et al.[54] reported that aspirin doses of 325 mg and 650 mg per day clearly more effectively altered aggregation of platelets than did 41 mg per day. A daily dose of oral aspirin improved aggregation more than a dose every other day or every 3 days. The antiaggregation response occurred with greater doses of aspirin in the patients who were hyperaggregable at baseline. Advances in the development of analytical tools to quantitate the dose dependence and time dependence of the effect of aspirin on platelet biochemistry and function led to progressive reduction in the dose in clinical trials. A level of aspirin dose exists in which no effect is seen. It was reported that 10 mg of aspirin does not alter platelet function.[55] However, a single administration of a small dose, from 12 mg of aspirin, causes an incomplete inhibition of platelets.[56] The cumulative effects of doses as low as 20 mg per day are sufficient for attaining complete inhibition of TxT_2 in all platelets, and it takes between 3 and 12 days to reach a steady state of complete TxT_2 suppression by use of doses between 20 and 40 mg.[56–58] In other words, 20 mg of aspirin is the minimum daily dose (in terms of TxA_2 suppression) needed to acetylate the fraction of new platelets formed each day (10%–15%).[56]

The studies that have demonstrated complete suppression of TxA_2 by daily doses of aspirin between 20 mg and 50 mg have included not only volunteers[55,59–62] but also patients with TIA[56] or myocardial ischemia.[62,63] It was shown[64] that aspirin at doses of 25–75 mg per day during long-term treatment is sufficient to inhibit platelet aggregation in patients with cerebrovascular disease. Aggregation of platelet-rich plasma induced by a stroke was significantly reduced after 40 mg per day of aspirin ($p < 0.005$).[50] This dose did not decrease the urinary concentration of prostaglandin-containing products, in contrast to higher aspirin doses. In another study,[51] it was shown that a loading dose of 40 mg of aspirin in combination with 40 mg as a maintenance dose was less effective in the inhibition of platelet aggregation and of thromboxane synthesis than a loading dose of 300 mg combined with 40 mg of aspirin. Also, a low loading dose of aspirin (40 mg) in combination with 40 mg of aspirin as a maintenance dose reached its maximal effect very late—at day 7 of the observation period—compared with other combinations.

In healthy persons, in vivo and ex vivo studies showed that a single dose of at least 160 mg had a profound antiplatelet effect within 1 hour of administration.[59,65] A loading dose of at least 100 mg of aspirin may have a complete antiplatelet effect that can be reached within 1 hour.[62,65] This degree of inhibition can then be sustained by daily administration of doses between 20 mg and 40 mg. If enteric-coated aspirin is used instead of the regular form, the required minimum dosage for complete inhibition of TxA_2 may increase because prolonged contact with the intestinal juice enhances hydrrolysis of the drug. For a slow release preparation, the necessary dose was 50 mg[66] and 80 mg for a granular form.[67]

Clinical Experience

Although the experimental data concerning the antithrombotic effect of low-dose aspirin on platelet activity may be convincing, the correlation between platelet aggregation with in vivo efficacy for patients with cerebrovascular disease is unclear. In reviewing the randomized clinical trials that were conducted since the late 1970s, it becomes clear that several issues were critical elements in the aspirin-dose controversy: (1) The "aspirin-dilemma," which led to the hypothesis that arterial thrombosis might occur more frequently with the higher dose of aspirin, and (2) the link between higher dose and absolute rate of serious side-effects (i.e., major hemorrhage). The main problem with a meta-analysis conducted in order to evaluate the usefulness of aspirin in stroke prevention[18,42] is the lack of direct comparison between a low (100 mg) and a high (1000 mg) dose of aspirin in a large randomized controlled trial. It is likely that the relative efficacy of aspirin for stroke prevention varies between patient populations with different spectra of stoke mechanisms regardless of aspirin dose, thereby confounding indirect comparisons.

Nevertheless, the relative risk reduction for stroke and death was 25% to 42% in the higher dose trials compared to only 7% to 18% for the lower dose trial.[68] There are also several clinical observations suggesting that higher doses of aspirin may confer a greater benefit in patients with high risk for stroke.[22,32] On the other hand, an assessment of benefits and risks should be taken in consideration as well. A direct comparison of GI bleeding was conduction in the U.K. TIA study[33]: it occurred in 1.6% of the patients on placebo, 2.6% on 300 mg of aspirin, and 4.7% on 1200 mg of aspirin. Minor side effects were reported by 24% of the placebo patients, 29% of those on 300 mg of aspirin, and 39% of those on 1200 mg of aspirin. In the Dutch TIA Trial Study,[34] a dose of 30 mg/day was compared to 283 mg/day. There were small absolute increases in major hemorrhage (0.3% per year) and fatal bleeding (0.15% per year) that were not statistically significant. In absolute terms, the incremental increase in major hemorrhage with higher doses of aspirin is small, although minor side effects are more common in higher doses of aspirin. Therefore, if a 30% in risk reduction exists with higher doses of aspirin vs. approximately 20% by lower doses[69] in a high risk group (10% risk of stroke or death in 1 year), 100 patients would need to be treated per year with higher doses to prevent one additional event effect by about one additional hemorrhage. One issue in the "aspirin dilemma" was recently solved (i.e., the optimal dose of aspirin to reduce the risk of stroke, myocardial infarction and death after carotid endarterectomy).[70] In a randomized double-blind, controlled trial, 2849 patients scheduled for carotid endarterectomy were randomly assigned to received 81 mg, 325 mg, 650 mg, or 1300 mg of aspirin prior to and for 3 months after this procedure. The risk of stroke, myocardial infarction, and death was lower in patients taking 81mg or 325 mg of aspirin, therefore, the recommended dose of aspirin after carotid endarterectomy is 325 mg for the prevention of a perisurgical complication.

CONCLUSION

In conclusion, assuming that our clinical practice should be conducted on the basis of evidence, no scientific data are available to recommend with confidence either high or low dose aspirin for the prevention of stroke. The definitive way of solving this problem is to have a head-to-head comparison of the two doses in a randomized clinical trial. In practical terms, surveys around the world and among experts show that 300 to 325 mg is the most widely used dose of aspirin.[71,72] According to interviews, 45% of participants at the European Stroke Conference recommended 100 mg, 45% favored 300 mg, but only 5% favored > 1000 mg of aspirin.[73] The Ad Hoc Committee on Guidelines for Management of Transient Ischemic Attacks of the Stroke Council of the American Heart Association[74] favors the dosage of 325 mg per day since this "promotes compliance and minimized gastrointestinal side effects," although they accept a dose range as wide as 30 mg to 1300 mg per day as recommendable treatment.

Acknowledgments

The author thanks Madeleine Bianco and Esther Eshkol for secretarial and editorial assistance.

REFERENCES

1. Flower RJ, Moncada S, Vane JR. Analgetic-antipyretics and anti-inflammatory agents: Drugs employed in the treatment of gout. In: Gilman AG, Goodman IS, Rall TW, Murad F, eds. *Goodman and Gilman's The Pharmacological Basis of Therapeutics*, 7th ed. New York: Macmillan, 1985, 674–675.
2. Craven LL. Experience with aspirin (acetylsalicylic acid) in the non-specific prophylaxis of coronary thrombosis. *Mississippi Valley Med J* 1953;75:38–44.
3. Craven LL. Prevention of coronary and cerebral thrombosis. *Mississippi Valley Med J* 1956;78:213.
4. Blatrix C. Allongement du temps de saignement sous l'influence de certains medicaments. *Nouv Rev F Hematol* 1963;3:346.
5. Weiss HJ, Aledort LM. Impaired platelet-connective-tissue reaction in man after aspirin ingestion. *Lancet* 1967;2:495–497.
6. O'Brien JR. Effects of salicylates on human platelets. *Lancet* 1968;1:779–783.
7. Majerus PW. Arachidonate metabolism in vascular disorders. *J Clin Invest* 1983;72: 1521–1525.
8. Weksler BB, Pett SB, Alonso D, et al. Differential inhibition by aspirin of vascular and platelet prostaglandin synthesis in atherosclerotic patients. *N Engl J Med* 1983; 308:800–805.
9. Jaffe E, Weksler B. Recovery of endothelial cell prostacyclin production after inhibition by low doses of aspirin. *J Clin Invest* 1979;63:532–535.

10. Patrono C. Aspirin as an antiplatelet drug: Review article. *N Engl J Med* 1994;330: 1287–1294.

11. Bjornsson TD, Scheider DE, Berger H. Aspirin acetylates fibrinogen and enhances fibrinolysis. *J Pharmacol Exp Ther* 1989;250:154–161.

12. Lekstram JA, Bell WR. Aspirin in the prevention of thrombosis. *Medicine* 1991;70: 161–178.

13. van Gijn J. Aspirin: Dose and indications in modern stroke prevention. In: Barnett HJM, Hachinski VC, eds. *Cerebral Ischemia: Treatment and Prevention.* Philadelphia: W.B. Saunders, 1992;10:1:193–207.

14. The Steering Committee of the Physicians' Health Study Research Group: Final report on the aspirin component of the ongoing Physicians' Health Study. *N Engl J Med* 1989;321:129–135.

15. Peto R, Gray R, Collins R, et al. Randomised trial of prophylactic daily aspirin in British male doctors. *BMJ (Clin Res Ed)* 1988;296:313–316.

16. Hennekens CH, Buring JE, Sandercock P, et al. Aspirin and other antiplatelet agents in the secondary and primary prevention of cardiovascular disease. *Circulation* 1989; 80:749–756.

17. Barnett HJM. 35 years of stroke prevention: challenges, disappointments and successes. *Cerebrovasc Dis* 1991;1:61–70.

18. The Aspirin Papers. Aspirin benefits patients with vascular disease and those undergoing revascularisation. Collaborative overview of randomised trials of antiplatelet therapy. I: Prevention of death, myocardial infarction, and stroke by prolonged antiplatelet therapy in various categories of patients. Antiplatelet Trialists' Collaboration. *BMJ* 1994;308:71–106.

19. Herbert P, Fuster V, Hennekens CH. Antiplatelet and anticoagulant therapy in evolving myocardial infarction and primary prevention. In: Fuster V, Verstraete M eds. *Thrombosis in Cardiovascular Disorders.* Philadelphia: W.B. Saunders, 1992:261–273.

20. Manson JE, Stampfer MJ, Colditz GA, et al. A prospective study of aspirin use and primary prevention of cardiovascular disease in women. *JAMA* 1991;266:521–527.

21. Kronmal RA, Hart RG, Manolio TA, et al. Aspirin use and incident stroke in the cardiovascular health study. *Stroke* 1998;29:887–894.

22. Hansson L, Zanchetti A, George S. Effects of intensive blood-pressure lowering and low-dose aspirin in patients with hypertension: Principal results of the Hypertension. Optimal Treatment (HOT) randomised trial. *Lancet* 1998;351:1755–1762.

23. Hart RG, Halperin JL, McBride R, et al. Aspirin for the primary prevention of stroke and other major vascular events. Meta-analysis and Hypotheses. *Arch Neurol* 2000; 57:326–332.

24. Cote R, Battista RN, Abrahamowicz M, et al: Lack of effect of aspirin in asymptomatic patients with carotid bruits and substantial carotid narrowing. *Ann Intern Med* 1995;123:649–655.

25. Ezekowitz MD, Cohen IS, Gornick CC, et al. Atrial fibrillation. In: Daniel WG, Kronson I, Mugge A, eds. *Cardiogenic Embolism.* Baltimore: Williams & Wilkins, 1996: 27–44.

26. Petersen P, Boysen G, Godtfredsen J, et al. Placebo-controlled, randomized trial of warfarin and aspirin for prevention of thromboembolic complications in chronic atrial fibrillation: The Copenhagen AFaspirinK Study. *Lancet* 1989;1:175–179.

27. Stroke Prevention in Atrial Fibrillation Investigators. Stroke Prevention in Atrial Fibrillation Study: Final results. *Circulation* 1991;84:527–539.

28. Boston Area Anticoagulation Trial for Atrial Fibrillation Investigators. The effect of

low-dose warfarin on the risk of stroke in nonrheumatic atrial fibrillation. *N Engl J Med* 1990;323:1505–1511.

29. Miller VT, Rothrock JF, Pearce LA, et al., on behalf of the Stroke Prevention in Atrial Fibrillation investigators. Ischemic stroke in patients with atrial fibrillation: effect of aspirin according to stroke mechanism. *Neurology* 1993;43:32–36.

30. Chesebro JH, Fuster V, Halperin JL: Atrial fibrillation—risk marker for stroke. *N Engl J Med* 1990;323:392–394.

31. Canadian Cooperative Study Group. A randomized trial of aspirin and sulfinpyrazone in threatened stroke. *N Engl J Med* 1978;299:53–59.

32. Bousser MG, Eschwege E, Haguemau M, et al. "AICLA" Controlled trial of aspirin and dipyridamole in the secondary prevention of atherothrombotic cerebral ischemia. *Stroke* 1983;15:5–14.

33. The United Kingdom Transient Ischemic Attack (UK-TIA) Aspirin Trial: Final results, UK-TIA study group. *J Neurol Neurosurg Psychiatry* 1991;54:1044–1054.

34. The Dutch TIA Study Group. A comparison of two doses of aspirin (30 mg vs. 283 mg a day) in patients after a transient ischemic attack of minor ischemic stroke. *N Engl J Med* 1991;325:1261–1266.

35. Swedish Aspirin Low-Dose Trial (SALT) of 75 mg aspirin as secondary prophylaxis after cerebrovascular ischemic events. The SALT Collaborative Group. *Lancet* 1991; 338:1345–1349.

36. Diener H, Cunha L, Forbes C, et al. European Stroke Prevention Study: Dipyridamole and acetylsalicylic acid in the secondary prevention of stroke. *J Neurol Sci* 1996;43: 1–13.

37. Van Gijn J, Algra A. Secondary stroke prevention with antithrombotic drugs: What to do next? *Cerebrovasc Dis* 1997; 7(suppl 6):30–32.

38. Hankey GJ. One year after CAPRIE, IST and ESPS 2. Any changes in concepts? *Cerebrovasc Dis* 1998; 8(suppl 5):1–7.

39. Wilterding JL, Easton JD. Dipyridamole plus aspirin in cerebrovascular disease. *Arch Neurol* 1999;56:1087–1092.

40. Hass WK, Easton JD, Adams HP, et al. A randomized trial comparing ticlopidine hydrochloride with aspirin for the prevention of stroke in high-risk patients. *N Engl J Med* 1989;321:501–507.

41. CAPRIE Steering Committee. A randomised, blinded trial of clopidogrel versus aspirin in patients at risk of ischemic events (CAPRIE). *Lancet* 1996;348:1329–1339.

42. Algra A, Van Gijn J. Aspirin at any dose above 30 mg offers only modest protection after cerebral ischaemia. *J Neurol Neurosurg Psychiatry* 1996;60:197–199.

43. Dyken ML. Meta-analysis in the assessment of therapy for stroke prevention. *Cerebrovasc Dis* 1992;2(suppl):35–40.

44. Robbins DC, Schwartz RS, Kutny K, et al. Comparative effects of aspirin and enteric-coated aspirin on loss of chromium. *Clin Ther* 1984;6:461–466.

45. Lanza FL, Rover GL, Nelson RS. Endoscopic evaluation of the effects of aspirin, buffered aspirin, and enteric-coated aspirin on gastric and duodenal mucosa. *N Engl J Med* 1990;303:136–138.

46. Kelly JP, Kaufman DW, Jurgelson JM, et al. Risk of aspirin-associated major upper-gastrointestinal bleeding with enteric-coated or buffered product. *Lancet* 1996;348: 1413–1416.

47. Adams HP, Bendixen BH. Low- versus high-dose aspirin in prevention of ischemic stroke. *Clin Neuropharmacol* 1993;16:485–500.

48. Jian H, Whelton PK, Ba BV, et al. Aspirin and risk of hemorrhagic stroke. A meta-analysis of randomized controlled trials. *JAMA* 1998;280:1930–1935.

49. O'Brien JR, Etherington MD. How much aspirin? (letter). *Thromb Haemost* 1990; 64:486.

50. Tohgi H, Konno S, Tamura K, Kimura B, Kawano K. Effects of low-to-high doses of aspirin on platelet aggregability and metabolites of thromboxane A2 and prostacyclin. *Stroke* 1992;23:1400–1403.

51. Buerke M, Pittroff W, Meyer J, et al. Aspirin therapy: Optimized platelet inhibition with different loading and maintenance doses. *Am Heart J* 1995;130:465–472.

52. Helgason CM, Tortorice KL, Winkler SR, et al. Aspirin response and failure in cerebral infarction. *Stroke* 1993;24:345–350.

53. Ackerman RH, Newman KL: Incomplete antiplatelet effects in patients on aspirin compounds (abstract). *Ann Neurol* 1990;28:224.

54. Hormes JT, Austin JH, James G, et al. Toward an optimal antiplatelet" dose of aspirin: Preliminary observations. *J Stroke Cerebrovasc Dis* 991;1:27–35.

55. Kallmann R, Nieuwenhuis HK, deGroot PG, et al. Effects of low doses of aspirin, 10mg and 30mg daily, on bleeding time, thromboxane reduction, and 6-keto-PG1 alpha excretion in healthy subjects. *Thromb Res* 1989;45:355–361.

56. Patrono C, Ciabattoni G, Patrignani P, et al. Clinical pharmacology of platelet cyclooxygenase inhibition. *Circulation* 1985;72:1177–1184.

57. Weksler BB, Kent JL, Rudolph D, et al. Effect of low dose aspirin on platelet function in patients with recent cerebral ischemia. *Stroke* 1985;16:5–9.

58. Toghi H, Tamura K, Kimura A, Kimura M, Suzuki H. Individual variation of platelet aggregability and serum thromboxane B2 concentrations after low-dose aspirin. *Stroke* 988;19:700–703.

59. Patrignani P, Filabozzi P, Patrono C. Selective cumulative inhibition of platelet thromboxane production by low-dose aspirin in healthy subjects. *J Clin Invest* 1982;69: 1366–1372.

60. FitzGerald GA, Oates JA, Hawiger J, et al. Endogenous biosynthesis of prostacyclin and thromboxane and platelet function during chronic administration of aspirin in man. *J Clin Invest* 1983;71:678–688.

61. Preston FE, Greaves M, Jackson CA, et al. Low-dose aspirin inhibits platelet and venous cyclo-oxygenase in man. *Thromb Res* 1982;27:447–456.

62. de Caterina R, Giannessi D, Bernini W, et al. Selective inhibition of thromboxane-related platelet function by low-dose aspirin in patients after myocardial infarction. *Am J Cardiol* 1985;55:589–590.

63. de Caterina R, Giannessi D, Boem A, et al. Equal antiplatelet effects of aspirin 50 or 324 mg/day in patients after acute myocardial infarction. *Thromb Haemost* 1985;54: 528–532.

64. Boysen G, Bottcher J, Olsen JS. Platelet cyclo-oxygenase inhibition by minimal doses of acetylsalicylic acid in patients with cerebrovascular disease. *Acta Neurol Scand* 1982;65(suppl. 90):178–179.

65. Patrono C, Ciabattoni G, Pinca E, et al. Low dose aspirin and inhibition of thromboxane B2 production in healthy subjects. *Thromb Res* 1980;17:317–327.

66. Roberts MS, Joyce RM, McLeod LJ, et al. Slow-release aspirin and prostaglandin inhibition. *Lancet* 1986;1:1153–1158.

67. Jakubowski JA, Stampfer MJ, Vaillancourt R, et al. Cumulative antiplatelet effect of ow-dose enteric coated aspirin. *Br J Haematol* 1985;60:635–642.

68. Barnett HJM, Meldrum EM. Drugs and surgery in the prevention of ischemic stroke. *N Engl J Med* 1995;332:238–248.

69. Matchar DB, McCrory DC, Barnett HJM, et al. Treatment for stroke prevention. *Ann Intern Med* 1994;121:41–53.

70. Taylor DW, Barnett HJM, Haynes RB, et al. Low-dose and high-dose acetylsalicylic acid for patients undergoing carotid endarterectomy: randomised controlled trial. *Lancet* 1999;353:2179–2184.
71. Dyken ML, Barnet HJM, Easton DJ, et al. Low-dose aspirin and stroke "It Ain't Necessarily So." *Stroke* 1992;23:1395–1399.
72. Hart RG, Harrison MJG. Aspirin Wars. The optimal dose of aspirin to prevent stroke. *Stroke* 1996;27:585–587.
73. Bogousslavsky J, Easton JD. Round table discussion: Assessment of benefit/risk of therapy in stroke prevention. *Cerebrovasc Dis* 1992;2(suppl 1):41–47.
74. Ad Hoc Committee on Guidelines for management of transient ischemic attacks of the stroke council of the American Heart Association. Guidelines for management of transient ischemic attack. *Stroke* 1994;25:1320–1335.

11

ANTIPLATELET THERAPY

J. Donald Easton

Platelet antiaggregation drugs help prevent atherothrombotic events, including transient ischemic attacks (TIA) and strokes. They inhibit the formation of intra-arterial platelet aggregates that can form on diseased arteries and induce thrombus formation, occlude the artery, or embolize into the distal circulation. Aspirin is the most widely prescribed drug for this purpose. Ticlopidine, clopidogrel, and dipyridamole also are used, though the implications of their efficacy, safety, and cost compared to aspirin are debated.

Because cost is a major factor in prescribing antiplatelet medication, it is important to assess the cost of treatments compared to the risk of stroke, myocardial infarction (MI), and vascular death. In general, individuals at relatively low risk for these events may be treated with relatively inexpensive medications that may be less beneficial than more expensive ones. High-risk patients may warrant high-risk and expensive procedures and medications.

The results of various trials of antiplatelet drugs for the prevention of stroke and other important vascular outcomes are sometimes confusing and difficult to apply to individual patients at risk. Some studies include all kinds of patients with various atherosclerotic diseases, while others include only patients with a recent stroke or TIA. Common terms used to describe trial results include hazard ratios, odds reductions, absolute and relative risk reductions, and numbers needed-to-treat to prevent one or more outcomes in one, two, three, or more years.

The primary outcomes, or endpoints, of studies vary enormously, and there may be more than one. The outcomes often include all strokes (including hemorrhagic), ischemic strokes only, major or disabling strokes, all deaths, vascular deaths, MI, and various combinations, or clusters, of these outcomes. The primary analyses of trials may be on an intention-to-treat or an efficacy basis, and the latter excludes various patients and outcomes for various reasons. This chapter reviews, assesses, and discusses the results of the important trials of antiplatelet drugs for the prevention of stroke and other important vascular outcomes in patients primarily with prior stroke or TIA and interprets them in a uniform context.

OVERVIEW OF ANTIPLATELET DRUGS

Aspirin for Secondary Prevention of Vascular Events

Aspirin is the most widely studied antiplatelet agent. Its antiplatelet effect is accomplished by acetylating the cyclooxygenase enzyme in platelets. This irreversibly inhibits the formation thromboxane A_2, a platelet aggregating and vasoconstricting prostaglandin. This effect is permanent and lasts for the 7- 10-day life of the platelet. Paradoxically, aspirin also inhibits the formation in endothelial cells of prostacyclin, an antiaggregating and vasodilating prostaglandin. This effect is transient. As soon as the aspirin is cleared from the cells, the nucleated endothelial cells again produce prostacyclin. Aspirin in low doses given once daily inhibits the production of thromboxane A_2 in platelets without substantially inhibiting prostacyclin formation. Most physicians recommend aspirin in doses of 325 mg or less daily for the prevention of atherothrombosis.

The Antiplatelet Trialists[1] conducted a major meta-analysis that assessed the effect of antiplatelet drugs in patients with various manifestations of atherosclerosis, such as unstable angina, MI, TIA and stroke, and other patients at risk for atherothrombotic events. They aggregated the 73,247 high-risk patients who had been in trials lasting longer than 30 days, that is, on long-term antiplatelet therapy. The Antiplatelet Trialists emphasized the composite outcome of stroke, MI, or vascular death. This outcome cluster included hemorrhagic stroke and death due to any hemorrhage. They also analyzed nonfatal stroke, nonfatal MI, vascular death, and death from any cause independently. They expressed the treatment effects for the various vascular outcomes as odds reductions. An ideal outcome cluster to analyze was stroke, MI, or vascular death (along with the individual outcomes of nonfatal stroke, nonfatal MI, vascular death, and death from all causes) because it included the important outcomes for all patients with atherosclerosis that can be prevented or caused by antiplatelet drugs.

Nevertheless, the final mechanism for stroke may differ from that for MI, and stroke patients may differ from MI patients in the pathophysiology of their strokes and MIs, although no evidence exists for the latter. Regulatory agencies require that specific outcomes be assessed in specific groups of patients. Thus, the focus will be on stroke alone, and the cluster of stroke, MI, or vascular death. These vascular outcomes will be considered in all kinds of patients with atherosclerosis, but will focus on patients with prior stroke or TIA.

The Antiplatelet Trialists found that overall (i.e., in all kinds of patients at high risk for vascular outcomes), antiplatelet drugs reduced the odds of the composite outcome of stroke, MI, or vascular death in secondary prevention by about 27% (Table 11.1). The odds reduction attributable to aspirin alone was 25%. They found that antiplatelet drugs reduce the odds of a nonfatal stroke by 31%, nonfatal MI by about 35%, and vascular mortality by 18%.

Whatever patients are analyzed across the spectrum of high risk (e.g., those with recent MI, prior MI, or prior stroke or TIA), they found a similar risk reduction in stroke, MI or vascular death of about 1/4. That is, no matter what vascular disorder brought these various patients to enter the various clinical trials that were analyzed, the relative effect of antiplatelet drugs on the prevention of stroke, MI, or vascular death was similar for all of them.

The Antiplatelet Trialists also analyzed the differences in patients over and under the age of 65 years, and also by gender. While some variation was seen, all patients benefited to a similar degree from antiplatelet therapy. The same was true for patients with and without hypertension and with and without diabetes.

The Antiplatelet Trialists Collaboration meta-analysis concluded that antiplatelet therapy typically prevents about 40 vascular events per 1000 patients with a past history of MI, stroke, or TIA when treated for 2 years. This presentation of the data emphasizes the absolute gain for these patients with various disorders, not just the odds reductions.

TABLE 11.1. The Odds Reductions in Risk of Vascular Outcomes Caused by Antiplatelet Therapy

VASCULAR OUTCOME	ODDS REDUCTION
142 randomized trials; 73,247 patients; all antiplatelet drugs in various patients at high risk of vascular events.	
Nonfatal stroke	31%
Nonfatal myocardial infarction	35%
Vascular mortality	18%
Overall vascular events	27%
46 randomized trials; 45,019 patients; aspirin only in various patients at risk of vascular events.	
Overall vascular events	25%

An important issue arising from the Antiplatelet Trialists' meta-analyses is whether the effect of various antiplatelet drugs on prevention of strokes, MIs and vascular deaths is the same in patients entering studies because of prior stroke or TIA as it is for patients entering because of prior MI or other vascular disorders. The Antiplatelet Trialists found that whereas "all antiplatelet agents" reduced the odds of stroke, MI, or vascular death in "all high-risk patients" by 27%, the odds reduction in patients with prior stroke or TIA was only 22% (Table 11.2).

Additionally, Algra and van Gijn[2] performed their own mini-meta-analysis that showed that in the 10 trials evaluating the benefit of aspirin alone in only prior stroke or TIA patients, aspirin reduced the odds for stroke, MI, or vascular death by only 16%. When they converted this odds reduction to the more conventional relative risk reduction, the reduction over placebo was only 13% (Table 11.2).

These analyses emphasize that the important points one must assess carefully are whether one is (1) evaluating all patients at high risk for vascular events, or specific patients (e.g., prior stroke or TIA), (2) evaluating the benefit of all antiplatelet drugs, individual drugs, or combinations of drugs, and (3) expressing the result in odds reductions or relative risk reductions. The importance of noting which outcome events are being measured (e.g., stroke, MI, vascular death, various combinations) is addressed below.

The Swedish Aspirin Low-Dose Trial[3] compared aspirin at 75 mg daily versus placebo in 1360 patients with minor stroke or TIA. The mean follow-up was 2.7 years, and the primary outcome measure was stroke plus all death. The 18% relative risk reduction of aspirin was statistically significant ($p = 0.02$). The relative risk reduction of stroke, MI or vascular death was 17% and was statistically significant also. This compares to the 13% that Algre and van Gijn found for all doses of aspirin in similar patients.

The Dutch TIA Trial[4] compared aspirin at 30 mg per day vs. 283 mg per day in 3131 patients with minor stroke or TIA. The mean follow-up was 2.6 years, and the primary outcome measures were stroke, MI or vascular death. The investigators found that aspirin at 30 mg daily was no less effective than 273 mg, and there were fewer bleeds occurred on the lower dose.

TABLE 11.2. Effect of Antiplatelet Therapy on TIA, Myocardial Infarction, and Vascular Death in Various Atherosclerotic Populations

PATIENT POPULATION	NO. OF TRIALS/PATIENTS/EVENTS			ODDS REDUCTION (95% CI)	RELATIVE RISK REDUCTION (95% CI)
High-risk, all drugs	142	73,247	9583	27%	—
High-risk, aspirin	46	45,019	6097	25%	—
Stroke or TIA, all drugs	18	11,707	2377	22%	—
Stroke or TIA, aspirin	10	6171	1474	16%	13%

By the early 1990s, these latter two trials,[3,4] along with the earlier U.K.-TIA Trial,[5] provided most of the data that led many clinicians to believe no important differences exist between 30 mg and 1300 mg of aspirin daily for preventing stroke. Also, low-dose aspirin is less gastrotoxic. Then, in 1996, the European Stroke Prevention Study-2[6] reported that 50 mg daily of aspirin per day given to patients following stroke or TIA reduced the risk of stroke, and stroke or death, by 18% and 13%, respectively. In 1999 the Aspirin in Carotid Endarterectomy (ACE) trial,[7] involving 2849 patients, investigated appropriate doses of aspirin for prevention of perioperative atherothrombotic events in patients undergoing carotid endarterectomy. ACE found that the risk of stroke, MI, and death between 30 days and 3 months after endarterectomy was lower for patients taking 81 mg or 325 mg of aspirin daily than for those taking 650 mg or 1300 mg. Finally, in 1998, the United States Food and Drug Administration (FDA) published their new recommendation that 50 mg to 325 mg of aspirin per day be used for prevention of ischemic stroke.[8] Consequently, the majority of clinicians worldwide recommend 325 mg or less per day for prevention of stroke.

It would be valuable to conduct a very large clinical trial to resolve the question of the ideal dose of aspirin for prevention of ischemic stroke. While definitive resolution of this question is not an important issue to some, many millions of people worldwide ingest aspirin daily to avoid atherothrombotic events. Small differences in important vascular events and gastrotoxicity could have an important effect on the absolute number of people benefiting from aspirin prophylaxis.

Aspirin gastrotoxicity is dose related, and more indigestion, nausea, heartburn and vomiting occur with higher doses.[3,5,9–15] Hemorrhages of many types, especially gastrointestinal, are caused by aspirin,[3,16] but the relationship to dosage is uncertain. It has been estimated conservatively that 16,500 nonsteroidal anti-inflammatory drug (NSAID)–related deaths occur among patients with rheumatoid arthritis and osteoarthritis every year in the United States. This figure is similar to the number of deaths from acquired immunodeficiency syndrome.[17] If deaths from the gastrointestinal toxic effects of NSAIDs were tabulated separately in the National Vital Statistics reports, they would constitute the 15th most common cause of death in the United States.[17] Additionally, an increase in hemorrhagic stroke has been reported.[3,9,16] While the optimal dose of aspirin for prevention of stroke remains somewhat unsettled, 325 mg or less daily is effective.

These important data show that aspirin reduces the risk of stroke, MI, and vascular death in all kinds of patients at high risk for these atherothrombotic outcomes. A trend exists toward patients with stroke or TIA benefiting less than other high-risk patients. A trend also exists toward stroke or TIA patients experiencing less reduction in nonfatal stroke than other high-risk patients. More data are necessary to determine if these trends are real. Nevertheless, these possible differences are worth considering as the benefits of ticlopidine, clopidogrel, and dipyridamole are reviewed and analyzed.

Ticlopidine

Ticlopidine hydrochloride is a thienopyridine. It is an adenosine diphosphate (ADP) receptor antagonist that inhibits ADP-induced fibrinogen binding to platelets, a necessary step in the platelet aggregation process. Ticlopidine is not a cyclo-oxygenase inhibitor (like aspirin) and thus has no effect on prostacyclin production. Also, it is not a phosphodiesterase inhibitor (like dipyridamole) and does not alter cyclic adenosine monophosphate (AMP) in platelets.

Ticlopidine has been evaluated for the prevention of vascular outcomes in several randomized studies.[1,18–21] Two large trials assessed ticlopidine for the prevention of stroke and other vascular events in patients presenting with cerebrovascular symptoms.[19,20]

The Ticlopidine Aspirin Stroke Study (TASS)[20] involved 3069 patients presenting with minor stroke or TIA. Half were treated with 650 mg of aspirin twice daily and half with 250 mg of ticlopidine twice daily. In the three-year event rate, ticlopidine effected a 21% greater relative risk reduction compared to aspirin in the primary endpoint of stroke, and a 13% greater reduction in the endpoint of all nonfatal stroke or death. Two percent of patients on ticlopidine were unable to tolerate the medication because of diarrhea and another 2% because of skin rash. Serious gastrointestinal adverse effects (e.g., ulcers and bleeding) were 2.5 times more common in the aspirin group, even though patients who had any history of gastrointestinal hemorrhage or dyspeptic symptoms were excluded from the trial. Bleeding from other anatomical sites was infrequent and about equal in the two treatment groups. Severe neutropenias occurred in 0.9% of patients in the ticlopidine-treated group. They reversed with cessation of treatment. Most occurred within two months after treatment began. Hence, it is important to perform blood counts at two-week intervals for the first three months on medication, that is, six blood counts in three months.

The Canadian American Ticlopidine Study (CATS)[19] involved 1072 patients with major stroke, rather than a minor stroke or TIA. The patients were randomly allocated to 250 mg of ticlopidine twice daily or placebo. The patients in this study treated with placebo had an event rate for stroke, MI, or vascular death of 15.3% per year, demonstrating the seriousness of stroke as a predictor of subsequent vascular events. Ticlopidine reduced the relative risk of stroke, MI, or vascular death, using the efficacy approach, by 30% ($p = 0.006$), down to 10.8%. The same outcome cluster using the intent-to-treat approach was reduced by about 23% ($p = 0.020$) in the ticlopidine group. Adverse effects were similar to those in TASS. Ticlopidine reduced the relative risk of ischemic stroke by 33.5% ($p = 0.008$). Bennett et al.[22] recently reported that ticlopidine occasionally causes thrombotic thrombocytopenic purpura.

Taken together, these data show that ticlopidine substantially reduces the risk of stroke and other vascular outcomes in patients at risk, and TASS showed ticlopidine to be better than aspirin. Ticlopidine is likely to be about 20% better than aspirin in reducing stroke, and the Antiplatelet Trialists concluded from direct comparisons[19,20,23] that, overall, ticlopidine is likely to be about 10% better than aspirin in reducing the composite outcome of stroke, MI, or vascular death.

Clopidogrel

Clopidogrel is a new thienopyridine derivative of the same chemical family as ticlopidine. It is an inhibitor of platelet aggregation induced by ADP. Its antithrombotic effects were recently evaluated in the Clopidogrel versus Aspirine in Patients at Risks of Ischemic Events (CAPRIE) Study.[24] CAPRIE was a randomized, blinded, multicenter trial designed to assess the relative efficacy of clopidogrel (75 mg once daily) and aspirin (325 mg once daily) in reducing the risk of the composite outcome of ischemic stroke, MI, or vascular death and to determine their relative safety. The three patient groups studied were those with recent ischemic stroke, recent MI, and symptomatic peripheral arterial disease.

The study involved 19,185 patients, with more than 6000 in each of the three clinical subgroups. They were treated during a mean follow-up of 1.91 years. There were 1960 validated first events in the primary outcome cluster. The intention-to-treat analysis showed that patients treated with clopidogrel experienced an annual 5.32% risk of ischemic stroke, MI, or vascular death, compared to 5.83% with aspirin, for an absolute risk reduction of 0.5% and a relative risk reduction of 8.7% (95% CI; 0.3–16.5; $p = 0.043$). The corresponding "on treatment" analysis showed a relative risk reduction of 9.4%. When serious hemorrhages were considered along with the primary outcome cluster in an intent-to-treat analysis, which provides a true "net benefit" assessment, the relative risk reduction with clopidogrel was 9.5% (95% CI; 1.2–18.5). Finally, when the results in CAPRIE were analyzed using the Antiplatelet Trialists' technique (i.e., intent-to-treat, all stroke, MI, or vascular death [including hemorrhagic]) and by odds reduction, a reduction of 10%, rather than 8.7%, was found favoring clopidogrel. For the 6431 patients entered into CAPRIE with a stroke as the qualifying condition, the relative risk reduction was 7.3% (95% CI; −5.7–18.7), and the odds reduction was 8.5%. For the outcome of stroke only, across the three qualifying conditions (patients with stroke, MI, and peripheral artery disease) a 6.0% relative risk reduction was detected favoring clopidogrel over aspirin. For the outcome of stroke only, in just the patients qualifying with a stroke, an 8.0% relative risk reduction was found favoring clopidogrel over aspirin.

While there were no major differences between aspirin and clopidogrel in terms of safety, and adverse experiences were minimal, more serious hemorrhages occurred in those patients on aspirin. Ten patients (0.10%) in the clopidogrel group suffered significant reductions in neutrophils (to <1,200/mm^3) compared to 16 (0.17%) in the aspirin group. The numbers of severe neutropenia (<450/mm^3)

numbered 5 and 4, respectively. The overall safety profile of clopidogrel is at least as good as that of 325 mg aspirin per day. Bennett et al. recently reported that clopidogrel rarely is associated with thrombotic thrombocytopenic purpura.[24a]

The CAPRIE Study data indicated that clopidogrel was more effective than aspirin in reducing the combined risk of ischemic stroke, MI, or vascular death in patients with atherosclerotic vascular disease. Clopidogrel's beneficial effects seem to be comparable to ticlopidine's, without the negative adverse effects profile. Its effect on reducing stroke seemed less striking than for ticlopidine. This result may have been simply the play of chance, ticlopidine and clopidogrel could conceivably prevent strokes differently, or perhaps its benefit in TIA patients is greater than that in stroke patients.

Dipyridamole

The Antiplatelet Trialists[1] analyzed trials involving dipyridamole (DP) alone vs. placebo, DP combined with aspirin vs. placebo, and DP combined with aspirin vs. aspirin. Ten trials compared DP alone vs. placebo (200 events in 1474 patients) and showed a 23% odds reduction in stroke, MI, or vascular death favoring DP. Thirty-four trials (1741 events in 13,718 patients) compared DP combined with aspirin vs. placebo and showed a 28% odds reduction in stroke, MI, or vascular death favoring the combination. It seemed clear that DP was effective and that the combination of DP plus aspirin might be more effective than either alone. However, more patients were needed to enhance these comparisons in the Antiplatelet Trialists' view.

The Antiplatelet Trialists analyzed 14 trials that compared the combination of DP plus aspirin vs. aspirin alone (628 events in 5317 patients) for prevention of the composite outcome of stroke, MI, or vascular death (Fig. 11.1). One trial involved patients entered because of prior MI, 3 involved patients entered because of prior stroke or TIA, 4 because of post–coronary artery bypass grafting, 3 because of intermittent claudication, 2 because of noncoronary grafting, and 1 because of diabetes. The odds reduction for all vascular events was −3%, indicating a slight (statistically nonsignificant) benefit favoring aspirin alone. The only outcome that was reduced by DP combined with aspirin was non-fatal stroke. This odds reduction was 12% and not statistically significant. Nevertheless, the Antiplatelet Trialists concluded that a moderate difference between DP combined with aspirin and aspirin alone could not be ruled out. They stated,

> Any real differences between two antiplatelet regimens are likely to be smaller than the differences between antiplatelet and no antiplatelet treatment. Hence tens of thousands of patients may need to be randomised directly between different antiplatelet regimens to ensure (by large numbers) small enough random errors and to avoid (by direct randomisation) important biases. Unfortunately, the numbers so far randomised between one antiplatelet regimen and another have been much smaller than this."

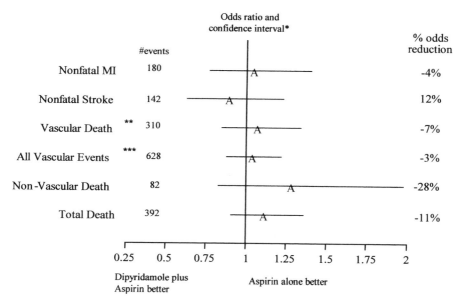

FIGURE 11.1. Direct comparisons of proportional effects on vascular events and nonvascular deaths of dipyridamole plus aspirin vs. aspirin.

In 1996, the results of the second European Stroke Prevention Study (ESPS-2) were published.[6] Patients who had experienced either an ischemic stroke or TIA were studied in a multicenter, randomized, blinded, factorial, placebo-controlled study with four treatment groups and a two-year follow-up for all patients. The four treatments were 25 mg aspirin, 200 mg DP, 25 mg aspirin plus 200 mg DP, and placebo, each given twice daily. DP was given as 200 mg of an extended-release formulation. A total of 6602 patients were included in the analysis, and the outcome event clusters were fatal or nonfatal stroke, stroke or death from any cause, and all-cause mortality. The investigators found that both extended-release DP at 200 mg twice daily and aspirin at 25 mg twice daily had an independent and significant effect in preventing the recurrence of stroke, and that the combination of DP plus aspirin was additive and produced highly significant benefits (Table 11.3). DP combined with aspirin vs. aspirin alone reduced the risk of stroke (nonfatal and fatal) by 23%. The absolute risk reduction was 3% at two years, or about 1.5% annually.

Are the results of ESPS-2 at odds with the results of earlier trials? When the results of ESPS-2 are added to the 14 previous trials of DP combined with aspirin vs. aspirin alone in various atherosclerosis patients, one finds a significant 23% reduction for DP plus aspirin in the odds of nonfatal stroke and a nearly significant 10% reduction in the odds of all vascular events, though all of the 10% is attributable to nonfatal strokes.[25]

TABLE 11.3. Number of Primary Outcome Events and Relative Risk Reductions after Two Years of Treatment in ESPS-2

	NUMBER OF EVENTS/RISK REDUCTION		
TREATMENT	STROKE[1]	DEATH	STROKE/DEATH
Dipyridamole + aspirin compared to placebo	157/37%	185/8%	286/24%
Dipyridamole compared to placebo	211/16%	188/7%	321/15%
Aspirin compared to placebo	206/18%	182/11%	330/13%
Placebo	250	202	378
Dipyridamole + aspirin compared to aspirin	157/23%	185/−3%	286/13%

[1]Nonfatal and fatal.

ESPS-2 was a cerebrovascular trial (i.e., it entered only patients with stroke or TIA). When the results of ESPS-2 are added to the three earlier cerebrovascular trials (Fig. 11.2 and 11.3),[26–29] one finds a significant 25% reduction in the odds of nonfatal stroke and a significant 18% reduction in the odds of all vascular events, though again all of the 18% is attributable to nonfatal stroke. These data provide evidence that DP combined with aspirin reduces the odds of nonfatal stroke by about 25% over aspirin alone ($p = 0.005$; CI 0.09–0.42). Also, the risk of stroke was reduced by 37% in ESPS-2 and 38% in ESPS-1.[30] This consistency

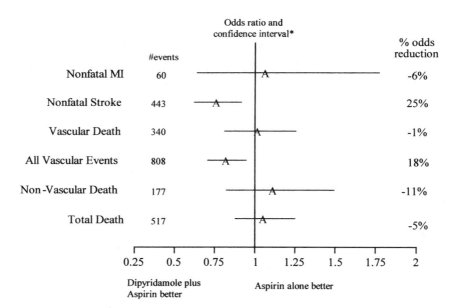

FIGURE 11.2. Direct comparisons of proportional effects on vascular events and nonvascular deaths of dipyridamole plus aspirin vs. aspirin.

is persuasive. It is odd that MI and vascular death were not reduced by DP combined with aspirin in ESPS-2, as they were by all antiplatelet drugs in the Antiplatelet Trialists' overview analysis.[1]

While the primary purpose of this overview is to focus on those antiplatelet trials involving patients with prior stroke or TIA, the totality of the evidence should be considered also. The two largest challenges to accepting combination DP and aspirin as more beneficial than aspirin alone in prevention of stroke (and MI and vascular death) lie in two facts: (1) some clinicians will view the combination's benefit as largely linked to a single trial, namely ESPS-2, and (2) the inconsistency in its effect on stroke, MI, and vascular death. The previous 14 trials were negative (i.e., there was no statistically significant benefit favoring combination DP and aspirin) for all important vascular outcomes, including stroke alone, though there was a trend favoring benefit for stroke alone. The same was true for the three cerebrovascular trials.

Nevertheless, these aggregate data provide strong evidence that the combination of DP and aspirin may be substantially better than aspirin alone in preventing strokes. Another trial of similar size to ESPS-2 (about 3,000 patients with stroke or TIA comparing DP plus aspirin at 325 mg to aspirin at 325 mg alone) may be required to confirm these findings and substantially alter clinical practice. The European and Australian Stroke Prevention in Reversible Ischemia Trial (ESPRIT)[31] may provide this confirmation. ESPRIT is a randomized clinical trial

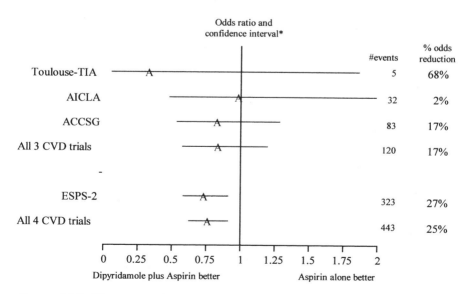

FIGURE 11.3. Direct comparisons of proportional effects on nonfatal strokes of dipyridamole plus aspirin vs. aspirin.

in which patients with cerebral ischemia of arterial origin will be randomized among oral anticoagulation (international normalized ratio [INR]: 2.0–3.0), a combination of aspirin (in any dose between 30 and 325 mg per day) plus DP (400 mg daily), and aspirin only (in any dose between 30 and 325 mg per day). The researchers plan to enroll 4500 patients, with a mean follow-up of three years. The primary outcome is the composite event of vascular death, stroke, myocardial infarction, or major bleeding complication.

DISCUSSION

Stroke is a major health problem, especially in terms of disability for patients and expense to patients and society. Ischemic strokes due to atherothrombosis and cardioembolism are the commonest causes of stroke. Additionally, patients at high risk for stroke are also at high risk for MI. Many of the atherothrombotic events resulting from these arterial and cardiac disorders are preventable.

Based on the clinical trial results available so far, the following statements seem reasonable:

1. Aspirin reduces the odds of the composite outcome of stroke, MI, or vascular death in patients with symptomatic atherosclerosis by about 25%, and it reduces the odds of stroke by about 30%.[1] In stroke or TIA patients, aspirin reduces the odds of the composite outcome of stroke, MI, or vascular death by about 16% (the relative risk reduction is about 13%).[2] Many patients have difficulty taking aspirin because of gastrointestinal discomfort, especially when high doses are taken, and aspirin sometimes causes serious bleeding.

2. Ticlopidine appears to reduce the same composite outcome by about a third in stroke or TIA patients, but there is a 5% incidence of bothersome adverse effects, a 0.9% incidence of severe neutropenia, and occasional thrombotic thrombocytopenic purpura.

3. Clopidogrel produces a benefit similar to ticlopidine but virtually without serious adverse effects. Clopidogrel is at least as safe as aspirin.

4. DP in combination with aspirin vs. placebo appears to reduce the risk of the composite outcome of stroke, MI, or vascular death in patients with symptomatic atherosclerosis by about 28%.[1] DP in combination with aspirin vs. placebo reduced the risk of stroke alone in patients with symptomatic atherosclerosis by 38% and 37% in ESPS-1 and -2, respectively. Finally, DP in combination with aspirin versus aspirin alone reduces the risk of the composite outcome of stroke, MI, or vascular death in patients with symptomatic atherosclerosis by about 10%;[25] it reduces the risk of (ischemic) stroke by about 23% over aspirin alone.[6,25]

CONCLUSION

Aspirin is inexpensive, can be given in low doses as infrequently as every other day, and could be recommended for all adults to prevent both stroke and MI. However, it causes adverse effects, including epigastric discomfort, gastric ulceration, and gastrointestinal hemorrhage. The gastric bleeding may be asymptomatic and detectable only by regular stool examinations. A life-threatening hemorrhage may occur without warning. Consequently, not every 40- or 50-year-old should be advised to take aspirin regularly because the risk of atherothrombotic stroke (and MI) is low and may be outweighed by the risk of adverse side effects. Conversely, every patient who has experienced an atherothrombotic stroke and has no contraindication should be taking an antiplatelet agent regularly because the average annual risk of another stroke is 5% to 15%, and the risk is another few percent higher for MI and vascular death. In this setting, the likelihood of benefit far outweighs the risks of treatment. The choice of antiplatelet agent and dose similarly must balance the risk of stroke against the benefit, risk, and cost of the treatments. These data are less definitive, and opinions therefore vary.

Aspirin reduces the odds of stroke, MI, or vascular death by about 25% in an aggregate group of high-risk patients. In patients with prior stroke or TIA, aspirin may reduce the relative risk of the same outcome cluster by only about 13%. Low-dose (30–75 mg daily) and high-dose (650–1300 mg daily) aspirin appear to be comparably effective, and low-dose is less gastrotoxic.

Ticlopidine is more effective than aspirin by about 10% for preventing stroke, MI, or vascular death and about 20% more effective for reducing stroke. The cost and risk of adverse effects of ticlopidine are higher, and it is given twice daily. Clopidogrel's benefit appears to be similar to ticlopidine's, but it has an excellent adverse-effect profile and is given once daily. Clopidogrel at 75 mg daily may be less effective for preventing stroke than ticlopidine at 250 mg twice daily.

The combination of DP and aspirin also is more effective than aspirin alone. Most of the benefit shown for this combination has been limited to stroke prevention in patients with prior stroke or TIA. It is given twice daily and the adverse-effect profile is good. In order to compare the relative benefits (efficacy and safety) of aspirin, ticlopidine, clopidogrel, and DP, it will be necessary to obtain more data from randomized clinical trials.

REFERENCES

1. Antiplatelet Trialists' Collaboration. Collaborative overview of randomised trials of antiplatelet therapy—I: Prevention of death, myocardial infarction, and stroke by prolonged antiplatelet therapy in various categories of patients. *BMJ* 1994;308:81–106.
2. Algra A, van Gijn J. Aspirin at any dose above 30 mg offers only modest protection after cerebral ischaemia. *J Neurol Neurosurg Psychiatry* 1996;60:197–199.

3. The SALT Collaborators Group. Swedish Aspirin Low-dose Trial (SALT) of 75 mg aspirin as secondary prophylaxis after cerebrovascular ischaemic events. *Lancet* 1991; 338:1345–1349.
4. The Dutch TIA Trial Study Group. A comparison of two doses of aspirin (30 mg vs. 283 mg a day) in patients after a transient ischemic attack or minor ischemic stroke. *N Engl J Med* 1991;325:1261–1266.
5. UK-TIA Study Group. United Kingdom transient ischaemic attack (UK-TIA) aspirin trial: Final results. *J Neurol Neurosurg Psychiat* 1991;54:1044–1054.
6. Diener HC, Cunha L, Forbes C, Sivenius J, Smets P, Lowenthal A. European Stroke Prevention Study 2. Dipyridamole and acetylsalicylic acid in the secondary prevention of stroke. *J Neurol Sci* 1996;143:1–13.
7. Taylor DW, Barnett HJ, Haynes RB, et al. Low-dose and high-dose acetylsalicylic acid for patients undergoing carotid endarterectomy: A randomised controlled trial. ASA and Carotid Endarterectomy (ACE) Trial Collaborators. *Lancet* 1999;353:2179–2184.
8. U.S. Food and Drug Administration. Internal analgesic, antipyretic, and antirheumatic drug products for over-the-counter human use: Final Rule for professional labelling of aspirin, buffered aspirin, and aspirin in combination with antacid drug products. *Federal Register* 1998;63:56802–56819,66015–66017.
9. Steering Committee of the Physicians' Health Study Research Group. Final report on the aspirin component of the ongoing Physicians' Health Study. *N Engl J Med* 1989; 321:129–135.
10. Weil J, Colin-Jones D, Langman M, et al. Prophylactic aspirin and risk of peptic ulcer bleeding. *BMJ* 1995;310:827–830.
11. Soll AH, Weinstein WM, Kurata J, McCarthy D. Nonsteroidal anti-inflammatory drugs and peptic ulcer disease. *Ann Intern Med* 1991;114:307–319.
12. Kelly JP, Kaufman DW, Jurgelon JM, Sheehan J, Koff RS, Shapiro S. Risk of aspirin-associated major upper-gastrointestinal bleeding with enteric-coated or buffered product. *Lancet* 1996;348:1413–1416.
13. Fuster V, Dyken ML, Vokonas PS, Hennekens C. Aspirin as a therapeutic agent in cardiovascular disease: Special Writing Group. *Circulation* 1993;87:659–675.
14. Laporte JR, Carne X, Vidal X, Moreno V, Juan J. Upper gastrointestinal bleeding in relation to previous use of analgesics and non-steroidal anti-inflammatory drugs: Catalan Countries Study on Upper Gastrointestinal Bleeding *Lancet* 1991;337:85–89.
15. Levy M, Miller DR, Kaufman DW, et al. Major upper gastrointestinal tract bleeding: Relation to the use of aspirin and other nonnarcotic analgesics. *Arch Intern Med* 1988; 148:281–285.
16. Peto R, Gray R, Collins R, et al. Randomised trial of prophylactic daily aspirin in British male doctors. *BMJ* 1988;1:313–316.
17. Wolfe MM, Lichtenstein DR, Singh G. Gastrointestinal toxicity of nonsteroidal anti-inflammatory drugs. *New Engl J Med* 1999;340:1888–1899.
18. Balsano F, Rizzon P, Violi F, et al. Antiplatelet treatment with ticlopidine in unstable angina: A controlled multicenter clinical trial. Circulation 1990;82:17–26.
19. Gent M, Blakely JA, Easton JD, et al. The Canadian American Ticlopidine Study (CATS) in thromboembolic stroke. *Lancet* 1989;1:1215–1220.
20. Hass WK, Easton JD, Adams HP, Jr., et al. A randomized trial comparing ticlopidine hydrochloride with aspirin for the prevention of stroke in high-risk patients: Ticlopidine Aspirin Stroke Study Group. *N Engl J Med* 1989;321:501–507.

21. Janzon L, Bergqvist D, Boberg J, et al. Prevention of myocardial infarction and stroke in patients with intermittent claudication: Effect of ticlopidine. Results from STIMS, the Swedish Ticlopidine Multicentre Study. *J Intern Med* 1990;227:301–308.

22. Bennett CL, Weinberg PD, Rozenberg-Be-Dror K, Yarnold PR, Kwaan HC, Green D. Thrombotic thrombocytopenic purpura associated with ticlopidine: A review of 60 cases. *Ann Intern Med* 1998;128:541–544.

23. Murakami M, Toyokura T, Omae T, Gotoh F, Tazaki Y, Ohtomo E. Effects of ticlopidine and aspirin on TIAs—a twelve month, double blind, comparative study. *Igaku no Ayumi* 1983;127:950–971.

24. CAPRIE Steering Committee. A randomized, blinded, trial of clopidogrel versus aspirin in patients at risk of ischaemic events (CAPRIE). *Lancet* 1996;348:1329–1339.

24a. Bennett CL, Connors JM, Carwile JM, Moake JL, Bell WR, Tarantolo SR, McCarthy LJ, Sarode R, Hatfield AJ, Feldman MD, Davidson CJ, Tsai HM. Thrombotic thrombocytopenic purpura associated with clopidogrel. *N Engl J Med* 2000;342:1773–1777.

25. Wilterdink JL, Easton JD. Dipyridamole plus aspirin in cerebrovascular disease. *Arch Neurol* 1999;56:1087–1092.

26. Bousser MG, Eschwege E, Haguenau M, et al. "AICLA" controlled trial of aspirin and dipyridamole in the secondary prevention of atherothrombotic cerebral ischemia. *Stroke* 1983;14:5–14.

27. Fields WS, American-Canadian Co-operative Study Group. Persantine aspirin trial in cerebral ischemia. *Stroke* 1983;14:99–103.

28. Fields WS, American-Canadian Co-operative Study Group. Persantine aspirin trial in cerebral ischemia. Part III: Risk factors for stroke. *Stroke* 1986;17:12–18.

29. Guiraud-Chaumeil B, Rascol A, David J, Boneu B, Clanet M, Bierme R. Prévention des récidives des accidents vasculaires cérébraux ischémiques par les anti-agrégants plaquettaires. *Rev Neurol (Paris)* 1982; 138:367–385.

30. The ESPS Group. The European Stroke Prevention Study (ESPS): Principal endpoints. *Lancet* 1987;2:1351–1354.

31. Gorter JW, De Schryver EL, Algra A. Secondary prevention after ischemic cerebral infarct. The ESPRIT Study: Low dose anticoagulation, combined therapy with acetylsalicylic acid/dipyridamole or monotherapy with acetylsalicylic acid? *Nervenarzt* 1999;70:368–370.

12

SURGICAL MEASURES TO PREVENT STROKE

H. J. M. Barnett and Heather E. Meldrum

Surgical repair of injured arteries on the battlefields of World War II set the stage for a surgical attack on arteries to the limbs, the heart, and the brain narrowed by arteriosclerosis. The cervical portion of the internal carotid artery had been shown by Egaz Moniz, the father of angiography, by the pathological studies of G.T.J. Hultquist, and by the dedicated studies by C. Miller Fisher of the neck arteries at post-mortem to be a commoner site of obstruction than had previously been accepted.[1-3] The middle cerebral artery, instead of being seen as the primary site of arteriosclerotic mischief, came to be regarded as the artery most commonly causing stroke from lodgment of cardiac and extracranial carotid embolic material. Except in Asian populations, the middle cerebral artery was no longer accepted as the primary site of obstruction due to arteriosclerosis.

As Goethe remarked, "What one knows, one sees." Quite quickly, an explosion of reports confirmed Moniz's, Hultquist's, and Fisher's observations. As more arterial lesions were identified in the neck, the phenomena of transient and recurrent ischemic events came to light. The stage was set for attempts to forestall, by antithrombotics and surgical methods, the strokes threatened by these transient events of cerebral and retinal ischemia. This chapter confines itself to the evolution of understanding of the appropriate use of surgical measures to prevent stroke.

DEVELOPMENT OF CAROTID ARTERY SURGERY

The credit for the first carotid surgical attempt to prevent ischemic stroke must go to Eastcott, Pickering, and Rob.[4] They were the first to publish a report in a peer-reviewed journal, the gold currency of scientific activity. Carotid endarterectomy (CE) quickly replaced localized carotid resection. Many surgeons learned the technique. Neurologists and other practitioners became aware of the significance of focal hemisphere and retinal events. By 1974, 15,000 carotid procedures had been done in the non-veteran hospitals of the United States. A small, randomized trial of 316 patients reported results in 1970 that were far from encouraging.[5] Too many patients (42%) had vertebral basilar, rather than carotid, symptoms, loss to follow-up was higher than desirable, and the perioperative complication rate was unacceptable (11%).

Despite this negative trial, enthusiasm persisted. It still appeared to be a logical procedure for preventing stroke. Other applications of the procedure were introduced that led to its expanded use. One application arose from the hypothesis that nonspecific symptoms, such as dizziness, vertigo, drop attacks, episodes of loss of consciousness, transitory memory difficulties, and even specific symptoms of vertebral basilar disease, might benefit from a general improvement in blood flowing to the brain by removing the accessible stenoses from diseased carotid arteries. As many as 10% of the increasing number of endarterectomies may have related to this improbable and unproven hypothesis. Another practice that became common was to remove an asymptomatic stenosing plaque as a prelude to major cardiovascular operations, particularly coronary artery bypass grafting. More importantly, the use of the procedure was extended to asymptomatic individuals with carotid artery stenosis. This custom is discussed in detail later in the chapter.

Another innovation was the introduction of ultrasound as an alternative diagnostic tool to be used instead of or with angiography. Safe and noninvasive, it became widely available and very extensively used. More will be said of this but its complete role in patient selection remains uncertain and in some dispute.

In the 11 years between 1974 and 1985, it was estimated that one million individuals worldwide had carotid endarterectomy.[6] Figure 12.1 illustrates that enthusiasm increased dramatically in this 11-year period. With doubts expressed about proof of its suitability for its widespread application, the numbers waned for a few years. They doubled again within two or three years of the completion of published trials because of an optimistic interpretation of the trial results. By 1999, it was quite certain that two million carotid endarterectomies had been performed worldwide and that a reasonably large number of these (probably at least one-third) were done without firm substantiating evidence, some in situations in which the harm may have exceeded benefit.

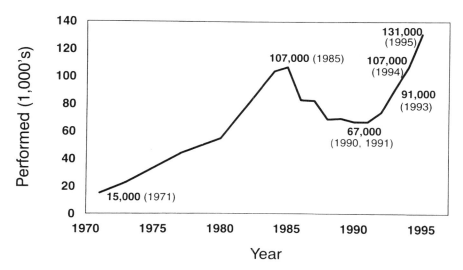

FIGURE 12.1. The number of endarterectomies performed annually from 1970 to 1995 indicates a decline after 1985, followed by a doubling after the publication of the first phase of NASCET and ECST and the final results of ACAS. Adapted from Pokras R., personal communication with permission.

LATER TRIALS OF CAROTID ENDARTERECTOMY

To fulfill the demands of modern scientific medicine, particularly when the course of a chronic disease is unpredictable and has protean outcomes, therapeutic data must be amassed from randomized trials that are designed, executed, and analyzed to answer the appropriate questions. Three such trials were launched and concluded to evaluate the role of CE in patients with symptomatic disease.[7–9] Two of these three trials prospectively followed the stroke outcomes relating to the stenosing lesions on the asymptomatic "other" side. Five were launched for asymptomatic individuals, of which four are concluded and published.[10–14] Finally, a study in which symptomatic patients and asymptomatic subjects were randomized to determine the optimum perioperative dose of aspirin allowed some observations to be made about asymptomatic disease.[15]

Symptomatic Trials

In 1981, Warlow and colleagues took up the challenge of the appropriateness of carotid endarterectomy and from the United Kingdom launched an ambitious trial. The European Carotid Surgery Trial (ECST)[7] required that patients have symptoms within 180 days and have angiographic proof of a stenosis caused by arteriosclerosis. Two patients were randomized to receive endarterectomy for every patient randomized to treatment with best medical care alone. Between 1981 and 1994, 3024 patients were randomized.

The other large trial, the North American Symptomatic Carotid Endarterectomy Trial (NASCET),[8] randomized 2885 patients between 1987 and 1996. All patients were required to have had recent (120 days for the first 30 months of the trial, 180 days thereafter) focal symptoms appropriate to an angiographically demonstrated stenosing lesion. Surgeons were required to produce evidence of experience and competence in the performance of CE. For each center, random-

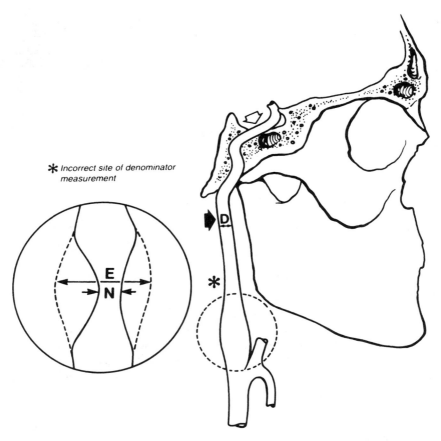

FIGURE 12.2. NASCET calculated the percentage of stenosis by using the narrowest linear diameter in two (or three) planes as the numerator, and the artery well beyond the carotid bulb (circled) and any poststenotic dilatation as the denominator (closed arrow) $(1 - N/D \times 100 = \%$ stenosis). Measurement of the artery too close to the bulb produced a misleading denominator (asterisk). The European Carotid Surgery Trial (ECST) used the same numerator but took the imagined site of the wall of the carotid bulb as the denominator. Reproduced with permission from Barnett et al. *Current Critical Problems in Vascular Surgery*, St. Louis, MO: Quality Medical Publishing, 1994.

TABLE 12.1. Correlation of NASCET and ECST
Measurements of % Stenosis

NASCET	ECST
30	65
40	70
50	75
60	80
70	85
80	91
90	97

NASCET found benefit from 50%–99%; greatest benefit 70%–99%. ECST found benefit at and above 80% (NASCET 60%).

ization balanced one medical to one surgical patient. The formula for measuring stenosis used the narrowest diameter of the stenosed segment as the numerator, and the artery diameter well beyond the disease, bulb, and post-bulbar dilatation as the denominator. Selected films were submitted for the central measurements used in all analyses. The formula used to calculate the measurement in ECST used a different denominator (Fig. 12.2). The differences have been sufficiently studied and rationalized so easy conversion is possible from the degrees of stenosis depicted in Table 12.1.

Best medical care included therapy to normalize blood pressure, cholesterol, and blood sugar and advice about the avoidance of tobacco. Enteric-coated aspirin was supplied to all NASCET patients at a recommended dosage of 1300 mg daily. Lesser amounts were discretionary, as was the use of other platelet inhibitors. Excluded were patients with symptoms due to nonarteriosclerotic disease of the carotid arteries, previous endarterectomy on the symptomatic side, heart disease likely to be associated with early cerebral embolic events, and organ failure or other morbid illnesses likely to cause death within five years. Outcome events in NASCET were adjudicated by independent clinicians blinded to the treatment arm. Data were gathered at entry and at the time of outcome events to assist the NASCET investigators in determining the cause, severity, and course of stroke and particularly in identifying the occurrences of hemorrhagic, large artery, lacunar, or cardioembolic stroke.

In neither ECST nor NASCET was ultrasound evaluation alone acceptable for randomization. It was encouraged in the preliminary screening of potential candidates, and in NASCET was performed at the first follow-up after CE and requested annually in all patients.

The third symptomatic trial, confined to 16 Veterans Affairs (VA) Medical Centers in the United States, randomized 189 symptomatic patients with ≥50% stenosis determined by angiography. The numbers were small, and the trial was discontinued after the declaration of benefit from CE for patients with 70%–99% stenosis.

The Results of the Trials for Symptomatic Patients

The benefit of CE was similar in the two large trials. Figure 12.3 demonstrates the five-year Kaplan-Meier survival curves from NASCET for any stroke and death and for disabling stroke and death in the patients in the 70%–99% and the 50%–69% stenosis range. It is clear that patients with focal symptoms who have severe (70%–99%) stenosis benefit most from the procedure. In the patients with moderate stenosis, the confidence intervals overlap, and the benefit, although present at a p-value of 0.045, is muted.

Several conditions were identified in post-hoc observations of perioperative risk from CE that led to a doubling, or near doubling, of the likelihood of postoperative outcome complications.[16] They included a hemispheric TIA compared with a retinal TIA as the qualifying event, a left-sided procedure, the presence of contralateral carotid occlusion, an ipsilateral ischemic lesion on the entry CT scan, and irregular or ulcerated plaque detected by angiography on the side of surgery and a lack of collateral circulation in the hemisphere beyond severe (70%–99%) symptomatic stenosis.[17] Despite imposing an increase in risk at the time of the procedure, none of these conditions contraindicate CE because, in the long-term follow-up of patients with both severe and moderate stenosis, these variables did not eliminate the benefit favoring surgery. The most unexpected of these observations was the increased complication rate for left-sided lesions. The initial impression was that this could be due to a statistical spin of chance. This probably is not the explanation, as it has been encountered in two other series of patients submitted to CE.[15,18] In patients who had contralateral occlusion ($n = 43$), the operative risk was tripled (14%) compared to those patients without contralateral occlusion. Treated medically, patients with this condition have a 69% risk of stroke in two years compared to 29% for patients without contralateral occlusion.[19]

FIGURE 12.3. (A) Kaplan-Meier curves for event-free survival of medical and surgical patients with severe (70%–99%) stenosis. The results favor endarterectomy for any ipsilateral stroke and disabling ipsilateral stroke ($p < 0.001$). The 95% confidence intervals are shown for each curve and there is no overlap. The number at risk annually are shown out to 8 years. (b) Kaplan-Meier curves for event-free survival of medical and surgical patients with moderate stenosis (50%–69%). The results favor endarterectomy ($p = 0.045$), but the confidence intervals overlap throughout, muting the importance of the statistical significance. The results for disabling stroke showed no benefit. Reproduced by permission of the *New England Journal of Medicine*.[8]

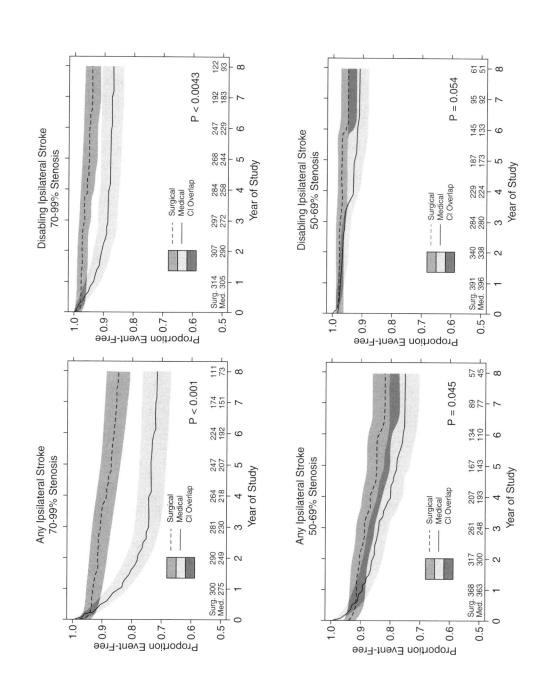

In the severe range (70%–90%), all risk subgroups benefited from the procedure. In the moderate range (50%–69%), best results were detected in males, in patients with tandem lesions (intracranial disease), in patients with hemisphere rather than retinal symptoms, and in patients presenting with a stroke rather than only transient ischemic attack (TIA). Below 50% stenosis, symptomatic patients received no benefit and were best treated with medical care; the ECST study found that these individuals were significantly worse off with CE than with best medical care.

For patients at ranges of stenosis of <60%, 60%–69%, and 70%–99%, outcomes were analyzed as to cause of stroke (large artery, lacunar, or cardioembolic in origin). The breakpoint at 60% was used because this was the minimal degree of stenosis in the Asymptomatic Carotid Atherosclerosis Study (ACAS) trial, and above it a benefit had been claimed for asymptomatic individuals from CE. In Figure 12.4, 83.6% of subsequent strokes were of large artery origin when the stenosis was severe (70%–99%). The combination of cardioembolic and lacunar ipsilateral strokes together constituted only 16.4% in patients with this severe degree of stenosis. Strokes of non–large artery origin rose to 40% in the patients with moderate stenosis. Lacunar strokes as outcome events were com-

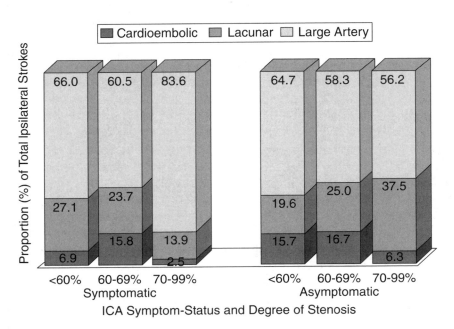

FIGURE 12.4. Kaplan-Meier proportion (%) of each cause (cardioembolic, lacunar, large-artery) of ipsilateral stroke in the symptomatic arteries and in the asymptomatic "other side." The cutpoints at 60% and 70% stenosis correspond to the current American Heart Association guidelines for recommending carotid endarterectomy to asymptomatic and symptomatic patients, respectively.[47]

moner than cardioembolic strokes. In large hospital-based and community-based stroke data banks, these two stroke causes are close to equal. The percentage of cardioembolic strokes in NASCET is lower because the protocol excluded patients who had evidence at entry of cardiac lesions likely to lead to cerebral embolization. The age of the patients in NASCET, however, determined that heart disease and small vessel disease became manifest in the long-term follow-up of these patients. The cause of strokes in asymptomatic patients is discussed in the next section.

The degree of stenosis proved to be the most important risk factor (Figure 12.5). The average annual risk of stroke peaked at 9.4% for those patients with 75%–94% stenosis. In the nearly occluded patients with a collapsing artery (95%–99%), the risk diminished again (6.5%). This decreased risk in the patients with very severe stenosis has been previously reported from NASCET.[20]

Asymptomatic Carotid Artery Disease

Angiography and noninvasive studies detect atherosclerotic plaque in the extracranial arteries, which increases in amount with the subject's age. From a small number of community surveys, it has been estimated that 2 million people above the age of 50 in the United States have an asymptomatic carotid artery steno-

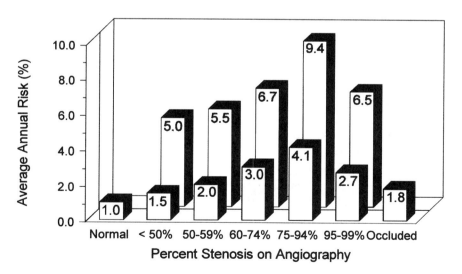

FIGURE 12.5. The average annual risk of stroke in the involved artery territory over a three-year period is depicted for increasing degrees of stenosis. The rear bars relate to the strokes of the symptomatic artery, the front bars to the territory of the asymptomatic artery on the other side. No symptomatic patient had normal arteries, and the NASCET protocol excluded patients with occlusion of symptomatic arteries. Reproduced by permission of REMEDICA.

sis.[21] This means that there are twice as many people living with this condition in the United States at the present time as were submitted to CE worldwide in the first thirty years of its application.

The question of appropriate treatment in the presence of asymptomatic lesions has been the subject of considerable enquiry. Uncertainty continues to surround the application of CE for these subjects, who in this discussion will not be described as "patients": they carry on normal lives with freedom from symptoms, and the likelihood is that a majority will never require aggressive therapy. The assumption that they are all "patients" requiring CE would increase by 10-fold the number currently being performed.

The risk of stroke facing these individuals was subjected to enquiry in large observational case-series. The best data came from approximately 1000 subjects in two studies who came under observation in two vascular ultrasound imaging laboratories and were examined at intervals over a five-year period.[22,23] These two studies concluded that the annual risk of stroke with lesions producing stenosis below 75% and 80%, respectively was less than 2% per year and rose to 5% only when the stenosis was above 80%. This risk for stroke decreased to 3% when only events ipsilateral to the lesion were included. Men were at higher risk than women. Some other observations about the risk came to light from the Toronto asymptomatic series. In a mean follow-up of 52 months involving 500 persons, Norris and Zhu detected a bi-modal distribution of ischemic events, observing a peak risk in the 75%–90% range of stenosis, and then a reduced risk in subjects with 91%–99% stenosis.[24] Fifty-one cerebral ischemic events were reported, most in the 75%–90% range. TIA, a harbinger of potential stroke, was four times as likely to occur ($n = 40$) as was ischemic stroke ($n = 11$). From this study and from other reports, evidence indicates that there is an increased likelihood of the development of symptoms when the lesion under observation increases rapidly in size. The postulate is that the increase in size is due either to rapid increase in atheromatous deposit or to intraplaque hemorrhage. More data are needed in this regard. It would appear to be an uncommon occurrence. NASCET has data indicating that the average rate of increase in stenosis is only 4% per year in long-term annual ultrasound observations.[25] The question remains unsettled about how often individuals with known stenosis should be reexamined for evidence of rapid increase while still asymptomatic. Studies at less than annual intervals appear to be excessive.

The gold standard of the randomized clinical trial has been applied in evaluating both medical and surgical therapy for asymptomatic subjects. The number of subjects has been smaller than ideal. The one medical trial, involving 372 subjects, was of meticulous design but was unable to determine any benefit from prophylactic aspirin therapy (325 mg daily) compared to placebo.[26] Larger studies are required to confirm or deny these observations, possibly using different dosages of aspirin.

Five randomized trials evaluating surgical treatment have been started, and four of these have been completed and published. Table 12.2 sets out the numbers admitted to the relevant trials and contrasts those with symptomatic disease to those with no symptoms. It identifies the outcome events of any stroke, vascular death, and other death extracted from the trials in which the information was available. Clearly, the symptomatic patients face an increasing annual risk of stroke and vascular death with the increasing degree of stenosis. The annual stroke risk in NASCET's medically treated symptomatic patients was 9.6% in those with severe disease and 4.7% in those with moderate disease. In ECST, the figures were 6.2% and 2.6% respectively. In asymptomatic subjects the annual risk varied between 2.6% and 2.9%. To improve on these medical risk figures with CE is realistic for the severe patients, as shown in ECST and NASCET, and for some moderate patients, as shown in NASCET. The challenge appears to be more daunting and may be impossible when the medical risk figures are below 3%, as they were in the asymptomatic trials and in the moderate patients in ECST. The trials involving asymptomatic subjects numbering in aggregate 2584 involved less than half the numbers in the trials of symptomatic patients ($n = 6092$). The lesser risk of stroke experienced in the asymptomatic artery suggests that larger trials would have been desirable. Perhaps as many as 10,000 subjects may be needed to establish efficacy with certainty. Whether seeking benefit by using such large numbers of subjects with such low risk of stroke is worthwhile remains in doubt.[27]

Two of the asymptomatic trials had sufficient design problems that they will not be further considered.[10,11] The Veterans Administration Cooperative Study trial randomized 444 men, and had it not been accompanied by a high perioperative risk, modest benefit in stroke reduction might have been shown. With a 4.4% complication rate, neither immediate nor long-term stroke-free survival resulted.

The ACAS study randomized 1662 individuals, 3 of whom in the surgical arm were not followed. Approximately 45% had previous symptoms or surgical procedures. The final publication reported a relative risk reduction of 53% favoring stroke-free survival for the subjects in the surgical arm compared to those in the medical arm. Unhappily, the absolute risk reduction was only 5.9% at five years, yielding little more than an annual risk reduction of 1%. The difference in the impact of relative and absolute risk reductions are seldom better demonstrated than in this differential of 53% and 1%. The relative risk reduction may be unduly optimistic. A statistically significant difference may not amount to an important clinical difference. For example, a relative risk reduction of 50% is obtained when the absolute risk is reduced from 50% to 25%. A 50% relative reduction also ensues when the absolute risk is reduced from 2% to 1%. In such low-risk situations, as in subjects who have asymptomatic carotid stenosis, attention should concentrate on the absolute reduction of risk.

The benefit claimed for CE based on the ACAS reports has not received universal acceptance.[6,28–33] The controversies of interpretation arise from a combi-

TABLE 12.2. Number of Patients and Outcomes in the Symptomatic and Asymptomatic Randomized Trials

| | TRIAL | TOTAL NUMBER OF PATIENTS | | AVERAGE FOLLOW-UP | ANY STROKE | | VASCULAR DEATH | | OTHER DEATH | | RATE PER 100 PATIENTS YEAR | |
| | | | | | | | | | | | STROKE AND VASCULAR DEATH PER YEAR (%) | STROKE PER YEAR (%) |
		MEDICAL	SURGICAL		MEDICAL	SURGICAL	MEDICAL	SURGICAL	MEDICAL	SURGICAL	MEDICAL	MEDICAL
Symptomatic Trials	ECST[7][†]											
	Moderate	1057	1533	6 yrs.	163	234	122	219	282	418	4.5	2.6
	Severe	154	274	6.6 yrs.	63	40	32	55	40	80	9.3	6.2
	NASCET[8,48]											
	Moderate	1118	1108	5 yrs.	264	233	123	130	108	88	6.9	4.7
	Severe	331	328	2 yrs.	64	34	14	10	7	5	11.8	9.6
	VA[9]*	98	91	1 yr.	7	3						
Total		**2758**	**3334**		**551**	**585**	**371**	**494**	**203**	**237**		
Asymptomatic Trials	ACAS[13]	834	825	2.7 yrs.	66	44	60	46	29	37	5.5	2.9
	VA Cooperative[12]	233	211	4 yrs.	25	17	51	45	27	25	8	2.6
	CASANOVA[10]	204	206	3 yrs.	0	3	0	0	0	0	0	0
	MACE[11]	35	36	2 yrs.	0	3	0	0	0	0		
Total		**1306**	**1278**		**91**	**64**	**111**	**91**	**56**	**62**		

*Data unavailable for detailed breakdown of outcome events.

†Additional data supplied from ECST by PM Rothwell using the NASCET Measurement Method, personal communication, 1999.

nation of what was shown, what was not shown, what has been extrapolated lacking good data, and what has been observed from other databases.

A major problem with ACAS was that too few patients were entered into the study to produce enough outcome events to answer pertinent questions. Neither the numbers entered nor the reliance on Doppler examinations alone for the analyses allowed a distinction in benefit among any deciles of stenosis. It is counterintuitive to believe that a person without symptoms, shown to have a 60% narrowing by ultrasound alone, can be given a green light to have CE, while a symptomatic patient with a 60% angiographic lesion is only to be considered for CE under certain circumstances.

Subgroup analyses were unable to declare benefit or lack of benefit for disabling stroke. This could be misleading again because of the small numbers. Women were not shown to benefit. This may be due to the better prognosis for recurrent ischemic events in women compared to men, or solely due to the higher perioperative complication rate in ACAS for women (3.3% compared to 1.7% for men). The reported combined perioperative complication rate of 2.3% for men and women would be a challenge to most institutions and surgical departments. The surgical complication rate is reduced to a daunting 1.1% when the inclusion of an unexpectedly high complication rate of 1.2% from angiography is subtracted from the 2.3%.

Large Medicare surveys report hospital mortality alone. They do not provide data about stroke morbidity nor distinguish between CEs performed for symptomatic patients or asymptomatic individuals. The latest mortality figures from the Medicare source indicate that 1.8% of patients submitted to CE under Medicare leave the hospital dead (Robert Pokras, personal communication, 1998). Because morbidity is 3 to 4 times this figure, no comfort can be taken from the possibility of a complication rate of stroke and death approaching 8%.

The databases of NASCET and ECST have been able to provide some useful information about asymptomatic arteries. Of 2377 NASCET patients from whom bilateral angiograms were available and who had never had symptoms on the other (asymptomatic) side, 509 had a stenosis of ≥50%, and 1330 had <50%, but a detectable amount of stenosis. The average annual risk of stroke over a three-year period from these asymptomatic arteries was calculated, and a comparison by different degrees of stenosis is depicted in Figure 12.5. At all degrees of stenosis, the annual risk is one-third, or at most one-half, that in the territory of the symptomatic artery. Only at the stenotic range of 75%–94% does the risk exceed what could be improved upon by good surgeons. The risk for subjects with nearly occluded arteries was less than for the two deciles below this. This seeming paradox was observed by Norris and Zhu in their case-series of asymptomatic subjects.[24] It appears that the flow beyond the stenosis in the severely narrowed artery is diminished to the point where the hemisphere is no longer dependent on it and emboli travel less frequently through the severely narrowed segment. Comparable observations have been reported from the symptomatic side of NASCET.[20]

NASCET prospectively recorded all strokes in the asymptomatic arteries. The causes of strokes were identified as related either to the large artery lesion or to be of cardioembolic or lacunar origin. Either cardioembolic or lacunar cause was ascribed to more than 40% of these strokes, and the high percentage of strokes not of large artery origin was observed at all degrees of stenosis (Figure 12.4). A figure of 50% is probably the accurate number in the series of endarterec-tomies not restricted by protocol to exclude threatening cardiac lesions. In any population of asymptomatic individuals, a recalculation of the annual risk of stroke must be made, accounting for the fact that approximately 50% of the risk is not subject to reduction by a carotid CE. For example in the 75%–94% steno-sis category, the highest risk group, only a 1.9% annual large-artery stroke risk would be predicted. This is not a risk that would be improved upon by CE.

The comparable ECST database contained 843 randomized patients with an asymptomatic (other side) artery with 30%–69% stenosis by ECST measurement, and 127 with 70%–99% stenosis.[34] During follow-up, 69 patients had a first stroke on the previously asymptomatic side lasting longer than 7 days, giving an esti-mated Kaplan-Meier stroke risk at three years of 2.1%. The risk for patients with 70%–99% stenosis was 5.7%. By degrees of stenosis there was a sharp gradient of risk when the stenosis reached 80%. The three-year risk was 9.8% for patients with 80%–89% stenosis and 14.4% with 90%–99% stenosis. Data were not avail-able identifying stroke by cause. There is no reason to believe that the distribu-tion of large artery, cardioembolic, and lacunar strokes differed from the percentages found in NASCET.

Additional data have become available from the Aspirin and Carotid Endar-terectomy trial (ACE), which ran parallel to NASCET in the NASCET centers. Altogether, 2804 CEs were performed, 1521 for asymptomatic subjects, and 1283 for symptomatic patients. The complication rate at 30 days was 6.4% for the symptomatic patients and 4.6% for the subjects without symptoms. Superim-posing the 4.6% obtained from ACE upon the Kaplan-Meier medical-surgical curves from ACAS, as Figure 12.6 demonstrates, no benefit was achieved from CE out to six years. This is of particular concern because the ACE trial submit-ted twice as many asymptomatic subjects to CE as did the ACAS trial. Harm was done, and medical therapy should become the preferred treatment.

A fifth asymptomatic trial is ongoing with a goal of 3200 individuals to be submitted to best medical therapy or to CE.[14] The larger numbers may confirm or deny the ACAS observations. This study may find a subgroup with convinc-ing evidence of benefit. A large, long-term observational study of risk factors is also being carried out that may identify the risk profile of asymptomatic indi-viduals more likely to benefit from CE than from the best contemporary medical care.[35]

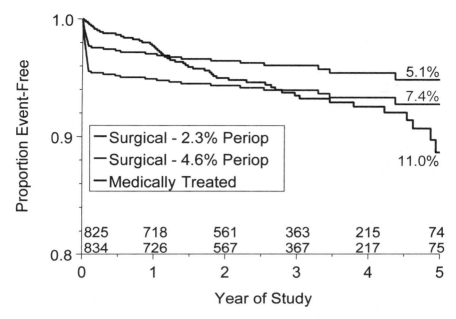

FIGURE 12.6. The medical and surgical five-year Kaplan-Meier freedom from ipsilateral stroke and perioperative stroke and death curves indicate a 5.9% difference (11.0% minus 5.1%) favoring endarterectomy at five years in the ACAS study. A marginal but definite statistical significance by Greenwood's formula ($p < 0.05$) can be claimed for this difference at five years, at which time only 149 patients were available for analysis. Superimposed on the curves is the outcome projected to five years for 1521 individuals receiving carotid endarterectomy for asymptomatic lesions in the ACE trial, based upon an actual 4.6% stroke and death rate at 30 days. The outcomes were then extrapolated beyond 30 days from the ACAS data. Using the projected 7.4% rate of outcomes at five years, the difference between the surgical and the medical group is 3.6% (11.0% minus 7.4%), only a 0.7% risk reduction per year ($p \approx 0.10$). Adapted from ACAS.[13] Reproduced by permission of Barnett HJM, Meldrum HE. Carotid Endarterectomy: A Neurotherapeutic Advance. *Arch Neurol* 2000;57:40–45.

In two other circumstances, a practice has developed to perform CE in subjects without carotid symptoms. The first has been based on the unsubstantiated hypothesis that "nonhemisphere" symptoms, including symptoms clearly of vertebral basilar origin, will benefit from CE. This has never been convincingly established. The second hypothesis was that the risk of stroke in the performance of major cardiovascular and aortic surgery would be reduced by performing CE on stenosing lesions incidentally found in the carotid arteries of these patients. Later studies have indicated, first that the strokes complicating the procedure occur as often in the territory of the nonstenotic artery or in the posterior circulation as in the territory of the stenosed artery. Second, the cause of the strokes complicating coronary artery bypass grafting (CABG) is most commonly related to the insertion of the shunt into the diseased aortic site. Finally, it has been recognized that these patients subjected to both CABG and CE have a morbidity and mortality equal to the sum of the two individual risks.[36] Neither of these applications of CE can be substantiated on the basis of scientifically evaluated evidence. Their use in these circumstances can be justified only if they are being done in a properly designed clinical trial.

CAUSES OF STROKE IN THE PRESENCE OF CAROTID STENOSIS

Therapeutic trials in stroke prevention have been justifiably criticized for regarding stroke as a generic phenomenon and not attempting to distinguish among stroke outcome events by cause.[37,38] A striking example was the huge (19,000-patients) International Stroke Trial (IST), which evaluated anticoagulants compared with platelet-inhibiting therapy.[39] Concern was expressed that a different type of protocol, designed to distinguish among outcomes of stroke by cause, may have found different results in the treatment for strokes of cardioembolic origin, lacunes, or those of large artery origin.[40] It requires a leap of faith to accept the contention that all of these causes of stroke will have comparable responses to identical medical therapy. To identify the cause of stroke outcomes is equally important in evaluating the benefit of CE. NASCET identified stroke events by cause. In patients with moderate disease and in strokes that occurred in the territory of the arteries of the asymptomatic "other side," the combination of lacunar and cardioembolic strokes was approximately 40% and occurred regardless of the degree of stenosis (Figure 12.4).[41]

Lacunar strokes were not excluded as entry phenomena into NASCET. The contention was that data did not exist at the time of writing the protocol for this trial to state with assurance that patients with lacunar stroke would or would not benefit from CE. At the conclusion of the trial, the nonlacunar patients were compared with the patients who entered with lacunar syndromes. Clear benefit was seen from CE for the nonlacunar patients, but less benefit was seen in the patients who entered the trial after a lacunar stroke.[42] Because the number of patients who came into NASCET with probable lacunar syndromes was small, further evaluation in other trials is desirable.

DECISIONS ABOUT CE BASED ON THE NUMBER-NEEDED-TO-TREAT CALCULATIONS

For symptomatic patients and asymptomatic subjects, it is possible from published randomized trials and from the observations made in the ACE trial to calculate the number needed to treat (NNT) by CE to prevent one additional stroke (in the case of symptomatic patients) or a first stroke (in asymptomatic subjects). These calculations, set out in Tables 12.3 and 12.4, are dependent particularly on

TABLE 12.3. Number Needed to Treat (NNT) by Endarterectomy: Symptomatic Patients

	NUMBER OF PATIENTS IN SPECIFIED TRIAL	MEDICAL RISK (%) AT 2 YEARS	SURGICAL RISK (%) AT 2 YEARS	RISK DIFFERENCE (%)	RELATIVE RISK REDUCTION (%)	NEEDED TO TREAT[1]	PERIOPERATIVE STROKE AND DEATH RATE (%)
Symptomatic 70–99% North American Symptomatic Carotid Endarterectomy Trial	659	24.5	8.6	15.9	65	6	5.8
Symptomatic 70–99% European Carotid Surgery Trial[2] (by NASCET Measurement)	501	19.9	7.0	12.9	65	8	5.6
Symptomatic 50–69% North American Symptomatic Carotid Endarterectomy Trial	858	14.6	9.3	5.3	36	19	6.9
Symptomatic 50–69% European Carotid Surgery Trial (by NASCET Measurement)	684	9.7	11.1	-1.4	-14	–	9.8
Symptomatic <50% North American Symptomatic Carotid Endarterectomy Trial	1368	11.7	10.2	1.5	13	67	6.5
Symptomatic <50% European Carotid Surgery Trial (by NASCET Measurement)	1822	4.3	9.5	-5.2	-109	–	6.1

[1]NNT = Number of patients needed to treat by endarterectomy to prevent one additional ipsilateral stroke for 2 years after the procedure, compared to medical therapy alone.

[2]Additional data supplied by Dr. P. Rothwell.

Reproduced by permission of Barnett HJM, Eliaszio M, Meldrum HE. Prevention of ischaemic stroke. *BMJ* 1999;318:1539–1543.

TABLE 12.4. Number Needed to Treat (NNT) by Endarterectomy—Asymptomatic Individuals

	NUMBER IN SPECIFIED TRIAL	MEDICAL RISK (%) AT 2 YEARS	SURGICAL RISK (%) AT 2 YEARS	RISK DIFFERENCE (%)	RELATIVE RISK REDUCTION (%)	NEEDED TO TREAT[1]	PERIOPERATIVE STROKE AND DEATH RATE (%)
Asymptomatic ≥ 50%, Veterans Affairs Cooperative Study, men only	444	7.7[2]	5.6[2]	2.1	27	48	4.4
Asymptomatic, Asymptomatic Carotid Atherosclerosis Study	1662	5.0	3.8[3] (actual)	1.2	24	83	2.6
Asymptomatic, Aspirin and Carotid Endarterectomy Trial	1521	5.0[4] (assumed)	5.8	-0.8	—	—	4.6

[1]NNT = Number of subjects needed to treat by endarterectomy to prevent one ipsilateral stroke for two years after the procedure, compared to medical therapy alone.

[2]Extrapolated from results. The perioperative risk is calculated on the 203 subjects who actually received surgery.

[3]Assigning a perioperative risk of 2.6% based on 724 of 825 subjects who actually received endarterectomy in the surgical arm of ACAS, and utilizing a 0.6% risk of stroke in each of the two years after endarterectomy. The same 1.2% risk is assumed for the ACE patients and VA patients.

[4]No medical arm—assumed from ACAS data.

Reproduced by permission of Barnett HJM, Eliasziw M, Meldrum HE. Prevention of ischaemic stroke. *BMJ* 1999;318:1539–1543.

the degree of stenosis and the presence or absence of symptoms. It was observed that only six patients in NASCET and eight patients in ECST needed to be treated by CE for symptomatic disease with a 70%–99% stenosis. The number reached 19 in NASCET for patients with 50%–69% stenosis. A higher postoperative stroke rate for patients in ECST with moderate disease did not permit an NNT calculation. The numbers in the Veterans Affairs (VA) asymptomatic trial and in ACAS were 48 and 83, respectively. In the ACE study a negative impact was shown and no NNT is calculable. These calculations for asymptomatic subjects do not take into account the fact that the medical risk should be cut in half to consider only likely strokes of large artery origin. When this was done, the NNT became incalculable for the VA and ACAS trials.

REQUIREMENTS FOR AN INSTITUTION PERFORMING CE

The appropriateness of CE in certain circumstances has been established. Expert surgeons, trained and capable of performing CE, and knowledgeable about how to deal with brain ischemia, working with a team of experts in intensive care, and whose anesthetists are familiar with the best neuroanesthetic methods for a brain with compromised circulation, must function as a cohesive team. This cooperation is required to keep the 30-day perioperative morbidity and mortality at a maximum of 7% for death and any stroke (regardless of site and severity). When the degree of disability is evaluated at 90 days, a death and disabling stroke rate of no more than 2% must be achieved. The team must be aware that the first 48 hours are more critical than all the rest of the days making up the 30-day postoperative period combined (Figure 12.7). The surgeons and intensive care staff must be prepared to cope with wound hematoma, wound infections, and the rare life-threatening injury to the vagus nerve that may cause acute dysphagia and aspiration.

Ideally, the team will include a stroke neurologist involved from the early selection of appropriate patients to the conclusion of long-term follow-up. In evaluation of stroke occurrence and in the assessment of its severity, neurologists provide the most reliable data.[43] Such data are necessary to obtain an accurate complication rate for the institution.

The team must be alert to the fact that the common nonstroke medical problems that arise in the postoperative period are of cardiac and respiratory origin.[44] Of 1415 patients treated with CE in NASCET, postoperative fatal and nonfatal myocardial infarction combined with sudden death occurred in only 1.1%. The figure will be higher in the routine practice of CE, where cardiac conditions threatening emboli are not necessarily excluded, as they were in NASCET. Rhythm disorders in this population occurred in 22 patients, of which 11 were nonvalvular atrial fibrillation. New or recurrent angina pectoris occurred in 19 patients. Respiratory complications were the next most common cause of med-

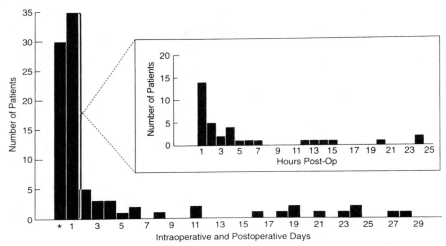

* events occurred intraoperatively

FIGURE 12.7. The time of onset of 92 perioperative outcome events in NASCET. Most strokes occurred during the endarterectomy and within the succeeding 24 hours. Reproduced by permission of *Stroke*.[16]

ical complications ($N = 11$) and most were pneumonia. Pulmonary embolism is a rare event as a sequel to CE. Patients are quickly mobilized. An alert for possible deep vein thrombosis must continue during the hospital period but will be expected in few post-CE patients.

CAROTID ARTERY IMAGING METHODS

The symptomatic patients who entered into the randomized trials were studied by conventional angiography, and diameter stenoses were assigned. It is against these well-defined levels of stenosis that decisions must be made about the potential benefit or lack of benefit from CE. Because no more powerful predictor of prognosis has been identified, and because the differences in prognosis are so striking for different degrees of stenosis, its accurate evaluation is of paramount importance.

Some progress has been made in efforts to determine which of the parameters of ultrasound measurements correspond to the levels of stenosis known from angiography to be within the range of benefit from CE. The correlations will never be exact, because angiography is a measurement to map the lumen, any intrusion into it, or any ulceration within the plaque, while ultrasound is a measurement of the velocity and volume of blood flowing through the artery. Approximations are achievable, but at two important levels of angiographically-measured stenosis, difficulties in correlation between ultrasound and angiography are still encountered: The first is in arteries narrowed by a substantial amount beyond severe stenosis and through which very little blood flows, and the second is in arteries with middle ranges of stenosis in which a close correlation between what is 70% or 50% by angiography and what is assessed by ultrasound would be desirable. In a patient with a severely narrowed artery and collapse of the distal segment, ultrasound may be erroneously misinterpreted because of modest velocity and volume, and the stenosis characterized as moderate. Such a patient would benefit from CE but may be denied the procedure on the basis of these measurements. This mistake is made less often with the additional use of B-mode and color, but it still occurs. In the second situation, the mid-range of stenosis, overreading frequently occurs, and the degree of disease is misinterpreted as sufficiently severe to benefit from CE. This mistake leads to a procedure being applied when the risk posed by the lesion is not sufficient to justify the risk of the operation.

Several reasons are advanced by some practitioners to persuade themselves and their colleagues that angiography can now be replaced by noninvasive studies. Poor angiograms are displayed that have failed to detect a severe stenosis because of failure to take oblique views of the site of the lesion. Such poor imaging is inexcusable, and expert neuroradiologists will not tolerate it. High risk of stroke from angiography is reported.[45] This too is unacceptable and denotes the need for proper training. The reports disclaiming the need for angiography make much of the complications from the procedure. They fail to report the fact that the majority (about 80%) of patients who suffer this complicating stroke make good to excellent recovery, and only one in five patients is left with a disabling stroke.[46] NASCET recorded nondisabling strokes throughout the trial from 2885 angiograms. The nondisabling stroke rate was 0.6%, from which may be extrapolated a risk of disabling stroke of 0.1%. This low risk is a small price to ask patients to pay so that none without an appropriate lesion be submitted to the 20-fold increase of risk from disabling stroke (2%) that confronts patients who undergo CE, even in the best centers.

Cost has been an argument supporting ultrasound as a replacement for conventional angiography. In some centers the cost attached to the performance of angiography and film interpretation is as much as the cost of CE. Moderate savings are not a reason to settle for the second-best in imaging methods. The economic cost of permanent disability resulting from stroke after CE exceed the savings by a wide margin.

Other methods may make conventional angiography obsolete in the future. Furthur improvements may occur in ultrasonography, so that the over-reading in the mid-ranges of stenosis is eliminated and the under-reading in the highest range is overcome. Angiography can then be replaced. To date, this remains a hope. Magnetic resonance imaging over-reads stenosis. When and if the problem of signal void is overcome, another possible replacement for angiography will have emerged. Meanwhile, ultrasound and magnetic resonance imaging are excellent screening tools, but conventional angiography remains desirable as a prelude to CE.

RECOMMENDATIONS

Symptomatic Patients

- CE prevents stroke in the territory of arteries with symptoms related to stenoses of 70%–99%, validated angiographically by the NASCET method of measurement.
- Surgeons who perform the procedure with ≤7% perioperative complication of stroke and death will achieve benefit in the presence of severely stenosed symptomatic lesions.
- Patients with <70% stenosis and appropriate symptoms cannot be assigned automatically to surgical therapy. Careful consideration must be given to all risk factors, as well as to the patients identified as likely to benefit the most.
- Conventional angiography must be seriously considered as a prelude to CE for most patients.

Asymptomatic Subjects

- Individuals with asymptomatic stenosis have not been shown convincingly to benefit from CE.
- The risk with medical therapy in asymptomatic individuals is less than one-third that for symptomatic patients with severe stenosis and one-half that for symptomatic patients with moderate stenosis.
- Approximately half the stroke risk facing the asymptomatic individual is for lacunar or cardioembolic stroke, neither of which are responsive to CE.
- The consensus statement provided by the American Heart Association interprets the data supporting CE for asymptomatic subjects in an optimistic fashion. This statement recommends that all patients with ≥60% asymptomatic stenosis be considered for CE, provided the surgical risk is <3%.[47]
- The authors regard CE for asymptomatic lesions as an overutilized therapeutic strategy. Future investigations of the highest risk subgroups may identify some patients who will benefit convincingly from CE.

REFERENCES

1. Moniz E, Lima A, de l'Acerda R. Hémiplegies Par Thrombose de la Carotide Intere. Presse Med 1937;1:977–980.
2. Hultquist GTJ. Uber Thrombose und Embolie der Arteria Carotis. Stockholm: Norstedt, 1942.

3. Fisher CM. Occlusion of the internal carotid artery. *Arch Neurol Psychiatr Chicago* 1951;65:346–377.
4. Eastcott HHG, Pickering GW, Rob CG. Reconstruction of internal carotid artery in a patient with intermittent attacks of hemiplegia. *Lancet* 1954;2:994–996.
5. Fields WS, Maslenikov V, Meyer JS, Hass WK, Remington RD, Macdonald M. Joint study of extracranial occlusion. V: Progress report of prognosis following surgery or nonsurgical treatment for transient cerebral ischemic attacks and cervical carotid artery lesions. *JAMA* 1970;211:1993–2003.
6. Barnett HJM, Eliasziw M, Meldrum HE, Taylor DW. Do the facts and figures warrant a 10-fold increase in the performance of carotid endarterectomy on asymptomatic patients? *Neurology* 1996;46:603–608.
7. European Carotid Surgery Trialists' Group. Randomised trial of endarterectomy for recently symptomatic carotid stenosis: Final results of the MRC European Carotid Surgery Trial (ECST). *Lancet* 1998;351:1379–1387.
8. Barnett HJM, Taylor DW, Eliasziw M. et al., for the North American Symptomatic Carotid Endarterectomy Trial Collaborators. Benefit of carotid endarterectomy in symptomatic patients with moderate and severe stenosis. *N Engl J Med* 1998:339:1415–1425.
9. Mayberg MR, Wilson SE, Yatsu F, et al. Carotid endarterectomy and prevention of cerebral ischemia in symptomatic carotid stenosis. *JAMA* 1991;266:3289–3294.
10. The CASANOVA Study Group. Carotid surgery versus medical therapy in asymptomatic carotid stenosis. *Stroke* 1991;22:1229–1235.
11. Mayo Asymptomatic Carotid Endarterectomy Study Group. Results of a randomized controlled trial of carotid endarterectomy for asymptomatic carotid stenosis. *Mayo Clin Proc* 1992;67:513–518.
12. Hobson RW II, Weiss DG, Fields WS, Goldstone J, Moore WS, Towne JB, Wright CB and the Veterans Affairs Cooperative Study Group: Efficacy of carotid endarterectomy for asymptomatic carotid stenosis. *N Engl J Med* 1993,328:221–227.
13. Executive Committee for the Asymptomatic Carotid Atherosclerosis Study: Endarterectomy for asymptomatic carotid artery stenosis. *JAMA* 1995;273:1421–1428.
14. Halliday AW, Thomas D, Mansfield A. The asymptomatic carotid surgery trial (ACST) rationale and design. *Eur J Vasc Surg* 1994;8:703–710.
15. Taylor DW, Barnett HJM, Haynes RB, Ferguson GG, Sackett DL, Thorpe KE, Simard D, Silver FL, Hachinski V, Clagett GP, Barnes RW, Spence JD, for the ASA and Carotid Endarterectomy (ACE) Trial Collaborators. Low-dose and high-dose acetylsalicylic acid for patients undergoing carotid endarterectomy: A randomised controlled trial. *Lancet* 1999;353:2179–2184.
16. Ferguson GG, Eliasziw M, Barr HWK, Clagett GP, Barnes RW, Wallace MC, Taylor DW, Haynes RB, Finan JW, Hachinski VC, Barnett HJM, for the North American Symptomatic Carotid Endarterectomy Trial (NASCET) Collaborators. The North American Symptomatic Carotid Endarterectomy Trial: Surgical results in 1415 patients. *Stroke* 1999;30:1751–1758.
17. Henderson R, Eliasziw M, Fox AJ, Rothwell P, Barnett HJM for the North American Symptomatic Carotid Endarterectomy Trial (NASCET) Group. Angiographically-Defined Collateral Circulation and the Risk of Stroke in Patients with Severe Carotid Artery Stenosis. *Stroke* 2000;31:128–132.
18. Kucey DS, Bowyer B, Iron K, Austin P, Anderson G, Tu JV, for the University of Toronto Carotid Study Group. Determinants of outcome after carotid endarterectomy. *J Vasc Surg* 1998;28:1051–1058.

19. Gasecki AP, Eliasziw M, Ferguson GG, Hachinski V, Barnett HJM, for the North American Symptomatic Carotid Endarterectomy Trial (NASCET) Group. Long-term prognosis and effect of endarterectomy in patients with symptomatic severe carotid stenosis and contralateral carotid stenosis or occlusion: Results from NASCET. *J Neurosurg* 1995;83:778–782.

20. Morgenstern LB, Fox AJ, Sharpe BL, Eliasziw M, Barnett HJM, Grotta JC, for the North American Symptomatic Carotid Endarterectomy Trial (NASCET) Group. The risks and benefits of carotid endarterectomy in patients with near occlusion of the carotid artery. *Neurology* 1997;48:911–915.

21. Bornstein NM, Norris JW. Management of patients with asymptomatic neck bruits and carotid stenosis. In: Barnett HJM, Hachinski VC, eds. Neurologic Clinics Cerebral Ischemia: Treatment and Prevention. Philadelphia: W.B. Saunders Company 1992:269–280.

22. Chambers BR, Norris JW. Outcome in patients with asymptomatic neck bruits. *N Engl J Med* 1986;315:860–865.

23. Hennerici M, Hulsbomer HB, Hefter H, Lammerts D, Rautenberg W. Natural history of asymptomatic extracranial arterial disease. *Brain* 1987;110:777–791.

24. Norris JW, Zhu CZ. Stroke risk and critical carotid stenosis. *J Neurol Neurosurg Psychiatry* 1990;53:235–237.

25. Cheung RTF, Chan RKT, Eliasziw M, Rankin RN, Hachinski VC, Barnett HJM, for the NASCET Group. Recurrent stenosis after carotid endarterectomy: How often should follow-up ultrasound be performed? Experience from the North American Symptomatic Carotid Endarterectomy Trial (NASCET). *Neurology* 1996;46(2):A281.

26. Cote R, Battista RN, Abrahamowicz M, Langlois Y, Bourque F, Mackey A. Lack of effect of aspirin in asymptomatic patients with carotid bruits and substantial carotid narrowing: The Asymptomatic Cervical Bruit Study Group. *Ann Intern Med* 1995;123(9):649–655.

27. Chambers BR, Norris JW. The case against surgery for asymptomatic carotid stenosis. *Stroke* 1984;15:964–967.

28. Foster DS. Endarterectomy for asymptomatic carotid artery stenosis (letter to the editor). *JAMA* 1995;274:1505.

29. Goldstein MR. Endarterectomy for asymptomatic carotid artery stenosis. (letter to the editor). *JAMA* 1995;274:1505–1506.

30. Oddone E. Endarterectomy for asymptomatic carotid artery stenosis (letter to the editor). *JAMA* 1995;274:1506.

31. Seiden SW. Endarterectomy for asymptomatic carotid artery stenosis (letter to the Editor). *JAMA* 1995;274:1506.

32. Gorelick PB, Sacco RL, Smith DB, Alberts M, Mustone-Alexander L, Rader D, Ross JL, Raps E, Ozer MN, Brass LM, Malone ME, Goldberg S, Booss J, Hanley DF, Toole JF, Greengold NL, Rhew DC. Prevention of a first stroke: A review of guidelines and a multidisciplinary consensus statement from the National Stroke Association. *JAMA* 1999;281:1112–1120.

33. Warlow C. Endarterectomy for asymptomatic carotid stenosis? *Lancet* 1995;345:1254–1255.

34. The European Carotid Surgery Trialists Collaborative Group. Risk of stroke in the distribution of an asymptomatic carotid artery. *Lancet* 1995;345:209–212.

35. Nicolaides AN. Asymptomatic carotid stenosis and risk of stroke. Identification of a high risk group (ACSRS). A natural history study. *Int Angiol* 1995;14:21–23.

36. Hertzer NR, O'Hara PJ, Mascha EJ, Krajewski LP, Sullivan TM, Beven EG. Early

outcome assessment for 2228 consecutive carotid endarterectomy procedures: The Cleveland Clinic experience from 1989 to 1995. *J Vasc Surg* 1997;26:1–10.

37. Caplan LR. Diagnosis and treatment of ischemic stroke. *JAMA* 1991;266:2413–2418.

38. Caplan LR. TIAs: We need to return to the question "What is wrong with Mr. Jones?" *Neurology* 1988;38:791–793.

39. International Stroke Trial Collaborative Group. The International Stroke Trial (IST): A randomised trial of aspirin, subcutaneous heparin, both, or neither among 19,435 patients with acute ischaemic stroke. *Lancet* 1997;349:1569–1581.

40. Bousser MG. Aspirin or heparin immediately after a stroke? *Lancet* 1997;349:1564–1565.

41. Barnett HJM, Gunton RW, Eliasziw M, Fleming L, Sharpe B, Meldrum H, for the North American Symptomatic Carotid Endarterectomy Trial (NASCET) Group. The causes and severity of ischemic stroke in patients with internal carotid artery stenosis. *JAMA* 2000;283:1429–1436.

42. Inzitari D, Eliasziw M, Sharpe BL, Fox AJ, Barnett HJM, for the North American Symptomatic Carotid Endarterectomy Trial (NASCET) Group. Risk Factors and Outcome of Patients with Carotid Artery Stenosis Presenting with Lacunar Stroke. *Neurology* 2000;54:660–666.

43. Rothwell PM, Slattery J, Warlow CP. A systematic review of the risks of stroke and death due to endarterectomy for symptomatic carotid stenosis. *Stroke* 1996;27:260–265.

44. Paciaroni M, Eliasziw M, Kappelle LJ, Finan JW, Ferguson GG, Barnett HJM, for the North American Symptomatic Carotid Endarterectomy Trial (NASCET) Collaborators. Medical complications associated with carotid endarterectomy. *Stroke* 1999;30:1759–1763.

45. Davies KN, Humphrey PR. Complications of cerebral angiography in patients with symptomatic carotid territory ischaemia screened by carotid ultrasound. *J Neurol Neurosurg Psychiatry* 1993;56:967–972.

46. Hankey GJ, Warlow CP, Sellar RJ. Cerebral angiographic risk in mild cerebrovascular disease. *Stroke* 1990;21:209–222.

47. Biller J., Feinberg WM, Castaldo JE, Whittemore AD, Harbaugh RE, Dempsey RJ, Caplan LR, Kresowik TF, Matchar DB, Toole JF, Easton JD, Adams HP, Brass LM, Hobson RW, Brott TG, Sternau L. Guidelines for carotid endarterectomy: A statement for healthcare professionals from a special writing group of the Stroke Council, American Heart Association. *Stroke* 1998;29:554–562.

48. North American Symptomatic Carotid Endarterectomy Trial Collaborators. Beneficial effect of carotid endarterectomy in symptomatic patients with high-grade carotid stenosis. *N Engl J Med* 1991;325:445–453.

13

ANGIOPLASTY AND STENTING

Martin M. Brown

The treatment of arterial stenosis by percutaneous transluminal angioplasty (PTA) and stenting to prevent stroke has the attraction of avoiding an invasive surgical incision and the general anesthesia usually used for surgical procedures. PTA and stenting are very widely used in the coronary and lower limb vessels to prevent angina, myocardial infarction, and the consequences of peripheral vascular disease. The acceptance of coronary and peripheral PTA reflects an acceptably low complication rate, similar to that of more invasive surgical procedures.

The pathology of atherosclerosis at these sites is very similar to that found in the carotid and vertebral arteries, and yet reluctance persists to recommend PTA for the prevention of stroke because of anxiety about the risks of cerebral embolism. Nevertheless, a number of centers have been using angioplasty and stenting in selected patients with carotid and vertebral stenosis over the last decade, and a large randomized trial comparing carotid surgery with carotid angioplasty, the Carotid and Vertebral Artery Transluminal Angioplasty Study (CAVATAS), has been completed. Most experience relates to the treatment of internal carotid artery stenosis at the carotid bifurcation, and only limited data are available about angioplasty at other sites relevant to the cerebral circulation.

The results of individual case series and the randomized trial suggest that the risks of angioplasty and stenting are similar to those of conventional carotid surgery. Surgery is well-established, while the techniques and devices available for angioplasty and stenting are still evolving, so more evidence is required from randomized trials before angioplasty and stenting will become widely used for stroke prevention. However, the techniques already provide a valuable option in experienced centers for the treatment of patients unsuitable for surgery.

DISADVANTAGES OF CAROTID SURGERY

Surgical endarterectomy has become the standard treatment for severe symptomatic carotid artery stenosis following the publication of the results of the European Carotid Surgery Trial (ECST) and the North American Symptomatic Carotid Endarterectomy Trial (NASCET), but significant morbidity and mortality are associated with carotid surgery. The combined stroke and death rate within 30 days of surgery in patients with severe stenosis was 7.5% in ECST and 5.8% in NASCET.[1,2] Surgery also risks myocardial infarction, deep vein thrombosis, and pulmonary embolism.

The systemic effects of the anesthetic and muscle relaxants and the discomforts of intubation and pneumonia are additional potential complications when general anesthesia is used. Some of these risks can be avoided by using local anesthesia, but this is not popular with many surgeons. Neck dissection and retraction needed to reach the carotid artery may injure cranial nerves, and the wound may be complicated by hematoma and infection. These complications affected 10% of patients after surgery in the ECST.[3] The incision also injures cutaneous nerves and frequently results in numbness around the scar, which may extend up to the face. Keloid scar formation may be troublesome in some patients. Fortunately, few of these complications lead to long-lasting complaints or permanent disability.

Some patients are not suitable for surgery because of severe ischemic heart disease, recent myocardial infarction, uncontrolled hypertension, or other medical risk factors that are contraindications to the procedure. The risk is also increased in women and in patients with contralateral carotid occlusion.[4] In Sundt et al.'s influential study, the presence of major medical risk factors increased the risk of surgery sevenfold.[5] Patients with major risk factors were therefore excluded from recent trials but may be included in routine practice.

Surgery is also more hazardous or impractical at sites such as the distal internal carotid and vertebral arteries, which are not easily or safely accessible to surgery. In these patients, angioplasty and stenting may provide the only alternatives to medical treatment.

Economically, carotid surgery has the disadvantage of being an expensive procedures requiring operating theater time, intensive postoperative care, and a stay in hospital of up to a week, even in uncomplicated cases. Even if discharged after a few days, patients rarely return to full activities until a month after surgery.

ADVANTAGES OF ANGIOPLASTY AND STENTING

The main advantages of the interventional radiology techniques for treating arterial stenosis are the avoidance of a neck incision and avoidance of general anesthesia. The discomfort and local neurological complications from an incision in
the neck, particularly cranial and superficial nerve injury, are avoided, although
hematoma can occur in the groin. Deep vein thrombosis, pneumonia, and myocardial ischemia have not been reported. From the patient's point of view, the
procedure is minor, and if all goes well, involves no more discomfort than a conventional angiogram. The patient is only required to stay in bed overnight after
the procedure and can usually be discharged after 24 hours, resuming normal activities almost immediately.

Angioplasty is usually cheaper than surgery in economic terms, mainly because of shorter hospital stays. However, the cost advantage of angioplasty compared to surgery is reduced if expensive devices, such as stents or protection
devices, are required or if further treatment is needed because of restenosis.

These advantages mean that patients often choose angioplasty over surgery
when given the choice, particularly if they have experienced angioplasty at other
sites. Clinicians offering angioplasty or stenting to a patient must be satisfied that
the complication rates in their unit are not significantly different from those of
surgery, or from medical treatment if the patient is unsuitable for surgery.

TECHNIQUES OF ANGIOPLASTY AND STENTING

Balloon Angioplasty

Standard balloon angioplasty technique consists of inflation of a balloon on the
end of a catheter across the stenosis, with access to the vessel through the femoral
artery in the groin after insertion of a sheath. A standard diagnostic catheter for
neurological procedures is then passed through the sheath, up the femoral artery,
and into the common carotid artery to take views of the stenosis. The diagnostic catheter is then exchanged for a guiding catheter, and a guidewire is carefully
placed across and beyond the stenosis. An inflatable balloon catheter is then
passed over the guidewire and maneuvered to straddle the stenosis. The diameter of the balloon is chosen to match the estimated diameter of the vessel, with
the aim of avoiding overdilation.

For lesions at the carotid bifurcation, the dilated balloon is usually 5–6 mm
(0.2–0.24 in) in diameter and 2 cm (0.8 in) long. The ideal catheter has a low-
profile tip and a rapid deflation time. It is inflated across the stenosis up to five
times to achieve satisfactory dilation. The inflation pressure should be monitored
during the procedure to avoid excessive pressures and overdilation; although there

is no consensus about the ideal pressure, usually less than two atmospheres is used. Inflation time should be less than 10 seconds. Brief total occlusion time limits the risk of hemodynamic ischemia unless the stenosis is so tight that the guidewire occludes the vessel for a longer time. This contrasts with carotid endarterectomy, in which, even if shunts are used, it may take several minutes to insert the shunt after the internal carotid artery has been clamped (see section on hemodynamic ischemia below).

Excellent anatomical results can be achieved after simple balloon dilation, even when the stenosis is very severe (Fig. 13.1), but fill dilation of the artery may not be achieved because of elastic recoil. Progressive spontaneous dilation of the artery over the next few weeks or months may follow the initial suboptimal resid-

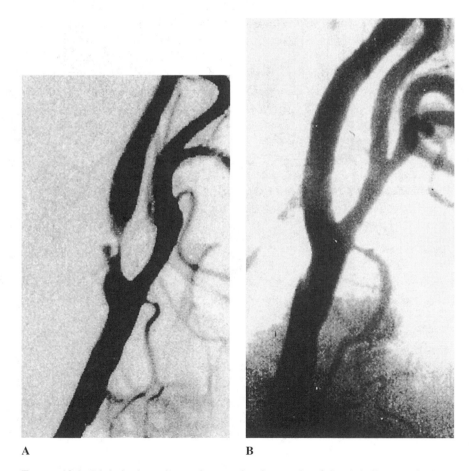

A   B

FIGURE 13.1. Digital subtraction angiogram showing results of simple balloon angioplasty in a patient with severe ulcerated internal carotid artery stenosis. *A*: immediately before angioplasty. *B*: immediately after angioplasty.

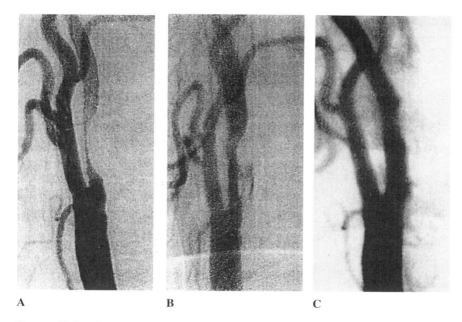

A   B   C

FIGURE 13.2. Digital subtraction angiogram showing remodeling of the arterial wall after a simple balloon angioplasty. *A*: immediately before angioplasty. *B*: immediately after angioplasty with suboptimal dilation and contrast medium within the atheromatous plaque, indicating plaque fissuring. *C*: one year after angioplasty demonstrating remodeling and a widely patent lumen.

ual lumen seen immediately after angioplasty ("remodelling"; Fig. 13.2). In the only angiographic study of this phenomenon after carotid PTA, remodelling was demonstrated in 7 out of 12 cases at one year follow-up.[6] Remodelling only occurred when at least 20% reduction in the severity of stenosis was achieved during the angioplasty procedure.

Stenting

A stent is a collapsed wire mesh inserted into the artery within a catheter or over a balloon and then expanded at the site of stenosis. Various designs of stents are available, including self-expanding and balloon-expandable models. Stents have the advantage of compressing flaps of intimal dissection against the arterial wall and so limiting the size of any embolic material released into the lumen. Stenting improves the appearance after balloon angioplasty, especially if the initial dilation is inadequate or produces dissection (Fig. 13.3). Initially, stenting was only used to "bail out" a poor result after a balloon angioplasty, but it is now the technique of choice in most patients. In primary stenting, no previous balloon dila-

FIGURE 13.3. Digital subtraction angiogram showing the results of stent deployment at the carotid bifurcation.

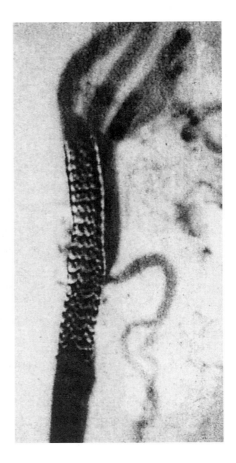

tion is needed, but with severe stenosis, predilatation with a balloon may be needed to allow the stent to cross the stenosis. After deployment of a stent, a balloon catheter can be placed in the stent and inflated if further dilation is required. In the coronary circulation, stenting improves the outcome of angioplasty, and, similarly, primary carotid stenting will probably prove safer than simple balloon angioplasty, since closure of the artery is less likely, especially when dissection or plaque rupture occurs because of the procedure.

Primary stenting aims to minimize the adverse consequencs of dissection or plaque rupture, maintain laminar flow, and prevent any free intimal flaps. In the long term, it is possible that restenosis will be less frequent after stenting than after simple balloon angioplasty. Because of these apparent advantages of stenting, it is likely that primary stenting will be increasingly used in preference to simple balloon angioplasty, even though there are no clinical trials demonstrating the superiority of the technique.

Protection Devices

Theron et al. designed a special triple lumen catheter for a carotid angioplasty to prevent cerebral embolism following disruption of plaque.[7] After introducing the catheter into the common carotid artery, a balloon is inflated beyond the stenosis to occlude the internal carotid artery distally. Next, a balloon dilatation catheter or stent is passed over this catheter and deployed across the stenosis to dilate the lumen. After the balloon or stent has been withdrawn, the third lumen of the introduction catheter is used to withdraw blood and irrigate with saline proximal to the occlusion and so remove any debris. Theron et al. reported cholesterol crystals up to 200 micrometers long in the aspirate using this technique.[7] A technique has also been described in which the carotid artery is occluded by a balloon below the stenosis.[8]

Theron's technique has the disadvantage of using a large introducer catheter, which may not be appropriate for the treatment of very severe stenosis, and the complexity of the procedure increases the hazards. The prolonged total occlusion time of more than 10 minutes increases the chances of hemodynamic ischemia, and the occlusion balloon may add to the risk of thrombosis. However, similar methods are currently undergoing clinical trials.

Carotid Filters

An alternative approach to the triple lumen catheter is to use a filter beyond the stenosis that opens like an umbrella, catching small particles of debris but allowing continuous flow of blood to maintain cerebral perfusion. Afterwards, the "umbrella" is collapsed, enclosing any debris, and then withdrawn across the dilated stenosis. Clinical experience with such filters is very limited, and their effectiveness remains to be determined.

Antithrombotic Regimes

Because of the risk of thromboembolism during carotid PTA and stenting, patients receive intravenous or intra-arterial heparin at the time of the procedure. In early studies, intravenous heparin was continued for at least 24 hours after the procedure, and an antiplatelet agent, often aspirin, was given 24 hours before treatment. Recently, it has been suggested that a combination of ticlopidine or clopidogrel with aspirin may replace heparin. It is possible that these regimes, in turn, will be replaced by more powerful drugs, such as glycoprotein IIb-IIIa antagonists. In some early series, complete anticoagulation was established with warfarin for some weeks before angioplasty to try to remove any thrombus that might be present within the atheromatous plaque. This is not currently recommended as a routine, but anticoagulation for two to four weeks may be a sensible precaution in patients who have had very recent symptoms.

Monitoring

One advantage of carotid PTA and stenting is that the patient remains awake during the procedure, and neurological complications can be easily detected. Simple neurological examinations, blood pressure monitoring, and pulse measurements at regular intervals during the procedure help to ensure that it is proceeding safely. Transcranial Doppler (TCD) to monitor blood flow velocity and to detect embolism in the middle cerebral artery has also been used.

MECHANISMS OF ARTERIAL DILATION

The increase in arterial diameter achieved by angioplasty results from an increase in diameter of the whole vessel, moving the walls outward,[9] and compression or redistribution of the atheromatous plaque does not occur. Experimental studies in animal models have shown that balloon inflation denudes the endothelium, splits atheromatous plaque so that it dehisces from the underlying media, and stretches the media and adventitia. Splitting of the atheromatous plaque appears to be essential for successful angioplasty and is the only way that concentric plaque can be dilated.

The arterial wall injury caused by angioplasty results in the stimulation of fibroblasts and smooth muscle cell replication, and this process continues throughout the following few weeks and possibly months. The process of repair may lead to remodelling of the artery, with an increase in diameter. Early absorption of hematoma within the wall and passive stretching of the artery over time may also contribute to an increase in diameter of the artery after the initial dilation. If the repair process is excessive, then restenosis may occur. Histological examination in one case of restenosis showed excessive smooth muscle proliferation narrowing of the lumen.[10] It is likely that similar pathological changes occur after stenting.

COMPLICATIONS

Splitting the atheromatous plaque, which is often required for successful dilation, produces mechanical complications (Table 13.1). Some intimal dissection is inevitable, usually localized to the area of plaque, but inadvertent subintimal insertion of the guidewire or catheter may produce extensive dissection, causing occlusion or pseudoaneurysm formation.

TABLE 13.1. Complications of Angioplasty and Stenting

ACUTE COMPLICATIONS

Mechanical

Intimal dissection
Aneurysm formation
Arterial spasm
Carotid sinus stimulation
Bradycardia and asystole
Hypotension
Vessel rupture
Balloon rupture

Neurologic

Hemodynamic ischemia
Cerebral embolism
Vessel occlusion

Angiographic

Groin hematoma
Puncture site pain
Contrast reactions
Hemorrhage from anticoagulation
Femoral artery thromboembolism

DELAYED COMPLICATIONS

Cerebral embolism
Vessel occlusion
Restenosis
Stent collapse
Cerebral hemorrhage
Hyperperfusion syndrome

Irritation of the wall of the artery by the guidewire or catheter causes arterial spasm, but this is usually symptomatic only if severe enough to result in thrombus formation. Vessel rupture is very rare but easily recognized by the sudden onset of severe pain in the neck associated with extravasation of contrast media outside the vessel. Balloon inflation or stent deployment at the carotid bifurcation frequently results in stimulation of the carotid sinus, leading to bradycardia and occasionally to brief periods of asystole. To prevent this complication, all patients should be pretreated with atropine to reduce the consequences of receptor stimulation. Hypotension may occasionally be troublesome for 48 hours after the procedure.

The major risks are cerebral embolism and carotid occlusion, occurring mainly in patients with unstable and very stenosed plaques. This present with "crescendo" transient ischemic attacks. Hemodynamic ischemia during the procedure may be responsible for a brief transient attack during balloon inflation, but this rarely leads to stroke.

Occlusion causes major stroke in about 50% of patients. Acute occlusion of the artery may follow hemorrhage into the plaque or be secondary to dissection after angioplasty. It is probable that this complication occurs less often after primary stenting than after simple balloon angioplasty. If occlusion does occur, options for management include immediate thrombolysis with or without stenting, emergency surgical endarterectomy, or conservative management with anticoagulation.

About half of patients experience some brief discomfort in the neck at the site of angioplasty or stenting at the time of the procedure, and occasionally this radiates to the eye and forehead or scapula (carotidynia). This pain is usually short lived and lasts only a few seconds during balloon inflation but occasionally may last up to 48 hours.

Despite the long list of potential complications, most tolerate angioplasty and stenting with little discomfort. Groin hematoma may cause problems, particularly if the stent requires a large introducer sheath, but this complication has been considerably reduced by devices that seal the artery and compress the groin after the procedure.

Occasional angiographic complications occur, including stroke from catheter or guidewire dislodgment of atheroma and thrombus in the aortic arch or major vessel on route to the site of stenosis. Delayed stroke may occur afterward due to either thrombosis on the stent or damaged intima, or as a sequel to dissection. Cerebral hemorrhage unrelated to anticoagulation may occur following successful angioplasty or stenting due to the reperfusion syndrome.[11,12] This occurs after treatment of very severe stenosis with subsequent marked increase in the velocities of flow in the ipsilateral carotid and middle cerebral arteries. Edema or hemorrhage of the ipsilateral cerebral hemisphere may also occur due to failure of autoregulation within the reperfused microcirculation. These delayed complications are unlikely to occur more than 10 days after the procedure.

Among the few long-term complications of angioplasty and stenting, the main concern is restenosis. Approximately 20% of carotid arteries treated by simple balloon angioplasty will have some degree of restenosis at one year by ultrasound examination.[13,14] However, few of those with restenosis become symptomatic, at least in the short term, because restenosis in these cases is due to smooth muscle proliferation and not atheromatous plaque. Restenosis is not, therefore, an indication for intervention, unless the patient is symptomatic. Symptoms are more likely to be caused by hemodynamic, rather than embolic, mechanisms, especially if associated with contralateral carotid occlusion.[10]

The restenosis rate of stenting is as yet unknown. Collapse of the stent may produce severe stenosis, possibly due to pressure on the neck deforming it, and new stents are being designed to avoid this complication.

Unlike surgery, with angioplasty and stenting the athermatous plaque remains, with its potential for recurrent ulceration and further growth, although the endothelial proliferative following the procedure may prevent this. There is insufficient long-term follow-up of patients treated by angioplasty or stenting beyond a few years, but available evidence suggests that, in the long term, recurrence of symptoms is unusual and probably no more frequent than after carotid surgery.

RESULTS IN CASE SERIES

Small case series of patients with athermatous carotid stenosis treated by balloon angioplasty first appeared nearly 20 years ago, but the procedure was limited to a small number of centers. Even in 1992, a review of all the published cases reported a total of only 123 patients with atheromatous internal carotid artery stenosis.[15] It was not until the 1990s that larger series were published[8,16–24] (see Table 13.2). Stroke and death rates from the procedure were similar to those of carotid

TABLE 13.2. Selected Series of Patients Treated by Carotid Angioplasty and/or Stenting

	NUMBER OF PATIENTS	STROKE OR DEATH RATE WITHIN 30 DAYS (%)
Balloon angioplasty		
Munari et al. 1992[16]	44	9.1
Eckert et al. 1996[17]	61	4.9
Gil-Peralta et al. 1996[18]	82	4.9
Balloon angioplasty with cerebral protection		
Kachel 1996[8]	74	3.1
Theron et al. 1996[19]	43	5.0
Stenting with cerebral protection		
Theron et al. 1996[19]	93	2.0
Stening alone		
Diethrich et al. 1996[20]	110	6.4
Wholey et al. 1997[21]	108	3.7
Waigand et al. 1998[22]	50	4.0
Henry et al. 1998[23]	163	3.1
Mathur et al. 1998[24]	231	6.9

Only series including more than 40 patients published in major peer reviewed journals are included.

surgery. At present, little evidence indicates that stents are superior to balloon angioplasty alone, with the possible exception of the study by Theron et al.[19] In a survey of 24 centers throughout the world up to 1998, a total of 2048 endovascular carotid stent procedures were reported, with a stroke and death rate of 5.8% within 30 days.[25] However, few case reports have been published that provide adequate information about long-term follow-up beyond 6 to 12 months. In the short term, very few recurrent strokes are described, suggesting that angiography and stenting are effective at preventing stroke after a successful procedure.

A number of potential biases are inherent in these data. Patients with carotid bifurcation lesions are likely to be highly selected, leading to a false underestimation of the risks. At least 40% of the cases in the stent studies were asymptomatic, while many had restenosis after carotid endarterectomy. Few studies adequately describe the degree of stenosis, and some patients may have had relatively mild narrowing. Also, case studies with poor results are unlikely to be reported. Conversely, patients referred for angioplasty and stenting because surgery was contraindicated may have above-average risks.[24]

Most reports of these procedures concern carotid bifurcation due to stenosis, either from atherosclerosis or restenosis following previous carotid endarterectomy. Other forms of carotid artery stenosis treated by PTA include fibromuscular dysplasia,[26] Takayasu's arteritis,[26,27] common carotid, external carotid artery stenosis, and distal internal carotid lesions too high in the neck to be surgically accessible.[28–30] Treatment of intracranial stenosis in the distal carotid, distal vertebral, basilar, and middle cerebral arteries is usually considered too hazardous, but has been attempted.[30–34]

Vertebral artery stenosis, particularly at the origin of the vertebral artery from the arch of the aorta, is relatively easy to treat by angioplasty or stenting. However, only a small number of case series have been reported in the literature, all with very low complication rates.[35] The limited number of cases presumably reflects the relative rarity of vertebrobasilar symptoms in comparison to carotid disease and the limited value of noninvasive investigations, such as ultrasound and magnetic resonance angiography, in detecting vertebral artery stenosis.[36] A larger series of patients with subclavian stenosis, sometimes associated with subclavian steal, have been treated successfully by angioplasty or stenting with a very low complication rate, but neurological details are almost universally lacking from these reports.

RANDOMIZED TRIALS

Only two randomized trials of angioplasty or stenting for stroke prevention have been reported. The first was a single-center study from Leicester, England, but the trial was stopped after only 17 patients had been treated because 5 of 7 treated by stenting had a stroke at the time of the procedure.[37] These poor results may reflect poor radiologic technique. The second trial was the Carotid and Vertebral Artery Transluminal Angioplasty Study (CAVATAS),[38] which compared carotid and vertebral PTA to conventional treatment in 560 patients in Australia, Canada, the United States, and other countries in Europe between 1992 and 1997. The published analysis was restricted to those with carotid stenosis suitable for surgery, randomized between PTA (balloon angioplasty or stenting, 251 patients) and carotid surgery (253 patients). Almost all the patients were recently symptomatic, and baseline variables were well matched (Table 13.3).

These patients had a high incidence of vascular risk factors and twice the prevalence of ischemic heart disease of those in the European Carotid Surgery Trial, and most patients had severe carotid stenosis. Because stents were introduced only during the last few years of the study, only 22% of patients received them; most patients were treated by balloon angioplasty. The rate of disabling stoke was virtually identical, at 5.9% in the surgical group and 6.0% in the angioplasty group, and, similarly, the rate of all strokes or death within 30 days of treatment was 9.9% in the surgical group and 10% in the angioplasty group (Table 13.4). CAVATAS counted only strokes lasting more than 7 days in order to match the criterion used in the European Carotid Surgery Trial and to avoid bias related to the fact that the majority of PTAs were carried out under local anaesthetic on neurological wards, while surgery was mostly carried out under general anesthesia on surgical wards without immediate neurological assessment.

PTA was found safer than surgery for minor morbidity, including cranial or peripheral nerve palsy (9% in the surgical group and none in the PTA group), as well as major adverse events, such as myocardial infarction and angina (2% in the surgical group and none in the PTA group). Hematomas prolonging hospital stay were more common in the surgical patients (7% compared to 2%).

TABLE 13.3. Baseline Variables in Patients with Carotid Stenosis Fit for Surgery, Randomized in CAVATAS ($n = 504$)

RISK FACTOR	PERCUTANEOUS TRANSLUMINAL ANGIOPLASTY	SURGERY
Mean age (years)	66.9	67.1
Male sex	69%	70%
Mean ipsilateral stenosis[1]	86%	85%
Smoker (at any time)	76%	76%
Hypertension	53%	58%
Ischemic heart disease	38%	37%
Previous MI	19%	17%
Peripheral vascular disease	24%	20%
Diabetes mellitus	14%	13%

[1]Common carotid method.

TABLE 13.4. Major Outcome Events in Patients with Carotid Stenosis Fit for Surgery Randomized in CAVATAS, Analyzed by Intention to Treat. (Values are percentages.)

	PERCUTANEOUS TRANSLUMINAL ANGIOPLASTY (n = 251)	SURGERY (n = 253)
Death	2.8	1.6
Disabling stroke	3.6	4.3
Nondisabling stroke[1]	3.6	4.0
Disabling stroke or death	6.4	5.9
All strokes[1] or death	10.0	9.9

[1]More than 7 days duration.
No difference were statistically different.

Long-term follow-up in CAVATAS showed no difference in stroke rate for up to three years after treatment. Survival analysis showed no difference in any major outcome events between the two groups, and the survival curves for ipsilateral stroke showed that both treatments were equally effective at preventing stroke over the time course of the studies, with virtually no ipsilateral strokes after the postoperative period (Fig. 13.4).

At a mean follow-up of 12 months, 19% of PTA patients had >70% stenosis or occlusion by ultrasound criteria, compared to only 5% of surgical patients, but

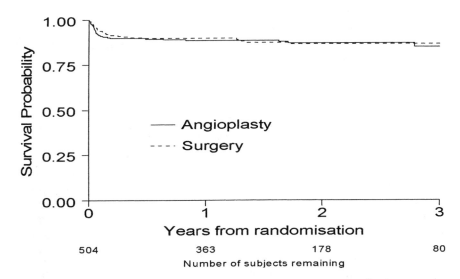

FIGURE 13.4. Kaplan-Meier survival curves in patients with carotid stenosis fit for surgery randomized in CAVATAS showing rate of ipsilateral stroke (>7 days duration). There is no significant difference between the curves.

this restenosis was rarely symptomatic. Some patients initially randomized to angioplasty but in whom the procedure was technically unsuccessful then went on to carotid surgery.

Little difference in quality of life resulted after these two procedures. Also, the procedural costs of these two techniques were similar, but angioplasty was more cost beneficial due to the shorter length of hospital stay.[39] The use of more expensive radiologic devices or shortening the length of surgical stay might abolish the cost advantages of stenting.

A relatively high rate of stroke or death occurred in the CAVATAS study, and although it was similar to the data of the ECST trial, it included patients with higher surgical risks than average, especially those with ischemic heart disease. There was some evidence in CAVATAS that stenting was safer than balloon angioplasty, but the numbers were small and further studies of stenting are needed.

The 30-day risk of stroke or death in CAVATAS was 10%, and the wide confidence limits of 5%–15% emphasize the imprecision of the findings. Although no evident difference was seen between surgery and stenting, with larger numbers a clinically important difference might emerge. Further trials of the procedure are therefore needed.

HEMODYNAMIC AND EMBOLIC CONSEQUENCES

Cerebral hemodynamics evaluations using transcranial Doppler (TCD) indicated a variety of effects following carotid stenting, and one study showed a 30% increase in CO_2 reactivity in the ipsilateral hemisphere, indicating improved vasodilator capacity secondary to improved perfusion pressure.[40] Severe reductions in middle cerebral artery blood flow at the time of PTA may be associated with hemodynamic symptoms.[41] This improvement was gradual over the first four weeks, presumably reflecting the process of remodelling occurring in the days after angioplasty.

Microembolic signals detected by TCD were frequent during carotid angioplasty,[42,43] although the cause of these signals is uncertain, varying from particulate matter to air bubbles. Numerous high-intensity signals occur during routine carotid angiography as a result of small bubbles in the contrast medium, and many of the embolic signals during carotid angioplasty are likely to represent similar air bubbles.[44]

More embolic signals are seen during and immediately after carotid angioplasty than after carotid surgery.[43] (Table 13.5). Although the duration of carotid occlusion and reduced blood flow in the middle cerebral artery to <30% were greater during surgery, no correlation was found between either this, the number of emboli, or clinical complications.

Microemboli are usually asymptomatic, and the duration of the signals suggests that most are very small and will only occlude the smallest capillaries,

TABLE 13.5. Randomized Comparison of Embolic Signals and Ischemic Time During Carotid Surgery and Percutaneous Transluminal Angioplasty Detected by Transcranial Doppler of the Ipsilateral Middle Cerebral Artery (Adapted from ref. 43.)

	SURGERY	PERCUTANEOUS TRANSLUMINAL ANGIOPLASTY
Number of patients	14	14
Mean occlusion time (sec $\pm$ SD)	337 $\pm$ 64	19 $\pm$ 8[1]
Number with reduced CBF[2]	7	6
Mean ischemic time (sec $\pm$ SD)	334 $\pm$ 83	23 $\pm$ 7[1]
Number of microemboli	53 $\pm$ 64	187 $\pm$ 117[3]

[1]$p < 0.0001$.
[2]MCA flow $<33\%$ of baseline.
[3]$p < 0.001$.

though they potentially could produce subclinical cerebral damage. However, in one study, no significant differences were detected in neuropsychological outcome after carotid surgery compared to carotid angioplasty.[44]

THE FUTURE OF ANGIOPLASTY AND STENTING

The risks of PTA and stenting are similar to those of carotid surgery but avoid the problems of surgical incision and anesthesia. Before this technique becomes accepted as routine treatment, however, data from randomized clinical trials are essential. Currently, several such trials are in progress or planned, and advances in technology, particularly the development of filter and other protection devices, are likely to improve the safety and applicability of PTA and stenting. Other potential advances in balloon technology include the local delivery of anticoagulant agents to reduce the chances of thrombosis and other drugs that may inhibit smooth muscle proliferation and limit restenosis.

Until the results of further clinical trials are available, interventional treatment should be restricted to specialised centers with demonstrated low complication rates and to the discipline of clinical trials. Despite understandable opposition from some vascular surgeons, it is likely that cerebrovascular PTA will eventually join coronary and peripheral PTA as a major first-line treatment for atheromatous cerebrovascular disease.

REFERENCES

1. European Carotid Surgery Trialists Collaboration Group. MRC European Carotid Surgery Trial: Interim results for symptomatic patients with severe (70–99%) or with mild (0–29%) carotid stenosis. *Lancet* 1991;337:1235–1243.

2. North American Symptomatic Carotid Endartectomy Trial Collaborators. Beneficial effect of carotid endarterectomy in symptomatic patients with high-grade carotid stenosis. *N Engl J Med.* 1991;325:445–453.

3. Rothwell P. Morbidity and mortality of carotid endarterectomy in the European Carotid Surgery Trial. *Cerebrovascular Diseases* 1995;4:226.

4. Rothwell PM, Slattery J, Warlow CP. Clinical and angiographic predictors of stroke and death from carotid endarterectomy. *BMJ* 1997;315:1591–1597.

5. Sundt TM, Sandok BA, Whisnant JP. Carotid endarterectomy: Complications and pre-operative assessment of risk. *Mayo Clin Proc* 1975;50:301–306.

6. F Crawley, A Clifton, H Markus, M M Brown. Delayed improvement in carotid ar-tery diameter after carotid angioplasty. *Stroke* 1997;28:575–579.

7. Theron J, Coutheouz P, Alachkar F, Bouvard G, Maiza D. New triple coaxial catheter system for carotid angioplasty with cerebral protection. *American Journal of Neuro-radiology* 1990;11:869–874.

8. Kachel-R. Results of balloon angioplasty in the carotid arteries. *J Endovasc Surg* 1996;3:22–30.

9. Castaneda-Zuniga WR, Formanek A, Tadavarthy M, et al. The mechanisms of bal-loon angioplasty. *Radiology* 1980;135:565–571.

10. F Crawley, A Clifton RS Taylor, MM Brown. Symptomatic restenosis after carotid percutaneous transluminal angioplasty. *Lancet* 1998;352:708–709.

11. Schoser BG, Heesen C, Eckert B, Thie A. Cerebral hyperperfusion injury after per-cutaneous transluminal angioplasty of extracranial arteries. *J Neurol* 1997;244:101–104.

12. McCabe DJH, Brown MM, Clifton A. Fatal cerebral reperfusion hemorrhage follow-ing carotid stenting. *Stroke* 1999;30:2483–2486.

13. Madrid A, Gil-Peralta A, Gonzalez-Marcos JR, Otero A, Crespo P. Restenosis and re-modeling after percutaneous transluminal carotid angioplasty. *Rev Neurol* 1998;27:649–652.

14. Schoser BG, Becker VU, Eckert B, Zeumer H, Thie A. Clinical and ultrasonic long-term results of percutaneous transluminal carotid angioplasty: A prospective follow-up of 30 carotid angioplasties. *Cerebrovascular Diseases* 1998;8:38–41.

15. Brown MM. Balloon angioplasty for cerebrovascular disease. *Neurol Res* 1992;14(suppl):159–173.

16. Munari LM, Belloni G, Perretti A, Gatti A, Moschini L, Porta M. Carotid percuta-neous angioplasty. *Neurol Res* 1992;14(suppl):156–158.

17. Eckert B, Zanella FE, Thie A, Steinmetz J, Zeumer H. Angioplasty of the internal carotid artery: Results, complications and follow-up in 61 cases. *Cerebrovascular Dis-eases* 1996;6:97–105.

18. Gil-Peralta A, Mayol A, Marcos JR, Gonzalez A, Ruano J, Boza F, Duran F. Percu-taneous transluminal angioplasty of the symptomatic atherosclerotic carotid arteries: Results, complications, and follow-up. *Stroke* 1996;27:2271–2273.

19. Theron JG, Payelle GG, Coskun O, Huet HF, Guimaraens L. Carotid artery stenosis: Treatment with protected balloon angioplasty and stent placement. *Radiology* 1996;201:27–36.

20. Diethrich EB, Ndiaye M, Reid DB. Stenting in the carotid artery: Initial experience in 110 patients. *J Endovasc Surg* 1996;3:42–62.

21. Wholey MH, Wholey MH, Jarmolowski CR, Eles G, Levy D, Buecthel J. Endovas-cular stents for carotid artery occlusive disease. *J Endovasc Surg* 1997;4:326–338.

22. Waigant J, Gross CM, Uhlich F, Kramer J, Tamaschke C, Vogel P, Luft FC, Dietz R.

Elective stenting of carotid artery stenosis in patients with severe coronary artery disease. *Eur Heart J* 1998;19:1365–1370.

23. Henry M, Amor M, Masson I, Henry I, Tzvetanov K, Chati Z, Khanna N. Angioplasty and stenting of the extracranial carotid arteries. *J Endovasc Surg* 1998;5: 293–304.

24. Mathur A, Roubin GS, Iyer SS, Piamsonboon C, Liu MW; Gomez CR, Yadav JS, Chastain HD, Fox LM, Dean LS, Vitek JJ. Predictors of stroke complicating carotid artery stenting. *Circulation* 1998;97:1239–1245.

25. Wholey MH, Wholey M, Bergeron P, Diethrich EB, Henry M, Laborde JC, Mathias K, Myla S, Roubin GS, Shawl F, Theron JG, Yadav JS, Dorros G, Guimaraens J, Higashida R, Kumar V, Leon M, Lim M, Londero H, Mesa J, Ramee S, Rodriguez A, Rosenfield K, Teitelbaum G, Vozzi C. Current global status of carotid artery stent placement. *Cathet Cardiovasc Diagn* 1998;44:1–6.

26. Mathias KD. Percutaneous transluminal angioplasty in supra-aorta artery disease. In: Roubin GS, ed. Internventional Cardiovascular Medicine: Principles and Practice. New York: Churchill Livingstone, 1994:745–775.

27. Tsai FY, Matovich V, Hieshima G, et al. Percutaneuous transluminal angioplasty of the carotid artery. *Am J Neuroradiol* 1986;7:349–358.

28. Rostmily RC, Mayberg MR, Eskridge JM, Goodkin R, Winn HR. Resolution of petrous internal carotid artery stenosis after transluminal angioplasty: Case report. *J Neurosurg* 1992;76:520–523.

29. O'Leary DH, Clouse ME. Percutaneous transluminal angioplasty of the cavernous carotid artery for recurrent ischemia. *Am J Neuroradiol* 1994;5:644.

30. Tsai FY, Higashida R, Meoli C. Percutaneous transluminal angioplasty of extracranial and intracranial arterial stenosis in the head and neck. *Interventional Neuroradiology* 1992;2:371–384.

31. Mori T, Mori K, Fukuoka M, Arisawa M, Honda S. Percutaneous transluminal cerebral angioplasty: Serial angiographic follow-up after successful dilatation. *Neuroradiology* 1997;39:111–116.

32. Takis C, Kwan ES, Pessin MS, Jacobs DH, Caplan LR. Intracranial angioplasty: Experience and complications. *Am J Neuroradiol* 1997;18:1661–1668.

33. Yokote H, Terada T, Ryujin K, Konoshita Y, Tsuura M, Nakai E, Kamei I, Moriwaki H, Hayashi S, Itakura T. Percutaneous transluminal angioplasty for intracranial arteriosclerotic lesions. *Neuroradiology.* 1998;40:590–596.

34. Eckard DA, Zarnow DM, McPherson CM, Siegel EL, Eckard VR, Batnitzky S, Hermreck A. Intracranial internal carotid artery angioplasty: Technique with clinical and radiographic results and follow-up. *Am J Roentgenol* 1999;172:703–707.

35. Higashida RT, Tsai FY, Halbach V, et al. Transluminal angioplasty for atherosclerotic disease for the vertebral and basilar arteries. *J Neurosurg* 1993;78:192–198.

36. Crawley F, Clifton A, Brown MM. Treatable lesions demonstrated on vertebral angiography for posterior circulation ischemic events. *Br J Radiol* 1998;71:1266–1270.

37. Naylor AR, Bolia A, Abbott RJ, Pye IF, Smith M, Lennard N, Lloyd AJ, London NJ, Bell PR. Randomized study of carotid angioplasty and stenting versus carotid endarterectomy: A stopped trial. *J Vasc Surg* 1998;28:326–334.

38. The CAVATAS Investigators. Carotid and Vertebral Artery Transluminal Angioplasty Study (CAVATAS): results in patients with carotid artery stenosis randomised between surgery and angioplasty. Submitted to Lancet

39. Davies A, Buxton M, Brown MM. An economic evaluation of the cost effectiveness of carotid angioplasty and stenting compared with surgery in patients with carotid

stenosis randomised in The Carotid and Vertebral Artery Transluminal Angioplasty Study (CAVATAS). Submitted for publication.

40. Markus HS, Clifton A, Brown MM. Carotid Angioplasty: Haemodynamic and embolic consequences. *Cerebrovascular Diseases* 1994;4:259.

41. Eckert B, Thie A, Valdueza J, Zanella F, Zeumer H. Transcranial Doppler sonographic monitoring during percutaneous transluminal angioplasty of the internal carotid artery. *Neuroradiology* 1997;39:229–234.

42. Markus HS, Clifton A, Buckenham T, Brown MM. Carotid angioplasty: Detection of embolic signals during and after the procedure. *Stroke* 1994;25:2403–2406.

43. Crawley F, Clifton A, Buckenham T, Loosemore T, Taylor RS, Brown MM. Comparison of hemodynamic cerebral ischemia and microembolic signals detected during carotid endarterectomy and carotid angioplasty. *Stroke* 1997;28:2460–2464.

44. Crawley F, Stygall J, Lunn S, Harrison M, Brown MM, Newman S. Comparison of microembolism detected by transcranial Doppler and neuropsychological sequelae of carotid surgery and percutaneous transluminal angioplasty. Stroke 2000;31:1329–1334.

III

PREVENTION: POLICY AND PRACTICE

14

STROKE PREVENTION: A GLOBAL PERSPECTIVE

Ruth Bonita

Cerebrovascular disease (stroke) is the second leading cause of death worldwide, responsible for approximately 9.5% of all deaths.[1] Despite almost 50 years of epidemiologic research and increasing knowledge about appropriate intervention, the global burden of stroke is still rising, with most of the stroke deaths now occurring in the poorer regions of the world. Although many lessons have been learned, the strategies adopted to date have been only partially effective in preventing and controlling the stroke epidemic.

Given the increasingly global nature of stroke, a global response is required. This chapter describes the dimensions of the global burden of stroke, its evolution, and its several patterns; summarizes current understanding of the determinants of stroke at both the individual and population levels; and identifies appropriate policies for the primary prevention and control of stroke, with a specific focus on developing countries.

THE GLOBAL BURDEN OF STROKE

Information on the global stroke burden that is of value for public health purposes comes from routine sources as well as specific epidemiologic and clinical studies. Despite many decades of research into stroke and cardiovascular disease

(CVD), there is still a surprisingly limited amount of reliable data on the global situation. In particular, there is a shortage of information from poorer regions and countries; most of the available data comes from developed countries. In addition, some difficulties remain in interpreting routine mortality data because of changes over time in national boundaries and in diagnostic, certification, and coding practices. However, good evidence indicates that the overall secular trends apparent in these data are real.[2]

A particular shortage of routine mortality information exists for much of Asia and Africa. Several eastern provinces of China are now collecting mortality data on a routine basis. A nationally representative system of 145 disease surveillance points covering about 1% of the Chinese population provides reliable statistics on death and disease.[3] In several countries, including India, the "verbal autopsy" method has been used by health workers who interview families of the deceased to estimate cause-specific mortality.[4] But for much of the world, it has been necessary to use extrapolation methods to estimate overall, age, sex, and cause-specific mortality rates. Most of the estimates of the global burden of stroke come from the Global Burden of Disease (GBD) study,[5] and the empirical data on which it is based are limited. However, less than one-third of the world's population is covered by national vital registration systems.

Mortality Patterns

Stroke was responsible for approximately 5.1 million of the total 16.7 million cardiovascular disease deaths in 1998.[1] Of these deaths, 4.2 million occurred in the poorer regions of the world, which are still experiencing a major burden of communicable diseases, the so-called "double burden" of disease. In Asian countries, such as Japan and China, stroke is the leading cause of death, in contrast to most developed countries where stroke is the third leading cause of death. In absolute numbers, almost as many strokes occur in China as in all developed countries combined.

The national burden of stroke and cardiovascular disease in general varies enormously depending on the social, economic, and cultural characteristics of the country. The tremendous variation in stroke mortality rates at the national level for 15 selected countries is shown in Figure 14.1.

The highest total mortality rates for both men and women are in central and eastern European countries, especially those of the former Soviet Union. In all countries, the total mortality rates are higher in men than in women. The ranking of countries is similar in men and women. The pattern is remarkably similar to the total mortality league tables, suggesting that stroke mortality variations are likely to be real and not explained by a shift from one category to another.

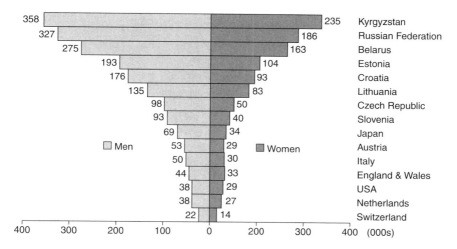

FIGURE 14.1. Age standardized (per 100,000) stroke mortality rates, selected countries, women and men aged 40–69 years, 1997.

Incidence and Case Fatality

The best international stroke incidence data comes from the WHO MONICA Project, which has used standardized methods to monitor the trends and determinants of CVD in 37 defined populations in 21 countries, all of which, except China, are developed countries.[6] As part of the MONICA Project, stroke incidence was monitored in 15 populations in 10 countries in the age group 35–64 years.[7] In a 10-year period, 86,000 acute strokes were registered. The highest stroke rates were found in Russia and Finland, which were more than three-fold higher than in Friuli, Italy, the population with the lowest rate. In half the populations studied, the stroke incidence was twice as high in men as in women.[8] For many MONICA populations, good agreement exists between stroke mortality statistics and fatal cases in the stroke register, although this is probably a reflection of "false positive" and "false negative" cases being of roughly equal numbers in the routine mortality statistics.[9] Case fatality at 28 days after a stroke in the MONICA populations ranged from 12% to 47%; the higher case fatality rates are probably a reflection of under-ascertainment of nonfatal strokes in the local register.

Disability

Various measures have been used to estimate the burden of stroke disability. Most recently, the GBD project used Disability Adjusted Life Years Lost (DALY) to

TABLE 14.1. Distribution of Deaths Due to Stroke by Region, 1990[5]

REGION		ESTIMATED STROKE DEATHS n (000s) 1990	ESTIMATED STROKE DEATHS % 1990	CARDIOVASCULAR	% OF ALL CARDIOVASCULAR
AFRO		449	8.8	998	45.0
AMRO	High income	281	5.5	1125	25.0
	Low and middle income	298	5.8	945	31.5
EMRO	Low and middle income	298,198	3.9	1097	18.0
EURO	High income	198,449	8.8	1802	24.9
	Low and middle income	449,817	16.0	2855	28.6
SEARO	India	557	10.9	2820	19.8
	Other low and middle income	325	6.4	1102	29.5
WPRO	High income	161	3.2	650	14.8
China		1467	28.7	2951	497
Other low and middle income		104	2.0	355	30.6
World		5106	100%	16,700	

World Health Report 1999: Making a Difference. Geneva: WHO, 1999.

AFRO, African region; AMRO, American region; EMRO, Eastern Mediterranean region; EURO, European region; SEARO, South East Asian region; WPRO, Western Pacific region.

estimate the global and regional burden of disease, including stroke. The DALY combines premature loss of life with years of life spent disabled to assess the overall and cause-specific burden of disease. The measured disease burden is the gap between a population's health status and that of an optimal, but perhaps unrealistic, reference population. The GBD study is a major advance, in that it has produced an internally consistent set of disease burden estimates for the entire world. At the same time, it has emphasized the extreme shortage of basic mortality and disease prevalence data for most of the world. In fact, because of the need to extrapolate from very limited data to whole regions, for example, Sub-Saharan Africa, it appears that some regional estimates of CVD burden may be misleading.[10] The GBD results have also given rise to criticism, especially concerning the use of DALYs rather than other types of quality adjusted life years.[11] The GBD study is revising estimates as data become available.

Overall, stroke is estimated to be the sixth leading cause of DALYs worldwide, responsible for 3.0% of all DALYs globally in 1998. The distribution of DALYs due to stroke by region for 1990 is shown in Table 14.2.[12] The contribution to DALYs by stroke varies by region, from 23% of the total in former socialist economies to 4% of the total in sub-Saharan Africa.

It has been projected that stroke will move from sixth place to fourth place as a cause of disability as measured by DALYs. These projections from the GBD study indicate that the coming epidemic of stroke disability will occur in the developing regions of the world.

As the CVD epidemic increases in developing countries, they will experience an economic burden comparable to that now experienced by developed countries. This economic burden will impose serious restrictions on the development capability of many developing countries, and they will be unable to afford the expensive, technological approach to CVD management already adopted by developed countries.

EVOLUTION OF GLOBAL STROKE EPIDEMICS

Health Transition

The health transition is a useful framework for describing the spectacular shifts in the patterns and causes of death that have taken place in all countries over the last few centuries. The health transition consists of three phases: the era of pestilence and famine (early), the era of receding pandemics (middle), and the era of noncommunicable diseases (late). A fourth stage has also been suggested, described as the era of delayed noncommunicable (or degenerative) disease. The health transition describes the changes in both overall pattern of causes of death and the changes within these broad categories. Four stages of the stroke transition are discernible.[13] In the early phase, stroke is more common than heart dis-

TABLE 14.2. Distribution of DALYs Due to Stroke by Region, 1998

REGION		ESTIMATED STROKE DALYS n (000s) 1990	ESTIMATED STROKE DALYS % 1990	CARDIOVASCULAR	% OF ALL CARDIOVASCULAR
AFRO		4894	11.8	11,744	41.7
AMRO	High income	1651	4.0	6109	27.0
	Low and middle income	2830	6.8	8763	32.3
EMRO	Low and middle income	2244	5.4	13,617	16.5
EURO	High income	2554	6.1	9553	26.7
	Low and middle income	5411	13.0	19,807	27.3
SEARO	India	4814	11.6	26,932	17.9
	Other low and middle income	3272	7.9	12,728	25.7
WPRO	High income	986	2.4	3670	26.9
China		11,906	28.6	24,824	48.0
Other low and middle income		1062	2.6	4269	24.9
World		41,624	100.0%	142,016	29.3%

AFRO, African region; AMRO, American region; EMRO, Eastern Mediterranean region; EURO, European region; SEARO, South East Asian region; WPRO, Western Pacific region.

ease, and hemorrhagic stroke more common than atherothrombotic. In the next
stage, one sees an increasing percentage of atherothrombotic stroke and the emer-
gence of heart disease. In the later phases of the health transition, heart disease
becomes more common than stroke. And in the final phase, which is now being
reached in developed countries, CVD death rates decrease, stroke becomes
concentrated in the age group over 65 years, and life expectancy increases into
the 80s.

Trends in Stroke Mortality

The best data on the recent evolution of the CVD epidemic come from the WHO
mortality database, which has reliable data for 35 (mostly developed) countries
since the early 1950s. These data cover less than one-third of the world's population. Based on data from the WHO database, stroke mortality rates have been
declining rapidly in most countries, especially since the mid-1970s (Figure 14.2).
Spectacular declines in mortality rates have occurred in Japan up to 7% on average per year. Stroke rates in Japan, which in the 1950s were the highest in the
world, are now similar to those in most western European countries.

Stroke rates in some eastern European countries were increasing until the
1980s. Within the region of the Americas, of 15 countries for which trend data
are available, stroke rates declined in all but four countries.[14] Declines in mortality are not necessarily associated with improvements in morbidity, disability,
and quality of life. In most populations, the mortality trends were similar or larger

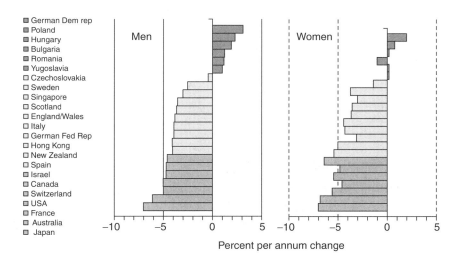

FIGURE 14.2. Change (% per year) in stroke rates, selected countries, men and women,
1970–1993.

TABLE 14.3. Ten Leading Causes of DALYs, 2020

RANK	CAUSE	DALY (% OF ALL DALYS)
1	Ischemic heart disease	5.9
2	Unipolar major depression	5.7
3	Road traffic accidents	5.1
4	Cerebrovascular disease	4.4
5	COPD	4.1
6	Lower respiratory infections	3.1
7	Tuberculosis	3.1
8	War	3.0
9	Diarrheal diseases	2.7
10	HIV	2.6

Source: World Health Report.

COPD, chronic obstructive pulmonary disease.

than the corresponding attack rate trends. In both men and women, mortality decreased in most of the populations from western Europe, while nearly all the populations from central and eastern Europe had an increasing mortality.

These declines in mortality in most developed countries are such that fewer stroke deaths occur now than 25 years ago, despite the growth of the older population during that time. For example, approximately 110,000 fewer stroke deaths now occur each year in the United States than was projected based on the rates in the mid-1970s (Figure 14.3).

The profile of stroke patients has also changed in those countries experiencing a decline in stroke mortality: fewer premature stroke deaths has shifted the average age at time of stroke death upwards. The other impact of these improvements in death rates is that an individual's risk of dying from a stroke has fallen con-

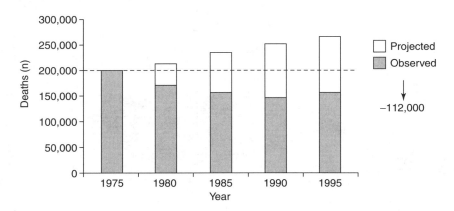

FIGURE 14.3. Decline in absolute number of deaths in the United States, 1975–1995.

siderably for both men and women; the lifetime risk of having a stroke is higher in women than in men because, on average, women live longer than men. The lifetime risk for men in the United States has declined from 11% in the 1950s to less than 6% in the 1990s. Although lifetime risk is higher among women, it has also decreased markedly, from 16% in the 1950s to 9% in the 1990s.

Trends in Incidence and Case Fatality

The major question concerning the trends in routine stroke mortality rates is the relative contribution to these trends of changes in incidence and case fatality rates. The WHO MONICA Project is the major international study investigating these trends. Stroke trends over a 7- to 10-year period across 15 MONICA populations in 10 countries indicate that annual stroke attack rates decreased in 8 populations in men and in 10 populations in women, with increased trends in 7 populations in men and 3 in women.[15] The average annual change in stroke attack rates was −1% in men and −1.3% in women. The average change in mortality was −0.7% in men and −2.1% in women. In most populations, trends in mortality were explained by both changes in incidence (one-third) and in case fatality (two-thirds).

The Demographic Transition

The changing age structure of populations will have an impact on the future burden of stroke. Great diversity exists in the pace and patterns of ageing among countries. Some will remain "young" in the foreseeable future, for example, sub-Saharan Africa, and it may be difficult to get stroke and other cardiovascular diseases on the agenda in the presence of continuing high levels of communicable disease. Countries undergoing rapid aging—especially those with large populations, such as China, India, and Indonesia—face a double burden, coping with both communicable and noncommunicable diseases. Areas with an already relatively high percentage of the population aged over 65 years, such as Europe, Japan, and Australasia, are experiencing shifts towards the very old.

One impact of an increasing percentage of people in the older age categories is the potential for an increasing burden of stroke. Population projections suggest that just seven countries—China, India, Brazil, Russia, the United States, Japan, and Indonesia—will dominate the world ageing scene in the future, with just two countries, China and India, making up almost half (44%) of the world's older population in the year 2020.

Figure 14.4 shows the projected increase in the older population between 1995 and 2025 for selected developing and developed countries. As the rate of increase in the latter is much slower, the impact of stroke in the developed countries in the future will be much less than in developing countries. Using the United States as an example, population-based incidence rates have been extrapolated to the

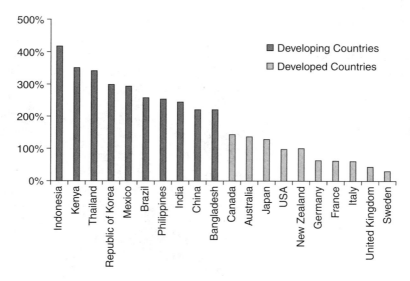

FIGURE 14.4. Projected percentage increase in the older population, 1995–2025.

entire U.S. population.[16] Figure 14.5 shows that if there is no change in incidence rates, there will, not surprisingly, be a corresponding increase in the number of acute strokes—from around 350,000 strokes each year in 1995 to 550,000 in 2030—because of the ageing of the population in that period.

Other estimates show the impact of a small annual percentage either increase or decrease in stroke incidence rates. In the United States and most other developed countries, only a small annual percent decline in stroke mortality, of around 1% per year, is necessary to hold the numbers steady into the foreseeable future. Small declines of around 2% to 3% per annum will lead to an ever-shrinking number of new stroke events each year. A future epidemic of stroke in the United States is therefore unlikely, even with a fall-off in the rate of decline, because up to a 6% decline each year has been achieved over the past few decades. The pattern is much the same for other developed countries: a continuing decline, even if not at the same level as in the past, seems achievable.

However, in countries where the pace of aging is much greater, as in China, a much greater preventive effort will be required to hold the numbers of new stroke events steady at around 2–3% (Fig. 14.6). Incidence rates based on a seven-county study have been extrapolated to the total Chinese population.[17] A small increase in rates of only 1% per year will have a major impact, increasing the absolute numbers of stroke from just under 2 million in 1990 to 5 million in 2020 and 7 million in 2030.

As per capita income increases, the social and economic conditions that allow for the widespread adoption of risky behaviors and habits gradually emerge. In particular, when disposable incomes increase sufficiently to produce a market for

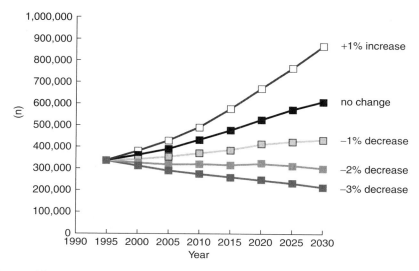

FIGURE 14.5. Projected number of new stroke cases in United States, 1990–2030, based on annual rate of change (%) in incidence.

the multinational tobacco, food, and beverages, the basic causes of future epidemics of noncommunicable disease become established. Combined with the aging of the population, changes in nutrition, the adoption of an atherogenic diet, and an increase in sedentary lifestyle are occurring much more rapidly than in many Western, developed countries. It is likely that the stroke epidemic will emerge faster in these middle income countries. Such estimated projections of future stroke burden and the need to alter it through preventive efforts are the most pressing challenge for the future.

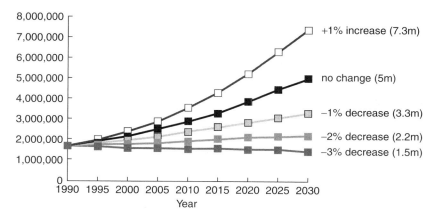

FIGURE 14.6. Projected number of new stroke cases (in millions) in China, 1990–2030, based on annual rate of change (%) in incidence.

Prevention of Stroke

Traditionally, the focus of stroke research, prevention, and control has been on the relationship between risk factors and disease and its management at the level of the individual. This body of research, much of it epidemiologic, has produced a rich source of information that has provided evidence for the public health and health sector responses to stroke and other cardiovascular diseases.

Prevalence of Risk Factors and Trends

In addition to heart disease and stroke registers, the WHO MONICA Project collected standardized risk factor information over a ten-year period. In summary, the prevalence of the major risk factors varies considerably across the study populations. In general, levels are highest in those populations with the highest heart disease and stroke rates. Over the three risk factor surveys conducted at baseline and then after approximately five and ten years, smoking rates have usually declined in men, but the trends are mixed in women; the mean diastolic blood pressure among populations differed by 15 mm Hg between the highest (Novosibirsk) and the lowest (Denmark). Smoking and elevated blood pressure explained 21% of the variations in stroke incidence among populations in men and 42% in women.[18] Obesity has generally increased in both men and women, particularly in men.

Risk Factor Levels in Developing Countries

Apart from the Beijing data collected as part of the MONICA Project, risk factor survey data are available from a number of other developing countries, including, Hong Kong, India, and Nigeria. In an Indian Council of Medical Research study conducted from 1989 to 1994, an urban population from New Delhi was compared with a rural population from Haryana province. Although rural women in this province have an unusually high rate of smoking, in general, risk factor levels are considerably higher in urban populations.[4]

Trend data in the level and proportion of standard risk factors is of most interest in predicting future patterns of stroke. In contrast to most developed countries in the MONICA Project, in which risk factors have moved in a favourable direction, the Beijing center registered increasing prevalence of smoking in both men and women.[19]

Effectiveness of Interventions to Reduce Risk Factor Levels

An increasing body of research indicates that interventions to reduce CVD risk factors is effective and in turn will reduce stroke mortality and morbidity. The best evidence comes from randomized, controlled trials of pharmacologic interventions to control blood pressure and cholesterol levels in individuals. These trials have demonstrated that pharmacologic lowering of blood pressure reduces the risk of both stroke and coronary heart disease, although the relative effect is greater for stroke and is apparent in people both with and without established disease. However, it has become increasingly obvious that this research has left the underlying social, economic, and cultural determinants of the epidemic largely unexamined, which has led to a rather narrow policy response to the epidemic.

Strategies to Reduce Risk

The debates on public health policy for CVD control have involved discussions of three issues: high-risk approach vs. population approach for prevention; single risk factor vs. multiple risk factor control strategies; and CVD control vs. integrated noncommunicable disease control programs. The debates have served to highlight the strengths and limitations of each strategy. These approaches are not mutually exclusive. Public health policy must incorporate all of these into an overall CVD control program.

High-risk strategy

The high-risk approach aims to identify persons with markedly elevated risk factors who are therefore at the highest risk of disease. These individuals are then targeted by interventions that aim to reduce the risk factor levels. If successful, the benefits to individuals are large, because the individual absolute risk is large. However, since the number of persons in this high-risk category is proportionately much smaller than in the moderate-risk group, the overall benefits to society may be limited in terms of death or disability avoided. The strategy reduces, but does not necessarily minimize, the risk for the individuals concerned. Although a fall of blood pressure from 160/95 to 150/90 does indeed reduce the risk of a major CVD event, even this attained value poses a greater risk than a lower level of blood pressure. Further, this strategy may be difficult to sustain.[20]

Population approach for prevention

The population approach aims at reducing the risk factor levels in the population as a whole through community action. Because there is a continuum of risk associated with most risk factors, widespread change will result in a large benefit across a wide range of risk. While individual benefits are relatively small, the cumulative societal benefits are large ("the prevention paradox").[20]

Blood pressure provides a good example because it is a key determinant of stroke risk, both in developed and developing countries. While the association appears to be stronger in Western populations, the Eastern Stroke and Coronary Heart Disease Collaborative Study Group, which analyzed data from 125,000 participants in 18 cohort studies from China and Japan, indicated that population-wide lowering of blood pressure has the potential to produce enormous declines in stroke in eastern Asia.[21] The study demonstrated that a small reduction in average diastolic blood pressure (by about 2%) would avert about a third of all strokes and one-sixth of all heart attacks. In the People's Republic of China alone this would result in about 370,000 fewer stroke deaths each year, with most of these averted events occurring in people who were not considered hypertensive. If similar benefits could be achieved throughout the Asia-Pacific region by 2020, about one million deaths from cardiovascular diseases would be averted by a population-wide intervention (Table 14.4).

The relative benefits of both strategies are similar to estimates made for U.S. and U.K. populations.[22,23] The absolute benefits, however, are many times greater due to the size of the predicted CVD burden in Asia.[24] Furthermore, the reduction in disability would be even more pronounced in China, as stroke tends to be more disabling than coronary heart disease. A population-wide approach to reducing blood pressure by 2 % would avert the loss of 10 million healthy life years, about 1.5% of the total disease burden.

The population-based, lifestyle-linked risk reduction approach is particularly relevant in the context of developing countries, where it is necessary to ensure that communities currently at low risk are protected from acquiring risk factors (sometimes referred to as "primordial prevention"). This is true for adults in the rural regions of most developing countries, as well as for children in all populations. Population-wide changes that lower blood pressure, such as reduced salt intake,[25–27] higher potassium intake,[28] more exercise, and less obesity,[29] all have the potential to produce large benefits. This approach is eminently applicable to moderate risk groups in urban areas, where lifestyle-based risk modification will help avoid drug therapy, with its attendant economic and biologic costs.

Health professionals must recognise the societal benefits of the population strategy and play a strong advocacy role for promoting appropriate health be-

TABLE 14.4. Estimated Number of Deaths Due to Coronary Heart Disease or Stroke Averted in Asia in 2020 by Two Blood Pressure Lowering Strategies[24]

	POPULATION-WIDE INTERVENTION[1]		TARGETED INTERVENTION[2]	
	n (000s)	**%**	**n (000s)**	**%**
India	300	9	380	11
China	450	12	530	15
OAI	200	10	220	11
Total	950	10	1100	12

[1]All individuals in the population reduce diastolic blood pressure by 2%.

[2]All individuals with usual diastolic blood pressure ≥95mmHg reduce diastolic blood pressure by 7%.

OAI, Other Asian islands.

haviors in the community. Policy makers who desire a national impact on the CVD burden can ill afford to ignore the imperatives of investing in a population approach, which will pay large long-term dividends in the control of what are, in effect, lifestyle diseases. Risk factors for CVD tend to cluster in individuals due to common determinants. It is appropriate, however, to adopt strategies that modify the total risk by reducing all or most of them.

The decline of CVD mortality rates in industrial countries is the collective result of population-based prevention strategies that improve the risk profile of communities, a high-risk approach of targeted interventions to protect individuals with markedly elevated risk factor levels, and case-management strategies to salvage, support, and sustain persons presenting with clinical problems.

CONCLUSION

Global prevention and control strategies need to be developed in tandem with surveillance systems to measure their impact on trends in stroke. The major challenge is to seize the opportunities and act now in the face of developing epidemics of stroke in particular and CVD in general. Greater emphasis on the public health dimensions of coming epidemics and the solutions necessary to contain them are amply illustrated by the case study of lowering blood pressure as a major preventive strategy. It is now obvious that not all strategies are equally relevant in all contexts.

REFERENCES

1. World Health Organization. *The World Health Report 1999*. Geneva: WHO, 1999.
2. World Health Organization. *The World Health Report 1997*. Geneva: WHO, 1997.
3. Lopez AD. Counting the dead in China: Measuring tobacco's impact in the developing world. *BMJ* 1998;317:1399–1400.
4. Chandramohan D, Maude G, Rodrigues LC, Hayes RJ. Verbal autopsies for adult deaths: Issues in their development and validation. *Int J Epidemiol* 1994;8:314–355.
5. World Health Organization. *World Health Report 1999: Making a Difference*. Geneva: WHO, 1999.
6. Tunstall- Pedoe H, Kuulasmaa K, Amouyel P, Arveiler D, Rajakangas A, Pajak A. Myocardial infarction and coronary deaths in the World Health Organisation MONICA Project: Registration procedures, event rates, and case-fatality rates in 38 populations from 21 countries in four continents. *Circulation* 1994;90:583–612.
7. Thorvaldsen P, Asplund K, Kuulasmaa K, Rajakangas AM, Schroll M. Stroke incidence, case fatality, and mortality in the WHO MONICA project: World Health Organization monitoring trends and determinants in cardiovascular disease. *Stroke* 1995;26:361–367.
8. Stegmayr B, Asplund K, Kuulasmaa K, Rajakangas A, Thorvaldsen P, Tuomilehto J. Stroke incidence and mortality correlated to stroke risk factors in the WHO MONICA project: An ecological study of 18 populations. *Stroke* 1997;28:1367–1374.

9. Asplund K, Bonita R, Kuulasmaa K, et al. Multinational comparisons of stroke epidemiology: Evaluation of case-ascertainment in the WHO MONICA Stroke Study. *Stroke* 1995;26:355–360.

10. Cooper RS, Osotimehin B, Kaufman TS, Forrester T. Distribution of burden in subsaharan Africa: What should we conclude from the absence of data? *Lancet* 1998; 351:208–210.

11. Williams A. Calculating the global burden of disease: Time for a strategic reappraisal? *Health Econ* 1999;8:1–8.

12. Murray CJL, Lopez AD. Mortality by cause for eight regions of the world: global burden of disease study. *Lancet* 1997;349:1269–1276.

13. *The Institute of Medicine (IOM) Report on Control of Cardiovascular Diseases in Developing Countries: Research, Development and Institutional Strengthening.* National Academy Press, Washington DC, 1998.

14. Kalache A, Aboderin I. Stroke: The global burden. *Health and Planning* 10:1–21.

15. The XV International Scientific Meeting of the International Epidemiological Association. Abstract book, volume I, 1999.

16. Sacco RL, et al. Stroke incidence among white, black, and Hispanic residents of an urban community: The Northern Manhattan Stroke Study. *Am J Epidemiol.* 1998;147: 259–268.

17. Cheng Xue-Ming, et al. Stroke in China, 1986 through 1990. *Stroke* 1995;26:1990–1994.

18. The XV International Scientific Meeting of the International Epidemiological Association. Abstract book, volume II, 1999.

19. Molarius A, Parsons RW, Dobson AJ, Evans A, Fortmann SP, Jamrozik K, Kuulasmaa K, Moltchanov V, Sans S, Tuomilehto J and Puska P. Trends in cigarette smoking in 36 populations from the early 1980s to the mid 1990s: Findings from the WHO MONICA Project (in press).

20. Rose G. Strategy of prevention: Lessons from cardiovascular disease. *BMJ* 1981;282: 1847–1851.

21. Eastern Stroke and Coronary Heart Disease Collaborative Research Group. Blood pressure, cholesterol, and stroke in eastern Asia. *Lancet* 1998;352:1801–1807.

22. Law M, Morris J, Wald N, Robinson D. The change in average blood pressure in Western countries, and its effect on the fall in stroke mortality. (in press).

23. Cook NR, Cohen J, Herbert PR, Taylor JO, Hennekens CH. Implications of small reductions in diastolic blood pressure for primary prevention. *Arch Intern Med* 1995; 155:701–709.

24. Rodgers A, MacMahon S. Blood pressure and the global burden of cardiovascular disease. *J Clin Exp Hypertension* 1999;21:531–542.

25. Elliott P, Stamler J, Nichols, et al. Intersalt revisited: Further analyses of 24-hour sodium excretion and blood pressure within and across populations. *BMJ* 1996;312: 1249–1253.

26. He J, Whelton PK. Role of sodium reduction in the treatment and prevention of hypertension. *Curr Opin Cardiol* 1997;12:202–207.

27. Cappucio FP, Markandu ND, Carney C, Sagnella GA, MacGregor GA. Double-blind randomised trial of modest salt restriction in older people. *Lancet* 1997;350:850–854.

28. Whelton PK, He J, Cutler JA, et al. Effects of oral potassium on blood pressure—meta analysis of randomised controlled trials. *JAMA* 1997;227:1624–1632.

29. Fagard RK. The role of exercise in blood pressure control: Supportive evidence. *J Hypertens* 1995;13:1223–1227.

15

FROM CLINICAL TRIALS TO CLINICAL PRACTICE

Geoffrey A. Donnan

> "Be delightfully surprised when any treatment at all is effective, and always assume that a treatment is ineffective unless there is evidence to the contrary."
>
> A. L. Cochrane, 1971[1]

In its endless quest for health into old age, the human race has been constantly searching for forms of therapy that will minimize the impact of disease processes. One of the interesting qualities of many therapeutic compounds is that they occur as natural products of our environment (e.g.,aspirin), sometimes in a ubiquitous fashion, and need to be identified, concentrated, and applied in a highly specific manner (e.g., intravenously) to produce benefit in terms of reducing morbidity or mortality. Other therapies need to be specifically manufactured (e.g., clopidogrel), but often their genesis lies in an understanding of the biological basis of the disease or the effect of a naturally available compound. Regardless of their origins, the real test of any form of therapy is efficacy. From early times the history of medicine has been riddled with therapies that have sometimes existed for centuries but have ultimately proven to be ineffective. Conversely, other therapies have been discarded without ever being adequately tested. The concept of adequate proof of efficacy has been gradually evolving since early in the twentieth century. Only simple experiments were required for such dramatically effective agents as penicillin, sulphonamides, and insulin, but for less markedly beneficial therapies, more specific proof is required.

One of the champions of a more scientific approach to the introduction of therapies in medicine was Archie Cochrane. Before working in the National Health

Service of Britain, Cochrane was a prisoner of war in Germany for about four years. As medical officer for about 20,000 prisoners of war inmates, he noted:

> Under the best conditions one would have expected an appreciable mortality; there in the gulag I expected hundreds to die of diptheria alone in the absence of specific therapy. In point of fact there were only four deaths, of which three were due to gunshot wounds inflicted by the Germans. This excellent result had, of course, nothing to do with the therapy they received or my clinical school. It demonstrated, on the other hand, very clearly, the relative unimportance of therapy in comparison with the recuperative powers of the human body.

While this point is perhaps a little overstated, it does illustrate the need for making a distinction between the natural history of disease processes and the effect of therapy per se. Understandably, most people (particularly physicians) wish for a beneficial outcome of therapy. This inherent bias has bedeviled observational literature on medical therapies over the centuries. The need to eliminate this positive (and negative) bias led to the simple concept of the randomized controlled trial (RCT) in the United Kingdom during the 1950s, which has been developed into more sophisticated forms during the last 30 years. One of the earliest such trials was published by Daniels and Hill,[2] who described three trials of the use of chemotherapy for pulmonary tuberculosis using a randomized approach to test bed rest, streptomycin PAS, or a combination of both chemotherapies. Trial methodology has been further refined and the "double blind" technique is now considered the gold standard for evidence against which all other forms should be measured. A boom in clinical trials has occurred in all branches of medicine and surgery, and, fortunately, stroke medicine has been not immune to its influence; so much so that Caplan called the 1980s "the era of clinical trials."[3]

This chapter addresses the problem of translating the burgeoning mass of knowledge about cerebrovascular disease prevention from clinical trials into clinical practice. In doing so, it is necessary to describe how trials are conducted and then discuss the various ways in which information from these trials can be converted into better clinical outcomes (Fig. 15.1). The process must involve physician, patient, and community acceptance of the information contained in the trial, so that generalized clinical usage is embraced by all stakeholders. Unfortunately, barriers to these processes abound, as will be shown.

HOW TRIALS ARE CONDUCTED

Types of Trials

A large variety of clinical trial types have been designed for testing of either pharmaceutical agents or surgical procedures.[4] These range from single-patient studies to mega-trials and include single or multiple groups of patients with par-

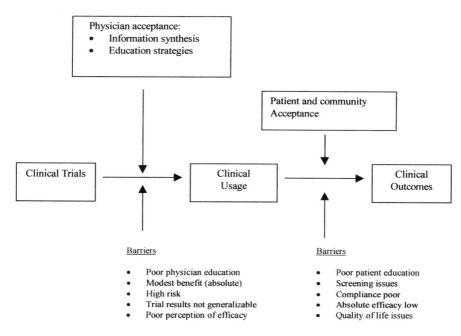

FIGURE 15.1. The pathway from clinical trial information to clinical outcomes, with the key elements of physician, patient, and community acceptance. Barriers to these elements abound.

allel, cross-sectional, longitudinal, cross-over, and other approaches. During the conduct of these trials, issues such as placebo effect, placebo and monitoring effects, and the importance of a background of "best medical therapy" all need to be taken into consideration. Within the study design, inclusion and exclusion criteria always form the "front door" to trial entry. In setting these criteria, the investigators make a conscious decision (usually based on the practicalities of recruitment and appropriateness of patient sample) as to the representative nature of the patients to be studied. Hence, the trial environment can range from artificial to realistic depending on the criteria for selection and the environmental setting of the trial (for example, hospital cases at a tertiary, or even quaternary, referral center, compared to community-based subjects). There is an increasing trend in many countries for a larger proportion of trials to be more community based (often involving general practices) to improve the generalizability of the results.

For trials of pharmaceutical compounds, the process is usually tiered from phase I through phase IV, as shown in Table 15.1.[5] In some instances, pharmaceutical companies may conduct a number of phases simultaneously or there may be some overlap between phases. Trials of surgical procedures (for example,

TABLE 15.1. Phases of Clinical Trials of Drug Therapy

Phase I	The effect of the drug as a function of dosage is established in a small number of healthy volunteers. Phase I trials are carried out to determine whether animals and humans show significantly different responses to the drug and to establish the probable limits of the clinical dosage range. These trials are nonblind, i.e., both the investigators and the subjects know what is being given. Pharmacokinetic measurements of absorption, half-life, and metabolism are often done in phase I. Such studies are usually performed in clinical research centers by specially trained clinical pharmacologists.
Phase II	The drug is evaluated in much larger numbers of patients with the target disease to determine safety and efficacy. A small number of patients (1–150) are studied in great detail. A single-blind design is often used, with an inert placebo medication and an older active drug (positive control) in addition to the investigational agent. Phase II trials also are usually done in special clinical centers.
Phase III	The drug is evaluated in much larger numbers of patients, sometimes thousands. Using information gathered in phases I and II, trials are designed (optimally) to minimize errors caused by placebo effects, variable course of the disease, etc. Therefore, double-blind and cross-over techniques are frequently employed. Phase III trials are usually carried out in clinical settings similar to those anticipated for the ultimate use of the drug. Phase III studies are difficult to design and execute and are usually very expensive because of the large numbers of patients involved and the masses of data that must be collected and analyzed. The investigators are usually specialists in the disease being treated.
Phase IV	This constitutes an attempt to monitor the safety of the new drug under ordinary conditions of use in much larger numbers of patients. The importance of careful and complete reporting of toxicity after marketing approval can be appreciated by noting that many important drug-induced effects have an incidence of 1:10,000 or less. Such low-incidence drug-effect associations will not generally be detected in phase I to III studies, no matter how carefully executed. Phase IV has no fixed duration.

Modified from reference 5.

carotid endarterectomy and angioplasty) usually involve pilot studies followed by a large pivotal trial (phase III, in pharmaceutical terms).

Sample Size and Statistical Power Considerations

A key issue in the design of any clinical trial is that of sample size. A design fault of many of the earlier randomized controlled trials was that of inadequate power to test the hypotheses proposed. Directly or indirectly, this has led to the phenomenon of pooled analyses, or meta-analyses, to generate greater power and avoid of type II error. The relationship between power and therapeutic effect is shown in Figure 15.2.[6] The most common mistake made by investigators in study design is to overestimate the likely therapeutic effect. Hence, sample sizes are often too small; the power of the study is thereby reduced, and a potentially positive effect may be missed (type II error). A good example of this is in trials of antiplatelet agents for the secondary prevention of stroke.[7–9] In general, early trials of therapy were underpowered,[7,10] resulting in confidence intervals that were wide and included unity (nonsignificant effect), although point estimates did suggest that a beneficial effect was possible. It was not until sample sizes were significantly increased that positive trial results were demonstrated.[8,9,11]

Funding for Clinical Trials

An inevitable accompaniment of the growth of clinical trials in medicine has been an explosion of costs associated with their conduct. The two broad groups involved in the clinical trial "industry" are academic clinical investigators and pharmaceutical companies. Each group has produced studies of varying quality as study design and trial conduct have improved over time. The agenda of the two

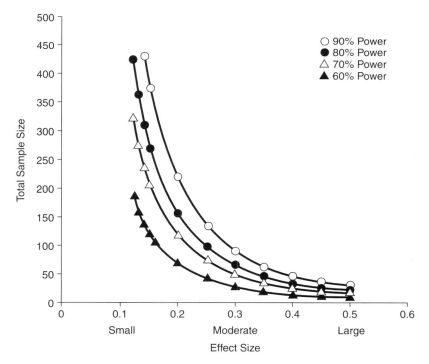

FIGURE 15.2. The relationship between effect size and power of trials of therapy. (Reprinted by permission of Kraemer, H.C. Sample size: When is enough? *Am J Med Sci.* 269:61;1986.[11])

groups is somewhat different: academic investigators pursue scientific truth (and academic advancement) while pharmaceutical companies seek both scientific truth and financial gain. Partnerships between the two groups are common (and are becoming increasingly so as trial costs escalate), usually to mutual benefit.

Categories of these relationships are shown in Table 15.2, and, as can be seen, the most highly regarded trials are those in which adequate funding is achieved through national research organizations or a collaborative effort between investigators and the pharmaceutical industry. When such collaborations occur, the ideal arrangement is for the academic investigating group to be "hired" to con-

TABLE 15.2. Funding for Clinical Trials: Models of Relationships Between Academic and Commercial Groups

MODEL	COMMENTS
Investigator only–driven studies, either unfunded or funded from local sources.	Samples sizes often small because investigators less experienced and funding levels low. Modest peer review. Trial results reasonably credible.
Investigator-driven with national research organization funding.	Usually well-run studies with adequate sample size. Studies run to completion without external influence. High-quality peer review. Trial results highly credible.
Partnership between academic investigators and pharmaceutical company. Funds provided by national research organization and pharmaceutical company. Trial conducted entirely by investigators	High-quality peer review. Very adequate sample sizes with credible results because of "hands-off" approach by the pharmaceutical companies Trial results highly credible.
Investigator–pharmaceutical company partnership, but pharmaceutical company monitors trial, collects and analyzes data in-house. Independent steering and safety monitoring committees.	Data not often able to be checked by investigators. Trials sometimes not completed because of "futility analyses." Modest or nonexistent peer review. Trial results reasonably credible.
Pharmaceutical company alone conducts trial. No independent steering or monitoring committee.	All analyses done "in-house," participants unable to check data. Poor-quality peer review. Negative trial results often not published. Quality of study centers often less certain. Trials may not run to completion when "futility analyses" performed. Trial results least credible.

duct the trial in its entirety (particularly data analysis), so that analysis and interpretation can be totally separate from commercial concerns.

Interestly, it has been shown that randomized trials conducted with commercial sponsorship are more likely to report statistically significant advances.[12] Further, some trials may be stopped by commercial sponsors without explanation.[13,14]

Standards of Trial Design and Reporting

As a part of the effort to improve the standards of study trial design, several important initiatives have recently been developed. The journal *Lancet* now accepts protocols for review, so that alterations can be made to defective protocols before study commencement.[15] Another was the development of the Consolidated Standards of Reporting Trials (CONSORT) guidelines.[16–18] These guidelines outline a set of minimum criteria that should be followed when investigators submit manuscripts to journals for publication. Although the guidelines have been adopted by only a small number of high-profile journals to date (including *Lancet*, *JAMA* and *BMJ*), they should gradually become more widespread, so that there will be more consistency in the design, analysis, and reporting of clinical trials.[18]

As stated, clinical trial methodology has changed considerably over the past 20 years, with improvements and quality control mechanisms now in place that may allow observers to place greater credence in published results. However, this higher-quality evidence must be translated into clinical practice and, ultimately, into improved clinical outcomes. For this to occur, physician, patient, and community acceptance of the information must occur.

CLINICAL TRIALS: FROM EVIDENCE TO CLINICAL PRACTICE

Physician Acceptance

For physicians to accept new clinical trial information, it must first be gleaned and synthesized by the target group. Sources of information include original research articles, pharmaceutical company material, expert reviews, scientific meetings, and standard texts. The technique of meta-analysis has been increasingly used to advantage, so that data from a number of clinical trials can be reviewed. Information from these and other sources may then be used to produce clinical practice guidelines. Interpretation of data from a variety of sources may be improved by adhering to the principles of evidence based medicine (EBM).

Meta-analyses

While the boom in clinical trials has been of enormous benefit to stroke physicians and their patients, it has also created problems. How can the mass of data generated from these trials be assimilated and the information disseminated to physicians and, ultimately, to patients and the general public? One method that has been increasingly used is the overview, or meta-analysis, technique, whereby all available randomized controlled trial evidence is amassed to produce an overview statistic of the aggregate effect. The most active group in producing meta-analyses of this type is the Cochrane Collaboration[19] (Fig. 15.3). Clinical areas in which there is the most need for aggregate information are identified, and an database of meta-analyses is generated that can be readily accessed.[20] The stroke section of this collaboration is one of the most active, and, to date, 27 overviews of stroke have been produced, 7 of which are concerned with stroke prevention

The power of meta-analysis is best illustrated by the technique of cumulative meta-analysis.[21] Using this method, the results of new trials are sequentially included in the analysis to provide a new point estimate and a steadily diminishing 95% confidence interval because of an incrementally increasing sample size. When this approach was retrospectively applied to the use of streptokinase in acute myocardial infarction, it was found that a statistically significant reduction in mortality was achieved in 1973 after only eight trials involving 2432 patients (Fig. 15.4). The results of the 25 subsequent trials, which enrolled an additional 34,542 patients, had little or no effect on the odds ratio for mortality, but simply narrowed the confidence interval. When these results were compared to recommendations of reviewers (articles and textbooks) of the same era, significant discrepancies were found between the information available from the trials and current recommendations[22] (Fig. 15.5). One can conclude that, without meta-analyses to aid in trial aggregation and synthesis, significant delays in the introduction of important therapies into routine practice may occur.

One of the most important meta-analyses performed in the area of stroke prevention was carried out by the Antiplatelet Trialists Group (APT).[7-9] By aggregating data from some 140,000 patients with increased risk of vascular disease from more than 300 trials, this group gained information on a variety of outcomes using this form of therapy.[7-9] Specifically, the relative risk reduction of about 22% for patients with prior stroke or transient ischemic attack of devel-

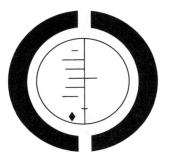

FIGURE 15.3. The Cochrane Collaboration logo showing how pooling data reveals the significance of treatment effects.

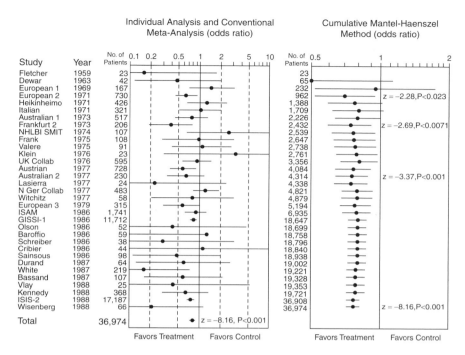

FIGURE 15.4. Conventional and cumulative meta-analysis of trials of intravenous strep-tokinase for acute myocardial infarction. The odds ratio and 95% confidence interval for an effect of treatment on mortality are shown on a logarithmic scale. From Lau et al.[21]

oping subsequent stroke or myocardial infarction or suffering vascular death is generally accepted as the benchmark level of effectiveness for aspirin therapy.[9]

However, the enthusiasm for meta-analyses is far from uniform. Critics emphasize that this approach involves the mixing of "apples and oranges," often causing clinical and statistical heterogeneity that may make correct interpretation of the results more difficult. On occasion, therefore, meta-analyses may provide misleading information, creating the need for more definitive proof from a "megatrial". An example of this was the use of magnesium in myocardial infarction. Meta-analyses of a large number of smaller trials had suggested that this approach might be effective.[23] However, a megatrial subsequently proved, to everyone's reasonable satisfaction, that this was not the case.[24] Issues such as variable protocols of differing quality and publication bias were probably responsible. In a formal comparison of meta-analyses and large trials, large trials differed from meta-analyses 10% to 23% of the time.[25] In other words, meta-analyses should not be taken as the absolute gold standard, but merely as guides based on, among other things, the quality of the input data.

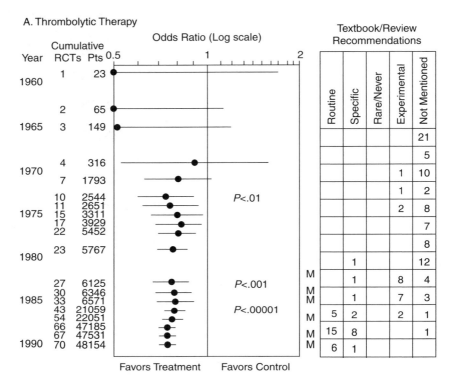

FIGURE 15.5. Results of meta-analysis and recommendations of reviewers (articles and textbooks of the same era). For each treatment for acute myocardial infarction, the cumulative meta-analyses by year of publication of randomized control trials (RCTs) are presented on the left. The cumulative number of trials and patients (PTs) are also presented. On the right, the recommendations of the clinical expert reviewers are presented in two-year segments (number of recommendations). The letter *M* indicates that least one meta-analysis was published that year. From Antman, et al.[22]

Even megatrials themselves are not without their critics. Charleton argued that megatrials tend to use simple protocols in multiple research centers rather than rigorous protocols in more clinically homogenous, smaller groups.[26] This trade-off between rigorous control of homogenous groups and large size to account for random fluctuations in trial entry criteria is a matter of ongoing debate. Further, megatrials may underestimate differences among groups ("null bias"), mainly due to poor compliance, but also perhaps due to poorly controlled additional therapies that can become unbalanced among groups, a phenomen that may have occurred in coronary artery disease studies.[27] To counter these problems, population-based strategies have been advocated, such as that instigated in the north of England, termed Population Adjusted Clinical Epidemiology (PACE). Here, concern had been expressed that progress in therapy among adults with leukemia had not paralleled similar advances in childhood leukemia therapy. One reason for this, it was felt, was a lack of rigor in clinical trial methodology, with large trials including many different forms of leukemia and many of the difficulties associated megatrials mentioned earlier. The PACE strategy was to establish region-wide mechanisms for recording the entire incident population of cases, followed by management options compared by using surveys, cohort studies, and clinical trials, as appropriate. The trials themselves were smaller and more focused, with homogenous groups. This approach certainly had merit, although in many countries it would be difficult to perform because of the lack of uniform health systems among regions. The PACE system has not, as yet, been adopted by investigators involved in stroke prevention.

Interpreting clinical trials and evidence-based medicine

Health policy is decided upon from a variety of sources, including observational studies, entrenched existing policies, and political expediency (often responding to high profile pressure groups). It has been estimated that less than 20% of clinical policies are based on randomized control trials.[28,29] A number of guidelines are available on how to interpret clinical trials. All follow the general principle of using a series of checkpoints to determine the nature of the population from which subjects are drawn, the randomization process, the stipulation of endpoints, and analysis techniques. Other guides have been published on how to decide on the applicability of clinical trial results to individual patients.[30]

The EBM approach to the interpretation of clinical information was developed during the 1990s.[31,32] It represents a sensible crystallization of an approach of searching for, and subsequently interpreting, data in the environment of clinicians. By structuring "levels of evidence" (Table 15.3), clinicians can quantify more readily the importance and reliability of the data they are examining. Increasingly, this approach is being used throughout the English-speaking world, although this process, also, is not without its critics.[33] The most common criticisms of EBM are that the process is "not new," that information is derived too heavily from randomized controlled trials and meta-analyses, and that it excludes specific patient problems. Further, the authoritative aura given to the collection of evidence under EBM may lead to major abuses that produce inappropriate guidelines or doctrinaire dogmas for clinical practice.

Clinical practice guidelines

A flurry of activity has occurred in the production of clinical practice guidelines, including those for stroke prevention.[34–39] While these have been extremely useful and widely published, particularly by the Scottish Intercollegiate Guidelines Network (SIGN), which receives government funding,[37–39] major problems remain in disseminating these guidelines among medical practitioners.

TABLE 15.3. Levels of Evidence

LEVEL	QUALITY OF EVIDENCE RATINGS
I	Evidence is obtained from a systematic review of all relevant randomized controlled trials.
II	Evidence is obtained from at least one properly designed randomized controlled trial.
III	Evidence is obtained from well-designed controlled trials without randomization; from well-designed cohort or case controlled analytic studies, preferably from more than one center or research group; from multiple time series with or without intervention; or from dramatic results in uncontrolled experiments.
IV	Opinions of respected authorities based on clinical experience, descriptive studies, or reports of expert committees.

Clinical trial interpretation, EBM, and clinical practice guidelines are intimately connected with the issue of continuing medical education (CME) and its effectiveness. Concerns have been raised about the effectiveness of traditional continuing medical educational strategies, an issue that has been examined in recent studies. For example, Davis et al.[40] reviewed educational approaches used from 1975 to 1994. Reassuringly, they showed that about two-thirds of the studies (70%) displayed a change in physician performance, while almost half (48%) of interventions produced changes in healthcare outcomes. The most effective strategies were community- and practice-based methods, such as reminders and patient-mediated strategies with multiple interventions. Poorer outcomes were demonstrated by audit and educational materials. The weakest approach was formal CME conferences. Fortunately, an increasing amount of research is being directed toward monitoring and improving the effectiveness of translating original research data into better clinical outcomes.

Patient and Community Acceptance

Even though the medical fraternity may accept a particular form of therapy, patient and community acceptance must be generated for favorable outcomes to be achieved. For example, when the evidence for aspirin as an effective antiplatelet agent emerged in the 1970s and 1980s, patient and community resistance to its use had to be overcome. The community needed to be convinced that an agent that had been used as a simple analgesic for 70 years would be effective in its new role as an anticoagulant. The main mechanism by which patient and community acceptance of new forms of therapy occurs is by education via the print and electronic media. Acceptance may be facilitated when there is ease of oral administration (in most instances), and a favorable side effect profile. As a result, quality of life is improved, rather than hampered.

Barriers to Physician Acceptance of Clinical Trial Information

While most worthy new information is introduced eventually into regular clinical practice, the rate and extent of adoption of new approaches varies enormously. This may be due to a number of factors, including the following.[41]

1. Failure of information transfer, based on the system outlined in the preceeding sections (Figure 15.1).
2. Misleading use of risk reductions by pharmaceutical companies or others (relative vs. absolute risk reduction).
3. Relatively small benefit balanced by high risk.
4. Trials not relevant to the general population because of restrictive inclusion/exclusion criteria.

Risk reductions

A particularly important issue in interpreting clinical trials is the difference between relative and absolute risk. Relative risk is always much greater and is often quoted by pharmaceutical companies in their promotional material to emphasize a positive clinical effect to the unwary physician. Absolute risk reduction is a better index of the effect of a drug. It can be translated readily into number needed to treat (NNT), a useful conceptual figure for physicians when assessing whether a particular form of therapy may be worthwhile. The method of calculating these figures from a hypothetical trial of stroke prevention conducted over five years is shown in Table 15.4.

Some good examples in the stroke prevention literature of the importance of understanding the relationship among relative risk, absolute risk, and NNT may be found in the Clopidogrel versus Aspirin in Patients at Risk of Ischaemic Events (CAPRIE)[42] and Asymptomatic Carotid Artery Surgery (ACAS)[43] trial reports. In the CAPRIE trial, a relative risk reduction of 8.6% was achieved in vascular endpoints for clopidogrel vs. aspirin. However, the absolute risk reduction was only 0.5% hence the NNT to obtain benefit was 200. It can be seen that the relative risk reduction of 8.6% was *statistically* significant, but it is open to discussion whether this was *biologically* significant. About a 50% relative risk reduction was achieved in vascular endpoints for patients treated with carotid endarterectomy in the ACAS trial. However, because the control population had only about a 2% stroke risk per year, the absolute risk reduction was only about 1% and the NNT 100. When put in this context, the 50% relative risk reduction does not appear to be as biologically important: it must be debated whether endarterectomy is appropriate on an individual patient basis.

TABLE 15.4. Calculation Method for Relative and Absolute Risk Reductions and Number Needed to Treat (NNT) in a Hypothetical Trail of Stroke Prevention Conducted Over Five Years

THERAPY		NUMBER OF PATIENTS		
		STROKE/DEATH	EVENT FREE	TOTAL
Treatment		1323	6458	7781
Placebo		3574	4208	7782
Control event rate	$=$	$\dfrac{3574}{7782}$ $=$	45.9%	(1)
Treatment event rate	$=$	$\dfrac{1323}{7781}$ $=$	17.0%	(2)
Relative risk reduction	$=$	$\dfrac{(1)-(2)}{(1)}$ $=$	63.0%	(3)
Absolute risk reduction	$=$	$(1)-(2)$ $=$	28.9%	(4)
Number needed to treat to prevent 1 event	$=$	$\dfrac{1}{(4)}$ $=$	$\dfrac{100}{28.9}$ $=$ 3.5	

Risks and benefits

The issues of risk vs. benefit and the generalizability of trial results are well illustrated in the use of anticoagulants as a form of primary stroke prevention in patients with atrial fibrillation. Atrial fibrillation (AF) has been investigated fairly thoroughly over the last few decades and has been established as one of the more important risk factors for stroke. The stroke risk in subjects with nonvalvular atrial fibrillation (NVAF) is about five times that of those who have no NVAF.[44] As discussed in Chapter 6, this risk is stratified depending on associated risk factors. The risk of stroke per year is only about 1% to 2% among those with "lone" AF, but rises to around 5% with the addition of one risk factor (e.g., hypertension, diabetes, age greater than 65 years, or recent-onset cardiac failure or thromboembolism elsewhere). With two or more risk factors, the stroke risk per year rises to around 7% to 8%.[45] Effective forms of therapy for the prevention of stroke in patients with atrial fibrillation are warfarin and aspirin. Based on pooled analyses, treatment with warfarin is associated with a relative risk reduction of stroke of around 70% (absolute reduction 3.1%, NNT 32).[45] Sudlow et al.[46] screened a random sample of 4843 people from a community aged 65 years and older for atrial fibrillation. Participants who were found to have AF received further investigations to stratify their eligibility for anticoagulation based on the pooled analysis of all trials of warfarin therapy for NVAF,[45] the SPAF[47] and SPAF III[48] trials. Of the participants, 228 (4.7%) had AF. Of these, 61% would have bene-

TABLE 15.5. Percentage of Patients with Atrial Fibrillation Eligible for Anticoagulation and Those Anticoagulated by Risk Classification (adapted from Sudlow et al.[46])

ANALYSIS TYPE	NUMBER OF PATIENTS	PERCENT (95% CI)
Pooled analysis	74/163	49% (41–57)
SPAF analysis	81/136	61% (53–69)
SPAF-3 analysis	49/127	41% (33–49)
Currently on warfarin	44/207	23% (17–29)

fited from anticoagulation according to the results of pooled analysis, but anticoagulants were used in only 1114 (23%) of all patients (Table 15.5).

The reasons for the low level of penetration of this form of anticoagulants in primary prevention of stroke risk are complex and probably relate to the difficulty in detecting cases (the majority are asymptomatic), together with a reticence by physicians to use a therapy that, although in use for around 40 years, is perceived to be difficult to manage (repeated INR estimations required) and is associated with significant risk of bleeding. While the latter is certainly an important issue, in the pooled analysis the rate of major bleeding was only 1.0% among controls and 1.3% among patients with AF. This figure is likely to be higher among nontrial patients in the community. While the ratio of benefit to risk is certainly in favor of therapy, physicians are clearly less willing to use warfarin unless they are convinced of its efficacy (and low risk).

An effect converse to the problem of delayed and limited acceptance of information from clinical trials was seen after the Extra-Cranial to Intra-Cranial (EC/IC) bypass trial results were published.[49] This procedure was logical in that blood was bypassed to a presumably under-perfused or hemodynamically at-risk cerebral hemisphere by anastomosing the external carotid artery branches to the middle cerebral artery branches through a skull burr hole. However, when formally tested by a randomized controlled trial, the procedure was found to be ineffective in minimizing subsequent stroke or death. A procedure that had become increasingly accepted among neurosurgeons over the preceding decade plummeted in frequency almost as soon as the trial results were published. Indeed, EC/IC bypass is now rarely performed. The transfer of clinical trial evidence to clinical practice was rapid and effective, probably because of the discrete, small number of clinicians involved (neurosurgeons), excellent communication within the group, and the relatively small number of procedures performed at baseline.

Barriers to Patient and Community Acceptance of Clinical Trial Evidence

As shown in Figure 15.1, issues that need to be considered in regard to patient and community acceptance of clinical trial data include community education strategies, problems with screening, poor compliance, low absolute efficacy, and quality-of-life effects. Some of these are considered in more detail below.

Screening problems

Screening for risk factors may seem a logical exercise, in that many risk factors are asymptomatic and may remain undetected unless some form of screening is undertaken. Examples in stroke prevention include screening for AF and asymptomatic carotid artery stenosis. In the latter case, a cost-benefit analysis was performed and the view was expressed that, given current screening costs and the level of effectiveness of surgery, routine screening programs should not be introduced.[35] This does not preclude the ongoing use of opportunistic screening, which occurs on many occasions when patients visit their doctor.

Compliance

Poor compliance remains a difficult issue for both physicians and their patients. The reasons are complex and involve drug side effects as well as cultural and societal resistance to taking medication. In a study of hypertension as a risk factor for intracerebral hemorrhage (ICH), cessation of antihypertensive medication (for whatever reason) was shown to increase the risk of ICH by more than two-fold (odds ratio 2.45, 95% CI 1.13–5.77).[50] Hence, compliance problems may significantly contribute to poor clinical outcomes.

Quality-of-life issues

A further barrier to therapy may relate to quality-of-life issues. While there is an increasing trend to include quality-of-life measures in clinical trials to reinforce (or otherwise) the efficacy of therapy, this was not always so. It is alleged that in some prophylactic trials, the clinical side effects (which affect quality of life) may have been measured inadequately. For example, when one antihypertensive agent was shown to be associated with a "better quality of life" than another, it was found that the investigators had performed an intention to treat analysis that did not evaluate compliance with therapy.[51,52] It has been suggested that with many antihypertensive agents, "quality of life" can be improved merely by stopping the drug.[51] While this might exaggerate the issue, the point is made.

WHAT TO DO IN THE ABSENCE OF EVIDENCE

While the emphasis of this chapter has been on the transfer of information from clinical trials to clinicians, patients, and the community as a whole, the problem remains that evidence from randomized, controlled trials (and other sources of evidence) does not provide guidance for every clinical situation. In these circumstances what does one do? In some areas, medical practice is ahead of clinical trial evidence. In these cases, lower levels of evidence, as well as common sense, must play a large part. For example, in the management of hypertension, it is not unusual to use combination therapies that have not been specifically tested for efficacy of stroke prevention.[53] Similarly, while there is, as yet, no evidence that combinations of antiplatelet agents are more effective than single agents alone (except for aspirin and dipyridamole[54]), various combinations are frequently used. Uncertainty remains as to which therapy to use in patients with ischemic stroke in whom the source of embolism to the brain is likely to be aortic arch atheroma.[55,56] Here, antiplatelet agents, warfarin, or both are used without clinical trial evidence of efficacy for any of these approaches. Other examples abound and serve to emphasize that, while we must (and do) live in a world of evidence-based practice, a place always will exist for the art of medicine and, above all, common sense.

REFERENCES

1. Cochrane AL. *Effectiveness and Efficiency: Random reflections on Health Services.* Cambridge: Cambridge University Press, 1971.
2. Daniels M, Hill A. Chemotherapy of pulmonary tuberculosis in young adults. An analysis of the combined results of three medical research council trials. *BMJ* 1952: 1;1162.
3. Caplan LR. How should a Clinician choose treatment for preventing stroke when therapeutic trials are not available to guide the situation? *Eur Neurol* 1995:35;293–303.
4. Spilker B. *Guide to Clinical Trials.* New York: Raven Press, 1991.
5. Berkovitz BA. Drug discovery and evaluation. In: Katzung BG, ed. *Basic and Clinical Pharmacology.* Lange Medical Publication, 1982.
6. Kraemer HC. Sample size: When is enough? *Am J Med Sci* 1986:296;361.
7. Antiplatelet Trialists' Collaboration. Secondary prevention of vascular disease by prolonged antiplatelet treatment. *BMJ* 1988:296;320.
8. Underwood MJ. Aspirin benefits with vascular disease and those undergoing revascularisation. *BMJ* 1994:308;71.
9. Antiplatelet Trialists' Collaboration. Collaborative overview of randomized trials of antiplatelet therapy - I: Prevention of death, myocardial infarction, and stroke by prolonged antiplatelet therapy in various categories of patients. *BMJ* 1994:308;81.
10. Candelise L, et al. Randomized trial of aspirin and sulfinprazone in patients with TIA (AITIAIS). *Stroke* 1982:13;175–179.
11. Canadian Cooperative Study Group. A randomized trial of aspirin and sulfinpyrazone in threatened stroke. *N Engl J Med* 1978:299;53–59.
12. Davidson RA. Source of funding: An outcome of clinical trials. *J Gen Int Med* 1986:1;155–158.
13. Good manners for the pharmaceutical industry (editorial). *Lancet* 1997:349;1635.
14. A curious stopping rule from Hoechst Marion Roussel (editorial). *Lancet* 1997:350; 155.
15. Horton R. Pardonable revisions and protocol reviews. *Lancet* 1997:349;6.
16. Begg C, Cho M, Eastwod S, Horton R, Moher D, Olkin I, et al. Improving the quality of reporting of randomized control trials. The CONSORT Statement (editorial). *JAMA* 1996:276;637–639.

17. Altman DG. Better reporting of randomized control trials: The CONSORT Statement (editorial. *BMJ* 1996:313;570–571.
18. CONSORT: An important step towards evidence based healthcare (editorial). *Ann Int Med* 1997:126;81–83.
19. Chalmers I, Dickensin K, et al. Getting to grips with trachie Cochranes Agenda. *BMJ* 1992:305;786–788.
20. Cochrane Database of Systematic Reviews. Oxford The Cochrane Library, Update Software Limited, issue 1, 1999.
21. Lau J, et al. Cumulative meta-analysis of therapeutic trials for myocardial infarction. *N Eng J Med* 1992:327;248–254.
22. Antman EM, et al. A comparison of results of meta-analysis of randomized control trials and recommendations of clinical experts. *JAMA* 1992:268;240–248.
23. Yusuf S, et al. Intravenous magnesium in acute myocardial infarction. An effective, safe, simple, and expensive intervention. *Circulation* 1993:897;2043–2046.
24. ISIS (Fourth International Study of Infarct Survival. Collaborative Group. ISIS-4: A randomized factorial trial assessing early oral captopril, oral mononitrate, and intravenous magnesium sulphate in 58,050 patients with suspected acute myocardial infarction. *Lancet* 1995:345;669–684.
25. Ioannidis JPA, Cappelleri JC, Lau J. Issues in comparisons between meta-analyses and large trials. *JAMA* 1998:279;1089–1093.
26. Charleton BG. The future of clinical research: From mega trials towards methodological rigour and representative sampling. *J Eval Clin Pract* 1996:2(3);159–169.
27. Woods KL. Mega trials and management of acute myocardial infarction. *Lancet* 1995:346;611.
28. Committee for Evaluating Medical Technologies in Clinical Use, Division of Health Sciences Policy, Division of Health Promotion and Disease Prevention, Institute of Medicine. *Assessing medical technologies*. Washington, DC: National Academy Press, 1985.
29. Hornberger J, Wrone E. When to base clinical policies on observational versus randomized trial data. *Ann Int Med* 1997:127;697–703.
30. Dans AL, Dans LF, Guyatt GH, Richardson S, for the Evidence-Based Medicine Working Group. Users guide to the medical literature XIV: How to decide on the applicability of clinical trial results to your patient. *JAMA* 1998:279;545–549.
31. Sackett DL, Rosenberg WMC, Gray JAM, Haynes RB, Richardson WS. Evidence based medicine: What it is and what it isn't. *BMJ* 1996:312;71–72.
32. Sackett DL, Richardson WS, Rosenberg WMC, Haynes RB. *Evidence Based Medicine: How to Practice and Teach Evidence Based Medicine*. Churchill-Livingstone, 1997.
33. Feinstein AR, Horwitz RI. Problems in the "evidence" of "evidence based medicine." *Am J Med* 1997:103;529–535.
34. National Health and Medical Research Council. *Prevention of stroke: The role of anticoagulants, anti-platelet agents and carotid endarterectomy*. Australian Government Publishing Service, Canberra: Commonwealth of Australia 1997.
35. *Prevention of Stroke: Clinical Practice Guidelines*. National Health and Medical Research Council, Canberra December 1996.
36. Lechtenberg R, Schutter AHS, *Neurology Practice Guidelines*. New York: Marcel Dekker, 1998.
37. *Clinical Guidelines: Criteria for Appraisal for National Use*. Edinburgh: Scottish Intercollegiate Guidelines Network (SIGN), September 1995.

38. *Clinical Guidelines: Management of Patients with Stroke. I: Assessment, Investigation, Immediate Management and Secondary Prevention.* Edinburgh: Scottish Intercollegiate Guidelines Network (SIGN), May 1997.

39. *Clinical Guidelines: Management of Patients with Stroke. II: Management of Carotid Stenosis and Carotid Endarterectomy.* Edinburgh: Scottish Intercollegiate Guidelines Network (SIGN), May 1997.

40. Davis D. Does CME work? An analysis of the effect of educational activities on physician performance or healthcare outcomes. *Int J Psychiatr Med* 1998:28;21–39.

41. Channer KS. Translating clinical trials into practice. *Lancet* 1997:349;645.

42. CAPRIE Steering Committee. A randomized, blinded trial of clopidogrel versus aspirin in patients at risk of ischaemic events. *Lancet* 1996:348;1329–1339.

43. Executive Committee for the Asymptomatic Carotid Atherosclerosis Study. Endarterectomy for asymptomatic carotid artery stenosis. *JAMA* 1995:273;1421.

44. Wolf PA, et al. Epidemiologic assessment of chronic atrial fibrllation and risk of stroke: The Framingham study. *Neurology* 1978:28;973–977.

45. Atrial Fibrillation Investigators. Risk factors for stroke and efficacy of antithrombotic therapy in atrial fibrillation: Analysis of pooled data from five randomized controlled trials. *Arch Intern Med* 1994:154;1449–1457.

46. Sudlow M, Thomson R, Thwaites B, Rodgers H, Kenny RA. Prevalence of atrial fibrillation and eligibility for anti-coagulants in the community. *Lancet* 1998:352;1167–1171.

47. Stroke Prevention in Atrial Fibrillation Investigators. Stroke Prevention in Atrial Fibrillation Study: Final results. *Circulation* 1991;84:527

48. Stroke Prevention in Atrial Fibrillation Investigators. Adjusted-dose warfarin versus low-intensity, fixed dose warfarin plus aspirin for high-risk patients with atrial fibrillation: Stroke Prevention in Atrial Fibrillation III randomized clinical trial. *Lancet* 1996:384;633–638.

49. The EC/IC Bypass Study Group. Failure of extracranial–intracranial bypass to reduce the risk of ischaemic stroke: Results of an intracranial randomized trial. *N Eng J Med* 1985:313;1191–1200.

50. Thrift AG, McNeil JJ, Forbes A, Donnan GA, for the Melbourne Risk Factor Study Group. Three important subgroups of hypertensive persons at greater risk of intracerebral haemorrhage. *Hypertension* 1998:31;1223–1229.

51. Croog SH, Levin S, Testa M, et al. The effect of antihypertensive therapy on the quality of life. *New Engl J Med* 1986:314;1643–1664.

52. Hansson L, et al. Effect of angiotensin-converting-enzyme in inhibition compared with conventional therapy on cardiovascular morbidity and mortality in hypertension: The Captopril Prevention Project (CAPP. randomized trial. *Lancet* 1999:353;611–616.

53. Joint National Committee on Detection, Evaluation, and Treatment of High Blood Pressure. The sixth report of the Joint national Committee on Prevention, Detection, Evaluation, and Treatment of High Blood Pressure (MNC VI). *Arch Intern Med* 1997: 157;2413–2146.

54. Diener HC, et al. European Stroke Prevention Study 2: Dipyridamole and acetylsalicylic acid in the secondary prevention stroke. *J Neurol Sci* 1996:143;1–13.

55. Jones EJ, et al. Proximal aortic atheroma: an independent risk factor for cerebral ischaemia. *Stroke* 1995:26;218–224.

56. Amarenco P, et al. Atherosclerotic disease of the aortic arch and the risk of ischaemic stroke. *N Engl J Med* 1994:331;1474–1479.

16

THE APPROPRIATENESS AND EFFECTIVENESS OF STROKE PREVENTION

Thomas E. Feasby

The recent introduction of tissue plasminogen activator (t-PA) for the treatment of acute stroke has energized the field of stroke care and directed attention toward acute treatment. This is long overdue. However, because of major access barriers, most eligible stroke patients will not be treated, and many other patients will not be eligible. Thus, stroke prevention is likely to remain the most important approach to decreasing its incidence and the disability resulting from stroke.

This chapter concentrates on carotid endarterectomy as a model of stroke prevention therapy. The general importance of quality of care and its measurement are discussed. One important quality process measure, appropriateness, is covered in detail. Finally, the measurement of effectiveness is introduced. It it illustrated with a new method to measure the effectiveness of carotid endarterectomy in series of clinical cases.

DEFINING QUALITY OF HEALTH CARE

Measurement of the quality of health care is becoming increasingly important to patients, providers, health care businesses, and employers.[1,2] Efforts to improve the quality of health care are critically dependent upon the measurement of quality.[3–5] Informed choice for patients requires readily available comparative quality data, not just efficacy data from randomized clinical trials. Patients, health care businesses, and payers need quality-of-care information to determine cost effectiveness.

The Institute of Medicine has defined quality of health care as "the degree to which health services for individuals and populations increase the likelihood of desired health outcomes and are consistent with current professional knowledge".[6] In this definition, *health services* refers to the broad range of services that affect health, including those that promote health, prevent disease, treat acute illness, and provide rehabilitation. The perspectives of *populations and individuals* must be considered, the latter including patients and health providers. *Desired outcomes* are those that patients value, not just the "objective" outcomes that clinicians have traditionally valued. The phrase *increases the likelihood* of good outcomes is a reminder that high-quality care does not always result in good outcomes, and patients may do well despite poor quality of care. This emphasizes the need to examine both the processes and the outcomes of care. The last qualifier, *consistent with current professional knowledge,* indicates the need for clinicians to continually update their knowledge of the current literature to be able to apply the best evidence in their management of patients.

Problems with the quality of health care may be classified into three categories, overuse, underuse, and misuse.[2] *Overuse* is when a health service is provided when its potential for harm exceeds its potential benefit. Clearly, it is *inappropriate*. An example relating to stroke would be the use of an EC/IC bypass to treat a transient ischemic attack (TIA) due to moderate carotid stenosis. The efficacy data suggest that this would be ineffective. *Underuse* is the failure to provide an *appropriate* service when it would be expected to produce a favorable outcome. For example, underuse would be the failure to provide TPA to an eligible acute stroke patient who was treatable under three hours from stroke onset. *Misuse* happens when an appropriate service is provided but an avoidable complication results in the patient receiving less than the full potential benefit. An example relating to stroke would be a patient receiving coumadin for atrial fibrillation who has a stroke because poor monitoring allowed the INR to fall too low.

Each of these types of quality-of-care problems is very common. Recent studies, for example, have shown that at least 21% of all U.S. antibiotic prescriptions given to ambulatory patients were used for upper respiratory infections in which they would not be expected to be effective.[7] The risks posed by this poor-quality practice include drug reactions, superinfections, and the development of antibiotic resistance. This is a serious problem of overuse.

Underuse is widespread and leads to lost opportunities to improve health and well-being. The undertreatment of hypertension, a proven preventive technique, results in many unnecessary strokes. β-blockers have been shown to reduce mortality after myocardial infarction but are grossly underused in practice.[8]

Unfortunately, *misuse,* the occurrence of *preventable* complications of treatment, is also frequent. Although misuse can be caused by error, not all errors are misuse because most do not result in harm and many are corrected before harm occurs. However, the wide range of perioperative complication rates reported for series of carotid endarterectomy cases not explained by differences in case mix suggests that misuse may be common. One study of U.S. Medicare patients hospitalized with congestive heart failure showed that those who received poor-quality care had a 74% greater mortality rate within 30 days than those who received good-quality care.[9]

In efforts to improve quality, sight must not be lost of the effects on cost, given the constraints on the health care system. Directives are frequently given to "do more with less." Is it possible? The answer in terms of the cost of quality improvement is "yes and no".[2] Reducing overuse clearly improves quality by reducing unnecessary risk and nuisance but also reduces costs by decreasing the number of procedures or treatments. Reducing misuse also improves quality by sparing patients misfortune and by improving outcomes. Cost will also be reduced. A recent study of patient harm showed that when preventable therapeutic drug errors occurred, the cost of each hospital stay was increased by almost $5000.[10] The conflict comes with underuse. There is no doubt about the improved health outcome, including stroke prevention, from the increased appropriate use of antihypertensive and anticholesterol treatment. Determining the effect on cost is more difficult. Most efforts to rectify underuse result in increased initial costs. Whether the costs of prevention or deferral of disease or disability will result in cost savings is unknown.

MEASURING THE QUALITY OF HEALTH CARE

For the purpose of measurement, the quality of health care can be separated into the domains of structure, process, and outcome.[11] *Structure* includes the physical facilities, such as hospital size and type, protocols, equipment, and the qualifications of the staff. These are the usual purview of accreditation boards, but they relate uncertainly to process and outcomes. *Process* includes all things that are actually done to and for patients. This involves the technical aspects of care and its competence, and also the "art" of medicine. That is, was the right choice of treatment made and how well was it done? One process measure that has been employed widely to examine whether the choice of treatment was right is appropriateness. This provides a contemporary measurement of process incorporating best evidence and informed opinion. It is discussed in detail in relation to stroke prevention below. Process measures are those most frequently used. They relate to evidence of best practice, and the deficiencies they reveal should be amenable to improvement.

Outcome is the most obvious quality measure, but not always the best. Even when the outcome measure is mortality, its assessment presents challenges. Mortality has been used frequently in monitoring coronary artery bypass surgery, but problems can arise in comparing results between series of cases because of insufficient risk adjustment to compensate for differences in case mix.[12] Mortality and morbidity, usually a combined stroke and death rate, have been used as outcome measures to assess quality in series of carotid endarterectomies. This approach ignores the expected good outcomes from the treatment (i.e., the prevention of stroke), probably because of the difficulty in measurement. For this reason, the rate of complications after carotid endarterectomy is not a sufficient outcome measure.

Bad outcomes may also be unsuitable outcome measures because bad outcomes due to misuse may be uncommon. Most patients survive mishaps in care. Also, overuse is not detected by measuring outcome. Healthy patients who do not need a treatment are likely to fare better than those who are ill or at risk and should receive the treatment. Thus, overtreatment can result in better results when only the negative outcomes are measured.

Aggregate population measures of outcome are insensitive for examining the effect of changes in process. Measures such as infant mortality, longevity, or even stroke rate are subject to so many influences that attributing improvement or worsening to changes made in any particular intervention is almost impossible. To some extent, this is a "signal and noise" problem.[13] If specific populations at risk are examined using specific outcome measures, the marginal benefits may be seen more easily.

Two quality measures are discussed in the following sections. The first is appropriateness, a process measure that has been applied widely to surgical procedures and to carotid endarterectomy, in particular. Its advantages and disadvantages will be considered. The second is effectiveness. This concept is defined and a new approach to its measurement is outlined using carotid endarterectomy as the example.

APPROPRIATENESS, A MEASURE OF PROCESS

A method to measure the appropriateness of medical interventions was developed at the RAND Corporation in the 1980s.[14] This work was motivated by concerns that the increasing complexity of medical care was resulting in many patients receiving unnecessary care and others not receiving necessary care.[15] The method was based on the following principles: timeliness to produce a contemporary measure; the best medical evidence from the literature; representation of a medical point of view (not one based on cost); and informed opinion from a multispecialty panel.

The first step in the process is a detailed review of the relevant literature to obtain and grade the evidence for the indications, efficacy, and effectiveness of the procedure being considered. Next, a list of indications for the procedure is compiled and transformed into scenarios incorporating the patient's age, symptoms, co-morbidities, etc., under which the intervention might be performed. An attempt is made to create enough scenarios with sufficient specificity that the patients in each scenario are reasonably homogeneous. The number of scenarios may exceed 1000 for some procedures. Reviewers assess the literature review and the compiled scenarios to detect and correct omissions or biases.

An expert panel of nine is recruited that includes experts in the procedure under study as well as those with general and related expertise. Members are often recruited by asking specialty societies for nominees, and an attempt is made to ensure geographic diversity. The panel is chaired by a physician trained in epidemiology, statistics, or research design. The panelists then read the literature review and suggest revisions to it and the list of scenarios. Next, the panelists go through two rounds in which they rate the scenarios on the basis of appropriateness. The first rating is done individually. Then, a group meeting is held to discuss and rate each of the indications. Discussion is encouraged to ensure thorough understanding of each scenario and the ratings.

The ratings are done on an ordinal, nine-point scale. Appropriateness is defined to mean that a procedure is worth doing if the expected medical benefit to the patient (e.g., health status, quality of life, longevity) exceeds the expected negative consequences (e.g., disability, pain, risk of death).[14] The scale contains three categories and allows a range within each category. Level 1 to 3 is inappropriate, 4 to 6 is uncertain, and 7 to 9 is appropriate. Using this system, each scenario is given a rating on the appropriateness scale. Cost is not considered.

The ratings are then applied to a series of real cases. The data is collected by chart review, and each case is categorized according to the list of scenarios. Since each scenario has a rating on the scale, the overall level of appropriateness for a series of cases can be determined. The method has been used to assess many therapeutic and investigative procedures, such as coronary artery bypass surgery, coronary angiography, coronary angioplasty, hysterectomy, colonoscopy, cholecystectomy, upper gastrointestinal endoscopy, and back manipulation.

THE APPROPRIATENESS OF CAROTID ENDARTERECTOMY

The rate of carotid endarterectomy (CE) was high in the 1980s, when the first study of the appropriateness of CE[16] was done. The wisdom of doing CE was almost unquestioned, but the evidence for efficacy was lacking; also, were marked regional variations existed in the rate of CE.[17] The surprising results of this study helped to fuel the drive for the randomized controlled trials of the 1990s, which truly determined the efficacy of CE.

Using the RAND appropriateness methodology, Winslow et al.[16] developed 864 scenarios under which CE might be performed. The scenarios included various categories of symptomatic patients, several categories of asymptomatic patients, and incorporated data about age, sex, comorbidities, and degree of carotid stenosis measured angiographically. These scenarios were rated on the nine point appropriateness scale. The ratings were then applied by chart review to a random sample of 1302 Medicare patients who underwent CE in three different geographic regions in the United States in 1981.

In this study, 35% of the procedures were found to be appropriate, 32% were uncertain, and 32% were inappropriate. Of the inappropriate cases, about half had carotid stenosis of less than 50%. Fifty-four percent of all the procedures were done in patients who did not have ischemic events in the carotid territory. The authors concluded that there was evidence of substantial overuse of CE in the regions studied.

Knowledge of CE and its efficacy improved markedly in the 1990s with the publication of the NASCET[18,19] and ACAS[20] trials. One would expect the appropriateness to have improved as well. Wong et al.[21] carried out an appropriateness study of CE in Edmonton, Alberta, on patients operated on in 1994 and 1995. They developed their appropriateness criteria in a different way; by reviewing the recent randomized controlled trials on CE and the clinical practice guidelines for CE published by the American Heart Association[22] and the Canadian Neurosurgical Society.[23] They then applied these criteria to 291 cases of CE by chart review. They improved their categorization of patients by remeasuring the carotid angiograms, allowing them to correct for misclassification. They found only a moderate agreement between the radiologists' original estimation of stenosis and the remeasured value (symptomatic stenosis: $\kappa = 0.72$; asymptomatic stenosis: $\kappa = 0.67$). They found that 33% of CEs were appropriate, 49% were uncertain, and 18% were inappropriate. These results are no better than those of Winslow et al. almost 10 years earlier, where 35% of CEs were considered to be appropriate.

Wong et al. put the method to an interesting test, trying to improve the level of appropriateness using an educational intervention.[24] They provided all the surgeons with the results of their first study as well as with current CE practice guidelines, and they let them know that there would be a prospective surveillance study. They then monitored the performance of CE for a year. The results of this study were 49% appropriate, 47% uncertain, and 4% inappropriate. This was a significant improvement in the proportion appropriate ($p = 0.0005$) and a significant drop in the proportion inappropriate. Forty per cent of the cases had asymptomatic carotid stenosis and represented the majority of those rated uncertain, as they had in the first study.

Two recent studies, one from Georgia and another from Oklahoma, illustrate how sensitive an appropriateness study of CE is to the criteria chosen for appropriateness.[25,26] The appropriateness study of CE from Georgia[25] found results strikingly different from those from Alberta. The authors did a retrospective review of the charts of 1945 CE Medicare patients from 1993. They found that 96.1% of CEs were done appropriately. The appropriateness study of 813 CEs on Oklahoma Medicare patients from 1993 and 1994 found an appropriateness level of 98%.[26]

Why are these results so different from the other studies? First, they used different appropriateness criteria. Both studies included as appropriate most patients who were asymptomatic. In fact, in the Georgia series, 51% of patients were asypmptomatic and in the Oklahoma series, 43%. This latter study accepted as appropriate both symptomatic and asymptomatic patients with ≥60% stenosis. Neither study included an "uncertain" category, and the authors did not independently remeasure the angiograms for validation. These factors, especially the decision to classify asymptomatic patients as appropriate rather than uncertain, had a large effect on the outcome. It is clear that the appropriateness criteria and ratings chosen have a major impact on the results of this type of study. The original RAND approach to the development of criteria still seems to be the most valid approach.

Many other procedures have been assessed for appropriateness, the most relevant for comparison being coronary artery bypass grafting (CABG). This procedure has been under intense scrutiny since the late 1980s, beginning first in New York state, where outcomes for surgeons and hospitals were measured and eventually published in the lay press as "report cards."[12] The development of risk adjustment methods to adjust for differences in case mix reflecting differing baseline risks between different case series has improved the credibility of this process. Appropriateness measurement has also been applied to CABG. A study using the RAND methodology on American patients from 1979 to 1982 found that 56% were appropriate, 30% uncertain, and 14% inappropriate.[27] More recent studies from the 1990s in the United States[28] and Canada[29] have shown levels of appropriateness (and necessity) of about 92%–95%.

It seems clear that appropriateness is a useful contemporary measure of process and quality of care, but it has limitations.[30] It is very sensitive to the criteria of appropriateness and their derivation. Even when the RAND method is used, the "gold standard" for appropriateness, the reproducibility between panels is deficient.[31] The ratings also vary depending on the specialty mix and background of the expert panels.[32] Naylor stated that these methods "are best regarded as rough screening tests for overuse and underuse of specific procedures."[30] In fact, these methods are not useful for detecting underuse. They are useful for assessing overuse, but their limitations are significant

EFFECTIVENESS AS AN OUTCOME MEASURE

In judging the quality of a medical intervention, effectiveness is the measurement of most value. However, when doctors discuss treatment options with patients, the measure of benefit usually cited is efficacy. Unfortunately, this is not a suitable quality measure for most situations.[15] Efficacy is the product of a randomized clinical trial (RCT), an *experiment* that tells us if a procedure works under ideal circumstances, and whether it is potentially useful.[33] Efficacy answers the question "Can it work?" Effectiveness is a better outcome measure, one which is similar to efficacy, except that it reflects the outcome of an intervention in the real world when it is applied by average physicians to average patients in average circumstances. Effectiveness answers the question "Does it work?" Efficacy is often employed as if it were effectiveness, but it is likely that efficacy is an overestimate of effectiveness under most circumstances. This is because (1) restrictive entry criteria of RCTs often exclude higher-risk and older patients; (2) restrictive entry criteria for physicians[18–20,33] may produce a higher quality of practice in an RCT; and (3) compliance with medical care is likely to be better in a trial. Underuse is the other major limitation to the realization of the full effectiveness of treatments. Although effectiveness is the outcome of most importance, it is difficult to measure for several reasons. In clinical practice, patients are not randomized, so that an equivalent untreated comparison group is lacking. Valid and reliable data are often unavailable. Outcomes of interest may be delayed.

Randomized clinical trials have shown that β-blockers can reduce the mortality of patients following acute myocardial infarction.[34,35] The Norwegian Multicenter Study, a RCT of timolol vs. placebo in 1884 patients after acute myocardial infarction, showed a 6.2% absolute risk reduction in sudden death rate in 33 months of follow-up.[34] The β-blocker Heart Attack Trial compared propranolol vs. placebo in 3837 patients after acute myocardial infarction. This study showed a 2.6% absolute risk reduction for mortality over 27 months of follow-up.[35] The results of both studies were statistically significant ($p < 0.005$). The evidence for the efficacy of β-blockers after myocardial infarction is thus clear, but what about its effectiveness, the "real world" equivalent of efficacy?

Soumerai et al.[8] performed a retrospective cohort study in New Jersey using a database that linked Medicare and drug claims data from 1987 to 1992. The database allowed them to determine all Medicare patients in New Jersey who had acute myocardial infarction, what drugs were prescribed, and mortality over the two years post–myocardial infarction. They found that only 21% of eligible myocardial infarction patients received β-blockers. However, in those who were prescribed the drugs, the absolute risk reduction was similar to that shown in the RCTs. Therefore, the effectiveness in the *treated* population was similar to the efficacy in the RCTs. However, on a population-wide basis, this treatment could not be considered effective because of underuse. A recent review of articles published on quality of care in the United States from 1993 to 1997 showed that for studies of disease prevention, only about 50% of eligible people received the necessary preventive care.[36] Underuse is the major reason why effectiveness of preventive care for an eligible population is less than efficacy.

Underuse also limits effectiveness in stroke prevention. A study of American health care plans showed that more than 50% of hypertensive patients did not have adequately controlled blood pressure.[37] This suggests underuse and, therefore, suboptimal effectiveness of a proven stroke preventative. Warfarin is also a proven stroke preventative in those with atrial fibrillation. A recent chart review study of Medicare patients hospitalized with ischemic stroke and atrial fibrillation in Connecticut showed that only 53% of the patients were prescribed warfarin at discharge, and 62% of those not given warfarin were not given aspirin, either.[38]

The ideal outcome measure of effectiveness should be objective and readily measured. It should also reflect the quality of care. An outcome that cannot be altered by changes in process is not useful as a measure of quality or effectiveness. Mortality has been used frequently in monitoring coronary artery bypass surgery, but its assessment presents challenges. Problems can arise in comparing results because of insufficient risk adjustment to compensate for differences in case mix.[12] Also, when only mortality is considered, the anticipated good outcomes of prophylactic care are often ignored, perhaps because they are more difficult to measure. This is especially so when the expected good outcomes may be considerably delayed, as in stroke prevention. An effectiveness measurement method that measures the outcomes of an intervention, incorporating both the complications and the good outcomes, and that is responsive to improvements in process is needed.

A METHOD TO MEASURE EFFECTIVENESS

This section describes a method to estimate the effectiveness of treatment interventions in case series. Of necessity, this measure deals only with the population actually treated. Measuring effectiveness in the population at risk is also important but requires different methods. The example of CE is used, but the method is suitable for other interventions, including other stroke prevention approaches. A more detailed description of the method is available.[39]

This method of measuring effectiveness incorporates the following principles and assumptions:

1. Randomized controlled trials are done with restricted categories of patients, unlike population-based case series (PBSs). For instance, a trial might enroll patients with a certain disease only if they were male and of a certain age. However, if there are sufficient categories of RCTs to account for the case-mix in the PBS, assuming that the baseline risk in the RCT category is similar to that in the PBS category, the efficacy data from the RCTs can then be applied to the corresponding categories of the PBS.
2. Efficacy results from RCTs must be adjusted for the difference in the intervention-induced mortality and morbidity between the RCT and the PBS before they can be applied to the categories of PBSs. Efficacy is a measure of the difference in outcome events between the control and the treated

(experimental) groups in a RCT. The outcome events caused by the intervention (e.g., surgical mortality/morbidity) are factored into the efficacy measurement, incorporated as part of the risk in the treated group. To apply efficacy results to a PBS with no control group, one must measure the rate of treatment-related events in the PBS, and use the difference between this rate and the rate in the RCT to adjust the efficacy results, so that an absolute risk reduction can be calculated for the PBS. Patients at high operative risk might receive surgery in a PBS, but would have been excluded from a RCT. This adjustment of efficacy for the PBS takes this into account by including the real perioperative mortality/morbidity, not just that from the RCT. It is assumed that the good outcome to be expected from the intervention (e.g., prevention of stroke) will be the same in the PBS as it was for the RCT, once this adjustment has been made. However, this assumption does not deal with the issue of possibly decreased life expectancy unrelated to the intervention in the PBS, because of treatment of patients of advanced age or with co-morbid conditions that may limit survival, patients who would not have been included in the RCT.

3. Patients are accurately classified according to prognostic criteria at entry into RCTs. Classification in PBSs is likely to be less accurate. If possible, misclassification should be measured and corrected in analyzing the PBS.

4. The adjusted efficacy estimates for the reclassified categories of the PBS can be combined proportionately to yield an overall estimate of the effectiveness of the intervention.

5. Efficacy can be expressed in several ways.[40,41] In epidemiologic studies, the relative risk (risk ratio, RR) is most commonly used. It is the ratio of the risk between the exposed (treated) and unexposed (control) groups. The relative risk reduction (RRR) is 1-RR and expresses the reduction in risk due to treatment. The importance of this measure in RCTs is highly dependent upon the baseline risk in the control group.[40,42] A large RRR is less impressive if the baseline risk in the control group is low. The absolute risk reduction (ARR, or risk difference) is the actual difference in risk between the control and intervention groups and is a more robust indicator of efficacy in RCTs. The reciprocal of the ARR, 1/ARR, is the number needed to treat (NNT). The NNT is the number of patients who must undergo the intervention to prevent one outcome event during the follow-up period of the study.[43] Effectiveness, like efficacy, can be expressed in all of the above ways, but the NNT is the most practical for clinical applications.

The major study of clopidogrel for prevention of stroke and other vascular events affords a useful example.[44] This RCT of 19,185 patients comparing the efficacy of clopidogrel to aspirin in preventing vascular events reported an RRR of 8.7%. However, the ARR was only 0.51% because the baseline risk in the aspirin-treated group was so low. Thus, the NNT to prevent one stroke over one year using clopidogrel rather than aspirin was 196 patients. This way of expressing the result is much more meaningful than using an RRR of 8.7%. The NNT will be used in the following example of CE.

EXAMPLE: THE EFFECTIVENESS OF CAROTID ENDARTERECTOMY

Many RCTs have examined the efficacy of CE in the last ten years, allowing division of cases from a PBS into four groups on the basis of the degree of carotid stenosis and whether they were symptomatic. Two major trials in symptomatic patients, the North American Symptomatic Carotid Endarterectomy Trial (NASCET)[18,19] and the European Carotid Surgery Trial[45] reported similar results. The results from NASCET will be used because they represent mostly North American patients and the measurement technique employed for carotid angiograms is the North American standard. NASCET reported on the efficacy of CE in symptomatic patients with ≥70% stenosis. The second phase of NASCET reported on efficacy in symptomatic patients with <70% stenosis.[19] The efficacy figures for surgery on those with asymptomatic carotid stenosis ≥60% are taken from the Asymptomatic Carotid Atherosclerosis Study (ACAS).[20] The ARR for the asymptomatic group with <60% stenosis is unknown. Given that the ARR in the those with stenosis of from 60% to 99% was 1.5%,[46] an assumption that the ARR was zero in the asymptomatic group with <60% stenosis seems reasonable. All figures are for two years of follow-up and are shown in Table 16.1.

The recent population-based series from the University of Alberta will be used to illustrate the "effectiveness" method. Wong et al.[21] reported on 291 consecutive patients receiving CE in Edmonton, Alberta, over 18 months in 1994 and 1995. The data were collected by chart review. The cases were classified as symptomatic and ≥70% or 50%–69% stenosis, or asymptomatic and ≥60% or <60% stenosis. Furthermore, the carotid angiograms were remeasured using the

TABLE 16.1. Results of Carotid Endarterectomy Clinical Trials

	ABSOLUTE RISK REDUCTION (%)	NUMBER NEEDED TO TREAT	PERIOPERATIVE MORTALITY/ MORBIDITY (%)
Symptomatic ≥70% stenosis	13.1	7.6	5.5
Symptomatic 50%–69% stenosis	4.9	20.4	6.8
Asymptomatic ≥60% stenosis[46]	1.5	67	2.3
Asymptomatic <60% stenosis	*0*	—	*2.3*

Figures in italics are estimates. Note that the ARR of 13.1% for the first category is the two-year estimate from the second NASCET paper[19] and is different from that in the first paper,[18] reflecting longer follow-up (Dr. M. Eliasziw, personal communication for NASCET, 1999).

TABLE 16.2. Alberta Endarterectomy Series Reclassified After Angiogram Remeasurement

ALBERTA SERIES	RECLASSIFIED %	PERIOPERATIVE MORTALITY/ MORBIDITY (%)
Symptomatic ≥70% stenosis	36.4	5.2
Symptomatic 50–69% stenosis	22.7	5.2
Asymptomatic ≥60% stenosis	27.8	5.1
Asymptomatic <60% stenosis	13.1	5.1

NASCET and ACAS criteria. This allowed detection of misclassification by degree of stenosis and permitted reclassification on the basis of the correct measurement (Table 16.2).

To calculate the effectiveness score (absolute risk reduction for the PBS, i.e., ARR_i^P) for each category (stratum), an adjustment is made in the efficacy score from the RCT (absolute risk reduction for the RCT, i.e., ARR^R), based on the difference between the perioperative mortality/morbidity rate (i.e., stroke and/or death) in the RCT (M^R) and the PBS (M^P). For the symptomatic ≥70% stenosis stratum in the Alberta series,

$$AAR_i^P = ARR^R - (M^P - M^R) = 13.1\% - (5.2\% - 5.5\%) = 13.4\%$$

The effectiveness in this stratum is higher than in the RCT because the perioperative stroke and/or death rate was lower in the Alberta series than in NASCET. The ARR^P for each stratum in each series is then calculated as shown in this example. The results are shown in Table 16.3.

The effectiveness scores (AAR_i^P) for each stratum are then weighted by the proportion of cases in each category and summed to produce an aggregate effectiveness score for the PBS:

$$AAR^P = \sum_{i=1}^{s} p_i^P(ARR_i^R + M_i^R - M_i^P) = \sum_{i=1}^{s} p_i^P(ARR_i^P)$$

$$= (0.364 \times 13.4\%) + (0.227 \times 6.5\%) + (0.278 \times (-1.3\%))$$
$$+ (0.131 \times (-2.8\%))$$

$$\therefore ARR^P = 5.6\%$$

The ARR for the entire Alberta series (including all four categories) is 5.6%. The NNT for the Alberta series is then derived by taking the reciprocal of the ARR^P:

$$NNT = 1/ARR^P = 1/0.056 = 17.9$$

TABLE 16.3. Efficacy and Effectiveness Results from All Categories and Studies

CLINICAL/STENOSIS CATEGORY	STUDY	ABSOLUTE RISK REDUCTION (%)	NUMBER NEEDED TO TREAT
Symptomatic ≥70% stenosis	NASCET	13.1	7.6
	Ohio	11.9	8.4
	Alberta	13.4	7.5
Symptomatic 50%–69% stenosis	NASCET	4.9	20
	Ohio	5	20
	Alberta	6.5	15.4
Asymptomatic ≥60% stenosis	ACAS	1.5	67
	Ohio	1.3	77
	Alberta	−1.3	(77)
Asymptomatic <60% stenosis	Ohio	−0.2	(500)
	Alberta	−2.8	(35.7)
Overall effectiveness	Ohio	5.2	19.2
	Alberta	5.6	17.9
	Calgary	8.7	11.5

ARR and NNT are for two years; NNTs in parentheses are, in fact, NNHs (numbers needed to harm).

Therefore, the estimated effectiveness of CE in the Alberta series can be expressed as an NNT of 17.9, meaning that one stroke was prevented in Alberta over 2 years for approximately every 18 CEs performed. Similar calculations for a recent Ohio[47] series of CEs extrapolating the proportions of stenosis categories from the Alberta series produced an NNT of about 19. The AARs and NNTs for each category in the two series are shown with the efficacy results from the RCTs for comparison in Table 16.3. Table 16.3 shows that the benefit (effectiveness) of operating on patients with asymptomatic carotid stenosis of ≥60% is extremely small, even in ACAS (AAR = 1.5%, NNT = 67).[46] It is worse in the Ohio series (ARR = 1.3%, NNT = 77) and is non-existent in the Alberta series (AAR = −1.3%, NNH = 77). In fact, in the Alberta series, the NNT is really an NNH, a number needed to harm, because the perioperative stroke/death rate was greater than in ACAS by an amount exceeding the AAR in ACAS. Operating on a sizable proportion of asymptomatic patients, even with a reasonable complication rate, reduces the overall effectiveness of a series of cases of CE.

This is illustrated by considering the result in a recent audit of CE cases in Calgary from 1994 to 1998[48] (see Table 16.3). The charts of 184 consecutive CE cases were reviewed, and 78% were symptomatic and 22% were asymptomatic cases. The perioperative stroke/death rate was 3.6% in the symptomatic cases. However, the rate in the asymptomatic cases was 12.7%, much higher than that in the ACAS trial.[20] Despite this deficiency, which in that category resulted in an

NNH of 11, the *overall effectiveness* of CE in this series was an NNT of 11.5 (ARR = 8.7%), largely due to the preponderance of symptomatic cases. The surgeons were operating on a higher proportion of patients where there was more to gain, namely symptomatic cases. Thus, it is possible for surgeons with higher complication rates to have greater overall effectiveness than those with lower complication rates if they choose to operate mainly on symptomatic patients. This is not to suggest that reducing the perioperative stroke and death rate is not an important way of improving effectiveness. Surgery performed with the lowest possible complication rate is extremely important, and some have suggested that those with higher complication rates should not be performing CE.[49] Nevertheless, the case mix will usually be a more important variable in determining the overall effectiveness of a series of CE cases.

It is possible to model the relationship between efficacy and case mix for CE. Figure 16.1 which demonstrates the effect of case mix on the ARR and NNT for CE. The efficacy figures are taken from the NASCET and ACAS trials. A series with 100% symptomatic cases will have an ARR of 13.1% and an NNT of 7.6 patients over two years as did NASCET, whereas one with 100% asymptomatic cases will have an ARR of 1.5% and an NNT of 67 patients. As the proportion

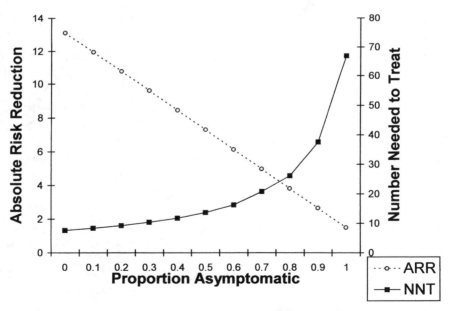

FIGURE 16.1. Model of the relationship between efficacy and case mix (proportion of cases that are asymptomatic) for carotid endarterectomy. Efficacy figures are from the NASCET (ref. 19) and ACAS (ref. 20) trials. The number needed to treat (NNT) and the absolute risk reduction (ARR) are for two years.

of asymptomatic cases increases, the efficacy declines. A similar relationship would apply to effectiveness in series of CE cases, measured to adjust from efficacy to effectiveness according to differences in the perioperative stroke/death rate between the case series and the RCTs, as in the method described above.

How does the effectiveness of CE compare with that of other stroke prevention interventions? Although they require long-term treatment, antiplatelet agents and anticoagulation for atrial fibrillation would appear to be much less cumbersome approaches, but are they more effective? Unfortunately, only efficacy data are available. For anticoagulation for patients with atrial fibrillation, the NNT to prevent one stroke over two years is 16.[50] For aspirin, the most widely used stroke prevention medication, 50 TIA patients must be treated for one year to prevent one stroke.[51] Clopidogrel is a new antiplatelet drug introduced to treat TIAs. However, only a marginal benefit ensues from using clopidogrel, rather than aspirin, requiring 196 patients to be treated over one year to prevent one more stroke than is prevented by aspirin treatment.[44] Almost certainly, the effectiveness of each of these prophylactic interventions is less than these efficacy figures, even in just the treated populations. The true effectiveness of these treatments must be measured to determine the quality of stroke prevention approaches. This is essential to enable a reduction in the incidence of stroke and to reduce its burden on society.

CONCLUSION

Quality problems, including overuse, underuse, and misuse, are widespread in clinical medicine. Both process and outcome measures are useful in detecting problems with quality. Appropriateness is the process measure most frequently applied to CE. It is very sensitive to the criteria used to determine appropriateness, and thus may vary widely between different studies. A more direct approach to measuring effectiveness has the advantage of incorporating both the adverse and good outcomes expected from an intervention such as CE. This may allow surgeons, hospitals, health regions, and health plans to monitor the health benefit of their treatment interventions.

REFERENCES

1. Chassin MR. Is health care ready for six sigma quality? *The Milbank Quarterly* 1998; 76:565–591.
2. Chassin MR, Galvin RW, and the National Roundtable on Health Care Quality. The urgent need to improve health care quality. *JAMA* 1998;280:1000–1005.
3. Hannan EL, Kilburn H, Racz M, et al. Improving the outcomes of coronary artery bypass surgery in New York State. *JAMA* 1994;271:761–766.
4. Epstein A. Performance reports on quality—prototypes, problems, and prospects. *New Engl J Med* 1995;333:57–61.

5. Brook RH, McGlynn EA, Cleary PC. Measuring quality of care: Part 2. *New Engl J Med* 1996;335:966–970.

6. Lohr KN, ed. *Medicare: A Strategy for Quality Assurance*. Washington, DC: National Academy Press, 1990.

7. Gonzales R, Steiner JF, Sande MA. Antibiotic prescribing for adults with colds, upper respiratory tract infections, and bronchitis by ambulatory care physicians. *JAMA* 1997;278:901–904.

8. Soumerai SB, McLaughlin TJ, Speigelman D, et al. Adverse outcomes of underuse of β-blockers in elderly survivors of acute myocardial infarction. *JAMA* 1997;277: 115–121.

9. Kahn KL, Rogers WH, Rubenstein LW, et al. Measuring quality of care with explicit process criteria before and after implementation of the DRG-based prospective payment system. *JAMA* 1990;264:1969–1973.

10. Bates DW, Spell N, Cullen DJ, et al. The costs of adverse drug events in hospitalized patients. *JAMA* 1997;277:307–311.

11. Donabedian A. *Explorations in Quality Assessment and Monitoring*. Vol. 1: *The Definition of Quality and Approaches to Its Assessment*. Ann Arbor, MI: Health Administration Press, 1980.

12. Green J, Wintfeld N. Report cards on cardiac surgeons: Assessing New York State's approach. *New Engl J Med* 1995;332:1229–1232.

13. Naylor CD. Assessing processes and outcomes of medical care. *Ann Roy Coll Phys Surg Canada* 1997;30:157–161.

14. Brook RH, Chassin M, Fink A, et al. A method for the detailed assessment of the appropriateness of medical technologies. *Int J Technol Assess Health Care* 1986;2:53–63.

15. Brook RH, Lohr KN. Efficacy, effectiveness, variations, and quality: Boundary-crossing research. *Med Care* 1985;23:710–722.

16. Winslow C, Solomon D, Chassin M, Kosecoff J, Merrick N, Brook RH. The appropriateness of carotid endarterectomy. *New Engl J Med* 1988;318:721–727.

17. Chassin MR, Brook RH, Park RE, et al. Variations in the use of medical and surgical services by the Medicare population. *New Engl J Med* 1986;314:285–290.

18. North American Symptomatic Carotid Endarterectomy Trial Collaborators. Beneficial effect of carotid endarterectomy in symptomatic patients with high-grade stenosis. *New Engl J Med* 1991;325:445–453.

19. Barnett HJM, et al. The benefit of carotid endarterectomy in symptomatic patients with moderate and severe stenosis. *New Engl J Med* 1998;339:1415–1425.

20. Executive Committee for the Asymptomatic Carotid Atherosclerosis Study. Endarterectomy for asymptomatic carotid artery stenosis. *JAMA* 1995;273:1421–1428.

21. Wong J, Findlay J, Suarez-Almazor M. Regional performance of carotid endarterectomy: Appropriateness, outcomes and risk factors for complications. *Stroke* 1997;228: 891–898.

22. Moore WS, Barnett HJM, Beebe HG, et al. Guidelines for carotid endarterectomy: a multi-disciplinary consensus statement from the Ad Hoc Committee, American Heart Association. *Stroke* 1995;26:188–201.

23. Findlay JM, Tucker WS, Ferguson GG, et al. Guidelines for the use of carotid endarterectomy: Current recommendations from the Canadian Neurosurgical Society. *Can Med Assoc J* 1997;157:653–659.

24. Wong J, Lubkey T, Suarez-Almazor M, Findlay JM. Improving the appropriateness of carotid endarterectomy: Results of a prospective city-wide study. *Stroke* 1999;30: 12–15.

25. Karp HR, Flanders D, Shipp CC, et al. Carotid endarterectomy among Medicare beneficiaries: A statewide evaluation of appropriateness and outcome. *Stroke* 1998;29: 46–52.

26. Bratzler DW, Oehlert W, Murray C, et al. Carotid endarterectomy in Oklahoma Medicare beneficiaries: Patient characteristics and outcomes. *J Okla St Med Assoc.* 1996;89:423–429.

27. Winslow CM, Kosecoff J, Chassin M, Kanouse D, Brook RH. The appropriateness of performing coronary artery bypass surgery. *JAMA* 1988;260:505–509.

28. Leape LL, Hilborne L, Schwartz J, Bates D, et al. The appropriateness of coronary artery bypass graft surgery in academic medical centers. *Ann Int Med* 1996;125;8–18.

29. Fox GA, O'Dea J, Parfrey PS. Coronary artery bypass graft surgery in Newfoundland and Labrador. *Can Med Assoc J* 1998;158:1137–1142.

30. Naylor CD. What is appropriate care? *New Engl J Med* 1998;338:1918–1920.

31. Shekelle PG, Kahan J, Bernstein S, et al. The reproducibility of a method to identify the overuse and underuse of medical procedures. *New Engl J Med* 1998;338:1888–1895.

32. Kahan JP, Park RE, Leape LL, et al. Variations by specialty in physician ratings of the appropriateness and necessity of indications for procedures. *Med Care* 1996; 34:512-523.

33. Wells KB. Treatment research at the crossroads: The scientific interface of clinical trials and effectiveness research. *Am J Psychiatr* 1999(Jan);156:5–10.

34. The Norwegian Multicenter Study Group. Timolol-induced reduction in mortality and reinfarction in patients surviving acute myocardial infarction. *New Engl J Med* 1981; 304:801–807.

35. β-Blocker Heart Attack Trial Research Group. A randomized trial of propranolol in patients with acute myocardial infarction. 1. Mortality results. *JAMA* 1982;247:1707–1714.

36. Schuster M, McGlynn E, Brook R. How good is the quality of health care in the United States? *The Milbank Quarterly* 1998;76:517–563.

37. Udvarhelyi I, Jennison K, Phillips R, Epstein A. Comparison of the quality of ambulatory care for fee-for-service and prepaid patients. *Ann Int Med* 1991;115:394–400.

38. Brass L, Krumholz H, Scinto J, Mathur D, Radford M. Warfarin use following ischemic stroke among Medicare patients with atrial fibrillation. *Arch Intern Med* 1998; 158:2093–2100.

39. Feasby TE. Measuring the effectiveness of carotid endarterectomy 2001, submitted for publication

40. Sackett DL, Haynes RB, Guyatt GH, Tugwell P. *Clinical Epidemiology. A Basic Science for Clinical Medicine.* Boston: Little, Brown & Co, 1991.

41. Sinclair JC, Bracken MB. Clinically useful measures of effect in binary analyses of randomized trials. *J Clin Epidemiol* 1994;47:881–889.

42. McQuay HJ, Moore, RA. Using numerical results from systematic reviews in clinical practice. *Ann Int Med* 1997;126:712-720.

43. Laupacis A, Sackett DL, Roberts RS. An assessment of clinically useful measures of the consequences of treatment. *New Engl J Med* 1988;318:1728–1733.

44. CAPRIE Steering committee. Randomized blinded trial of clopidogrel versus aspirin in patients at risk of ischemic events. *Lancet* 1996;348:1329–1339.

45. European Carotid Surgery Trialists' Collaborative Group. Randomized trial of endarterectomy for recently symptomatic carotid stenosis: Final results of the MRC European Carotid Surgery Trial (ECST). *Lancet* 1998;351:1379–1287.

46. Barnett HJM, Eliaziw M, Meldrum H, Taylor D. Do the facts and figures warrant a 10–fold increase in the performance of carotid endarterectomy on asymptomatic patients? *Neurology* 1996;46:603–608.
47. Cebul RD, Snow JR, Pine R, et al. Indications, outcomes, and provider volumes for carotid endarterectomy. *JAMA* 1998;279:1282-1287.
48. Janes E, Ghali W, Karbalai H, Feasby TE, Buchan AM. The risks of inappropriate carotid endarterectomy. *Ann Neurol* 1998;44:510.
49. Goldstein LB, Moore WS, Robertson JT, Chaturvedi S. Complication rates for carotid endarterectomy: A call to action. *Stroke* 1997;28:889–890.
50. Atrial Fibrillation Investigators. Risk factors of stroke and efficacy of anti-thrombotic therapy in atrial fibrillation: Analysis of pooled data from five randomized, controlled trials. *Arch Int Med* 1994;154:1449–1457.
51. Antiplatelet Trialists' Collaboration. Collaborative overview of randomized trials of antiplatelet therapy: Prevention of death, myocardial infarction, and stroke by prolonged antiplatelet therapy in various categories of patients. *BMJ* 1994;308:81–106.

17

POLICY AND PRACTICE IN THE PREVENTION OF STROKE: BETWEEN THE IDEAL AND THE AFFORDABLE

Graeme J. Hankey

This chapter applies the evidence presented in the preceding chapters to a hypothetical population of one million people and seeks to determine the most cost-effective strategies of stroke prevention, from which policy for the primary and secondary prevention of stroke can be developed that is somewhere between the ideal and the affordable. The primary goal of such a policy is to prevent stroke. The rationale for developing an effective policy of stroke prevention is that stroke is an enormous medical, social, and financial burden on the population, and that the burden is likely to increase as the population ages unless effective prevention strategies can be implemented. The development, implementation, and evaluation of such a policy therefore requires consideration of the size of the problem of stroke, the cost of stroke, the major causes of stroke, the major modifiable risk factors for stroke, the strategies of stroke prevention, the evidence of the effectiveness of each strategy, the relative and absolute costs of each strategy, and the methods of monitoring the effectiveness of each strategy (i.e., the incidence of stroke) in the population.

THE SIZE OF THE PROBLEM

In most Western populations, 0.2% of the population (2000 per million) suffer a stroke each year,[1] of whom one-third die over the next year, one-third remain permanently disabled, and one-third make a reasonable recovery.[2] The third who die (666 per million per year) make stroke the third most common cause of death (after ischemic heart disease and cancer), accounting for about 12% of all deaths. The two-thirds of individuals who survive a stroke (1300 per million) add to a large pool of stroke survivors (about 1% of the population, or 10,000 per million), of whom at least half are disabled,[4] making stroke the most important single cause of severe disability in people living in their own homes.[5]

THE COST OF THE PROBLEM

The cost of stroke is very difficult to assess because most estimates are based on what is currently spent on stroke and not necessarily on what actually needs to be spent. It has been estimated that in the United Kingdom, direct hospital and family doctor costs of stroke account for almost 5% of all health service costs,[6] and in the Netherlands about 3% of the annual health care budget is spent on stroke.[7] Despite the fact that only about 55% of stroke patients are admitted to hospital in the United Kingdom,[1] stroke constitutes about 2% of all hospital discharges, 7% of all hospital bed–days, and 6% of all hospital costs.[6] In other Western countries, where a greater percentage of stroke patients are hospitalised,[1] the percentage of hospital costs spent on stroke is even higher.[8] If the direct hospital costs of stroke are added to direct costs related to long-term care of disabled survivors and indirect costs, such as loss of family income and national productivity, the total cost of stroke may be as high as US$100,000 per patient in the United States at 1990 prices.[8]

A LOOMING EPIDEMIC

During the 1990s there was a considerable deceleration in the rate of decline in stroke mortality.[9] In some Western countries stroke mortality rates are stabilizing, and the absolute number of incident stroke cases is increasing because the populations are becoming older (and half of all strokes occur in people older than 75 years[2]). If the decline in stroke mortality (and presumably stroke incidence) cannot be maintained, the aging population will cause an increase in the absolute number of stroke patients, and probably an increase in the number of dependent stroke survivors. It is therefore crucial that effective strategies of stroke prevention and measurement of the effect of these interventions be developed, implemented, and monitored.

THE MAJOR CAUSES AND MODIFIABLE RISK FACTORS FOR STROKE

In order to develop strategies of stroke prevention it is necessary to consider the major causes of stroke and the prevalent, modifiable, and causal risk factors for stroke. About 85% of all strokes are ischemic, and 15% hemorrhagic, due to intracerebral hemorrhage (10%) or subarachnoid hemorrhage (5%). The proportion of stroke in the population that can be attributed to a particular risk factor is called the attributable risk (AR). The major modifiable causal risk factors for ischemic stroke are hypertension (AR: 26%, 95% CI: 12% to 41%), cigarette smoking (AR: 12%, 95% CI: 8% to 16%), atrial fibrillation (AR: 8%, CI: 4% to 12%), and diabetes (AR: 5%, CI: 2% to 9%).[10] The non-modifiable risk factors are transient ischemic attacks (TIAs) of the brain (AR: 14%, CI: 11% to 17%) and ischemic heart disease (AR: 12%, CI: 7% to 17%).[10] In addition, there are other probable causal and modifiable risk factors for ischemic stroke not mentioned here that remain to be established, such as hypercholesterolaemia[11] and possibly hyperhomocysteinaemia.

STRATEGIES OF STROKE PREVENTION

Two major strategies of stroke prevention exist. The "population," or "mass," strategy aims to reduce the prevalence, or shift the distribution to the left, of a causal risk factor (e.g., blood pressure) across a population by lowering the mean level of the causative risk factor in the entire population.[12] The "high-risk" strategy aims to identify and treat individuals who are at high risk of stroke, such as those with hypertension, atrial fibrillation, TIA, and carotid stenosis.[12] The strategies are complementary rather than mutually exclusive.

EVALUATING STRATEGIES OF STROKE PREVENTION

Types of Evidence

The optimal method of evaluating the effectiveness and safety of strategies of stroke prevention is the randomized controlled trial (level I evidence) (Table 17.1), particularly (1) when the intervention has a modest effect on patient outcome that could be hidden or diluted by modest differences in outcome in the other direction, for example, due to systematic bias in treatment allocation, for example (type II error), and (2) when the intervention has no effect that could be disguised by modest differences in outcome due to systematic bias in treatment allocation (type I error). Large numbers of individuals need to be randomized to ensure that there is a roughly equal prevalence of important prognostic factors in each group and a large enough number of outcome events to have the statistical power to produce reliable results in which the random play of chance (random error) is minimized.

Limitations of Randomized Trials

Although randomized trials are likely to provide the least biased and most reliable evidence of effectiveness of an intervention, they can be limited by insufficient sample size and generalizability.

Systematic Reviews

A systematic review (meta-analysis) of all similar, unconfounded, truly random-ized trials can help to overcome the limited sample size and generalizability of isolated, randomized trials, particularly if strict scientific principles are applied to reduce systematic and random errors and bias.[13] Even so, several potential sources of bias may arise in systematic reviews that can make the results unre-liable. These include publication bias, study quality bias, and outcome recording bias.[13] Furthermore, the interpretation of the results of systematic reviews can be difficult because the data are derived from diverse and heterogeneous studies. There may be diversity among the participants, the context of the background health services, the methodological rigor in which the trials were conducted, and the interventions themselves. However, the influence of such variations on the results of the review can be explored by subgroup or sensitivity analyses, which exclude trials that exhibit particular characteristics. In this way it is possible to examine to what degree the results are influenced by trials with particular char-acteristics.[13]

Outcomes

The major outcomes of a stroke prevention policy are the number of strokes pre-vented each year in the population, the proportion of strokes prevented by each strategy or specific intervention, the number of individuals needed to treat with each strategy or intervention to prevent one stroke each year, and the costs and risks of treating these individuals to prevent one stroke per year.

TABLE 17.1. Levels of Evidence About Health Care Interventions[14]

LEVEL	TYPE OF EVIDENCE
Ia	Evidence obtained from a meta-analysis of two or more randomized controlled trials that specifically address the question of interest in a group of patients comparable to the one of interest.
Ib	Evidence obtained from at least one randomized controlled trial.
IIa	Evidence obtained from at least one well-designed controlled study without randomization.
IIb	Evidence obtained from at least one other type of well-designed experimental study.
III	Evidence obtained from well-designed nonexperimental descriptive studies, such as comparative studies, correlation studies, and case studies.
IV	Evidence obtained from expert committee reports or opinions and/or experiences of respected authorities.

Based on guidelines published by the U.S. Department of Health Services. Agency for Health Care Policy and Research.[14]

THE EVIDENCE FOR EACH STROKE PREVENTION STRATEGY

The Population, or Mass, Approach

No randomized controlled trials of the population, or mass, approach to stroke prevention have been done because this strategy requires every person to be "treated," and it would be impracticable, if not impossible, to apply the "treatment" to a random half of the population. The potential effect and cost of this approach therefore needs to be evaluated from the results of observational epidemiologic studies and randomized trials of treatments that may lower risk factor levels.[15,16] For example, Ebrahim[17] used population data from Framingham to calculate that reducing the population mean systolic blood pressure by a mere 2–3 mm Hg would reduce the incidence of stroke by about 10% (Table 17.2), which is about 200 (10%) of the 2000 new strokes that occur each year in a population of 1 million people.[1] The data in Table 17.2 also show how most strokes occur in people at moderate risk (e.g., systolic blood pressure (SBP) of 140–159 mm Hg) and the enormous potential of preventing stroke events, not just among the small number of high-risk individuals (e.g., SBP >180 mm Hg), but among the much larger number of people at moderate risk (e.g., SBP 140–159 mm Hg). The effect of shifting the entire distribution of a continuously varying risk factor (such as blood pressure or cholesterol) in the population slightly to the left (i.e., slightly lowering everyone's blood pressure or cholesterol) would have the effect of not just reducing the mean level of the risk factor in a population but also of reducing the number of patients at particularly high risk who are therefore declared "diseased" and require treatment (Table 17.3).[18]

The mean population blood pressure *could* be lowered by several millimeters by any one of several nonpharmacological interventions: a reduction in salt intake by a tolerable 3 grams per day by means of a public health campaign and

TABLE 17.2. Estimated Effect of a Reduction in the Mean Systolic Blood Pressure in the Population by 2–3 mm Hg[17]

SYSTOLIC BLOOD PRESSURE (MM HG)	PREVALENCE BEFORE INTERVENTION (%)	PREVALENCE AFTER INTERVENTION (%)	EXPECTED NUMBER OF STROKES BEFORE INTERVENTION	EXPECTED NO OF STROKES AFTER INTERVENTION
>180	4	3	127	95
160–179	8	7	102	90
140–159	29	26	162	146
120–139	43	44	155	158
<120	16	17	27	29
Total			573	518

Net effect is a reduction in stroke numbers (and incidence) by (573–518)/573 = 10%.

TABLE 17.3. Estimated Effect of a Reduction in the Mean Level of a Risk Factor in the Population on the Prevalence of Disease (Abnormally High Values)[18]

RISK FACTOR	REDUCTION IN MEAN VALUE	PREDICTED FALL IN PREVALENCE OF HIGH VALUES (%)	
		FROM	TO
Systolic blood pressure	5 mm Hg	15	11
Alcohol intake	15 ml/week	17	15
Body weight	1 kg	6	4

insistence on the labeling of the salt content of processed and other foods, with a gradual reduction in the permitted concentration; facilitation of regular exercise by children and adults by discouraging car use and the provision of sports grounds and safe cycling facilities; reduced alcohol consumption by safe drinking campaigns; and a general emphasis on weight control by promoting exercise and calorie labeling of foods.[19–23] All these interventions depend on political action, legislation, and education.[24] The political initiative is the responsibility of the entire government (e.g., the treasury and departments of education, agriculture, transportation, and the environment) and not merely the department of health.[25] Countries such as Iceland, the United States, and Finland have already produced remarkable reductions in mean cholesterol, blood pressure, and smoking in their populations.[26–28]

Perhaps the major downside to this simple, presumably inexpensive, and theoretically sensible strategy is the so-called prevention paradox, in which an intervention that realizes large benefits for the community offers little benefit to each participating individual.[12] For example, in order to prevent a few serious head injuries among cyclists (which are extremely costly to the individuals affected and the community), every cyclist must wear a bicycle helmet. Similar analogies apply for stroke prevention: the whole population has to eat less salt and consume less alcohol to prevent a small number of strokes relative to the number of people changing their lifestyle. However, these interventions are no more invasive or prescriptive than providing a clean water supply or mass immunization. Another concern of this strategy is the uncertainty that moving an entire distribution of a risk factor to the left, and thus increasing the number of individuals at very low risk, might possibly systematically disadvantage the low-risk individuals in some way. For example, if mean population blood pressure were lowered, the larger number of patients with "low" blood pressure could become at risk of some unexpected disorder, such as depression or fatigue.[29] Similarly, if the mean alcohol and saturated fat intake of the population were reduced, the increased number of nondrinkers might have a higher mortality, particularly from coronary heart disease, than light drinkers,[30,31] and the increased number of people with very low cholesterol might increase the rate of hemorrhagic stroke, suicide, or cancer.[25,33,34] Despite these uncertainties, the argument in favor of the mass strategy of stroke prevention is persuasive, if not compelling.[12]

The High-Risk Approach

The high-risk approach aims to identify people who are at the highest risk of stroke (e.g. severe hypertension) and then reduce their individual risk. The first step in identifying the "cases" generally requires systematic screening of all potentially at-risk people (usually on a practice register) or by opportunistic case finding (e.g., by measuring blood pressure or degree of carotid stenosis of all adults over a certain age attending a practice).[35,36] The second step requires education and treatment of the cases at high risk of stroke by means of lifestyle modifications, medication and sometimes surgery, and ongoing monitoring and maintainance of compliance, often for the life of the patient.

Randomized trials to date have been disappointing, showing only a very limited effect of the high risk strategy on modifiable vascular risk and little, if any, reduction in all-cause mortality.[37-41] This may reflect methodological limitations, such as inadequate sample size, in the trials, but if this is not the case, it suggests that the high risk strategy may be flawed.[42] If so, one reason may be that compliance with treatment in real life is considerably less than it is in randomized controlled trials.[43] Another may be that the high-risk strategies studied have not confined themselves to those at particularly high risk. This is because the high-risk strategy becomes less cost effective with attempts to identify and treat those at lower risk but still clearly at risk (e.g., with moderate, rather than severe, hypertension); the number who have to be detected and treated to prevent one stroke increases. This leads to the paradox that the more the high-risk strategy is refined to make it cost effective (e.g., by focusing preventive efforts on those individuals at highest risk and so reducing the number of patients who need to be treated to prevent one stroke), the smaller becomes the proportion of *all* events that are prevented. This is because most events occur *not* in those at highest risk (because their numbers are small), but in those at moderate risk (because their numbers are very much greater, even though their absolute risk is less than that in individuals at highest risk) (Tables 17.2 and 17.4[44]). For example, if drug treatment for hypertension that lowers diastolic blood pressure by 5–6 mm Hg and reduces an individual's stroke risk by about 38%[45] could somehow be given to *all* people with a systolic blood pressure of 160 mm Hg or more, then stroke incidence would be reduced by 15% (Table 17.4). Although this is a greater potential effect than that achieved by lowering blood pressure by 2–3 mm Hg in the population (Table 17.2), it would be extremely costly to identify and treat the 11% of the population (110,000 in a population of 1 million) with systolic blood

TABLE 17.4. Estimated Effect of Treating All Hypertensive People (Systolic Blood Pressure >160 mm Hg) in the Population and Reducing the Risk of Stroke by 38%[17]

SYSTOLIC BLOOD PRESSURE (MM HG)	PREVALENCE (%)	EXPECTED NUMBER EOF STROKES BEFORE TREATMENT	EXPECTED NUMBER OF STROKES AFTER TREATMENT
Treated			
>180	3	127	79
160–179	8	102	63
Not treated			
140–159	29	162	162
120–139	43	155	155
<120	16	27	27
Total		573	486

Net effect is a reduction in stroke numbers (and incidence) by $(573 - 486)/573 = 15\%$.

pressure ≥160 mm Hg, probably undesirable in some of the very elderly, and probably impossible actually to achieve in practice.

Other high-risk strategies include identifying and treating all individuals with atrial fibrillation (AF) and asymptomatic carotid stenosis. However, because only about 20% of patients with first-ever stroke are in atrial fibrillation at or before presentation,[46] the treatment of fibrillating patients could only possibly prevent as few as one-fifth of all strokes. Indeed, the likely percentage prevented would be only about 5% if anticoagulation could be given to as many as half of the fibrillating patients under the age of 80. Aspirin for AF might also reduce stroke incidence by 5% to 8%, despite the fact it is relatively less effective than warfarin. This is because the risks and difficulties associated with aspirin use are less than with warfarin, and so it can be given to many more people.

Carotid endarterectomy (CE) for severe asymptomatic carotid stenosis does seem to halve the risk of stroke ipsilateral to the carotid stenosis, but only by about 1% per year (from 2% per year). Consequently, about 85 patients need to be operated on to prevent one stroke in one year, and the cost effectiveness of CE is highly questionable (see below). Furthermore, screening the population for carotid stenosis and then undertaking surgery in those who are fit and willing would be enormously expensive and harmful to some, without realizing much benefit. For example, in a hypothetical population of 1 million people, about 250,000 (25%) are 50–75 years of age (the population to be screened), of whom about 10,000 (4%) have asymptomatic carotid stenosis of 60%–99% and 240,000 do not.[25,47] If all 250,000 people aged 50–75 years were screened by carotid ultrasound (with an optimistic sensitivity of 95% and specificity of 95% for detecting 60%–99% stenosis[48]), then carotid ultrasound would accurately identify 9,500 (95% sensitivity) with disease and 228,000 without disease (95% specificity). It would also identify 12,000 false positives (5% of 240,000 without disease) and miss 500 false negatives (5% of 10,000 without disease). Performing CE (appropriately) on the 9,500 with disease would prevent about 114 strokes (1.2% absolute risk reduction) per year over the next five years.[49] However, performing CE (or angiography) inappropriately on the 12,000 false positives (without severe disease, but probably with mild or moderate disease) would immediately cause at least 180 (1.5%) perioperative strokes or deaths in a group that was at lower risk of stroke.[33,39] In addition, failing to perform CE in the 500 false negatives (with disease) would fail to prevent a further 6 strokes (1.2% absolute risk increase) per year over the next five years.[49] So, the net effect of screening for asymptomatic carotid stenosis in a population of a million people with a prevalence of severe carotid stenosis of only 4% is the cost and effort of performing 250,000 carotid ultrasounds, and 21,500 CEs (or angiograms), and an excess of about 72 strokes per year. Clearly, screening can be justified only in populations with a high prevalence (at least 20%) of severe carotid stenosis.

In summary, the high-risk approach to stroke prevention requires considerable resources (particularly in primary practice to identify the high-risk individuals), and many high-risk individuals may not benefit. This may be because many are treated unnecessarily (i.e., only a minority of high-risk invididuals actually go on to suffer a stroke), and some may be affected adversely by being labelled as "sick."[12] However, the high-risk approach can be a cost-effective strategy of stroke prevention among individuals at particularly high risk of stroke who readily identify themselves, such as those who present with high blood pressure, AF, or TIA or mild ischaemic stroke, and have more to gain than lose from treatment.

SECONDARY STROKE PREVENTION OF STROKE AMONG PEOPLE WITH TIA AND STROKE

In a hypothetical population of 1 million people, about 12,000 individuals have had a previous TIA (2,000), stroke (9,000), or both stroke and TIA (1,000).[4] About 2,500 will have suffered TIA (500) or stroke (2000) in the previous year. Among these 12,000 individuals with prevalent TIA/stroke, about 800 (7%) will suffer a stroke each year (600 recurrent strokes and 200 first-ever strokes among people with previous TIA only).[50,51] These 800 strokes (40% of the 2000 strokes that occur each year in a population of 1 million people) are those that are potentially preventable by effective secondary prevention strategies targeted to the 12,000 people with a previous history of stroke or TIA. The strategies for which there exist level 1 evidence of effectiveness (i.e., systematic review of randomized trials [Table 17.1]) include control of vascular risk factors (e.g., blood pressure reduction), antiplatelet therapy, anticoagulant therapy, and CE (Table 17.5).

TABLE 17.5. Summary of the Cost Effectiveness of the Different Strategies of Secondary Stroke Prevention for 12,000 TIA and Stroke Patients in a Population of 1 Million People

STRATEGY/ INTERVENTION	TARGET POPULATION	STROKE RISK PER YEAR		RELATIVE RISK REDUCTION (%)	ABSOLUTE RISK REDUCTION (%)
		CONTROL (%)	INTERVENTION (%)		
Blood pressure–lowering drug therapy	6000 (50%)	7.0	4.8	28 (15–39)	2.2
Smoking cessation	3600 (30%)	7.0	4.7	33 (29–38)	2.3
Cholesterol-lowering drug therapy	4800 (40%)	7.0	5.3	24 (8–38)	1.7
Antiplatelet therapy	7875 (75%				
Antiplatelet therapy overall	of 10500 TIA/	7.0	5.8	23 (9–33)[1]	1.2
Aspirin	ischemic	7.0	6.0	13 (4, 21)[2]	1.0
Clopidogrel	strokes)	7.0	5.5	8.7 (0.3, 16)	1.5
Aspirin + dipyridamole[3]		7.0	5.1	15 (5–26)[2]	1.9
Anticoagulant therapy	2100 (20% of 10500 TIA/ ischemic strokes)	12.0	4.0	67 (43–80)	8.0
Carotid endarterectomy					
Symptomatic	816 (8% of 10500 TIA/ ischemic strokes)	8.8	5.0	44	3.8
Asymptomatic#	10,000	2.2	1.0	53 (22–72)	1.2

[1]Odds reduction.

[2]Relative to aspirin.

[3]The size of this effect remains to be confirmed in ongoing trials.

[4]This estimate does not include the cost of inappropriate angiography and carotid endarterectomy in people with false positive carotid ultrasound (see text).

NUMBER OF STROKES AVOIDED PER 1000 TREATED PER YEAR	NUMBER OF STROKES AVOIDED PER YEAR IN TARGET POPULATION	% OF ALL STROKES AVOIDED EACH YEAR IN TARGET POPULATION	NUMBERS OF TIA/STROKE PATIENTS NEEDED TO TREAT TO PREVENT ONE STROKE PER YEAR	COST PER STROKE AVOIDED (AUS$)
22	132	6.6	45	$1350 (diuretic) $4,500 (beta blocker) $18,000 (ACE inhibitor)
23	83	4.1	43	$0 (voluntary) $<19,600 (patches for all)
17	81	3.4	59	$41,000
12	94	4.7	83	
10	79	3.9	100	$1,000
15	118 $(39)^2$	5.9	66	$66,000
19	188 $(70)^2$	9.4	53	$37,000
80	168	8.4	12	$1,200
38	31	1.5	26	$182,000
12	120	6^3	83	$580,000[3]

Blood Pressure Reduction

Among the 12,000 people who have had previous TIA or stroke (in a population of 1 million people), about 6,000 (50%) have hypertension.[51,52] Lowering the blood pressure of these 6000 hypertensive TIA/stroke patients by 5–6 mm Hg diastolic and 10–12 mm Hg systolic for two to three years would reduce the annual incidence of stroke in these people from about 7% ($n = 420$ strokes) to 4.8% ($n = 288$) (relative risk reduction: 28%, 95% CI: 15%–39%),[53] assuming they have the same rate of stroke as individuals who do not have hypertension (Table 17.5). This reduction of about 132 strokes per year is about 6.6% of all (2000) strokes occurring in the population each year. Treating 45 hypertensive TIA/stroke patients for one year (at least) would avoid one stroke each year.

The cost of diuretic therapy is about Aus$30 per patient per year for bendrofluazide at 5 mg daily and $50 per patient per year for hydrochlorthiazide at 50 mg/amiloride 5 mg, compared with $100 for metoprolol at 100 mg bd, $137 for atenolol at 50 mg daily, and about $400 per patient per year for angiotensin converting enzyme inhibitors such as enalapril, lisonopril, and perindopril.[54] If the least expensive antihypertensive treatment (bendrofluazide) were used (the best-case scenario), at a cost of about $30 per patient per year, it would cost about $1350 each year to prevent one stroke. If angiotensin converting enzyme inhibitors were used, at a cost of about $400 per patient per year, it would cost about $18,000 each year to prevent one stroke.

Cigarette Smoking

About 30% (3,600) of TIA/stroke patients are cigarette smokers.[51,52] Although there have been no randomized trials, observational studies suggest that if all 3,600 TIA/stroke patients who smoke were to stop smoking, the annual number of strokes could be reduced by at least one-third,[55] from about 7% (252) to 4.7% (169), avoiding about 83 strokes each year (4.1% of all strokes). This means that 43 people with TIA/stroke need to stop smoking to avoid one stroke of any type each year.

Aids to stop smoking may be required, such as counseling, nicotine gum, or skin patches. Nicotine patches cost about Aus$456 for 12 weeks ($1824 per patient per year).[54] If all smokers who have had TIA/stroke (3,600) wanted to use a nicotine patch daily for three months, it would cost as much as $ 1.64 million to prevent up to about 83 strokes, or $19,600 to treat 43 people to prevent one stroke.

Cholesterol Reduction

About 40% (4,800) of TIA/stroke patients have hypercholesterolemia.[51,52] Although there have been no randomized trials of cholesterol-lowering therapy in

TIA/stroke patients, trials in different patient populations suggest that lowering serum cholesterol over a few years years with hydroxymethylglutaryl coenzyme A reductase inhibitors (or "statin" drugs) could reduce the number of strokes by about 24% (95% CI: 8% to 38%), from 7% (336) to 5.3% (255) per year.[11] This reduction, of about 81 strokes, would be 3.4% of all (2000) strokes in the population each year. About 59 TIA/stroke patients with hypercholesterolemia would need to be treated effectively to avoid one stroke each year.

If simvastatin at 20 mg day (or pravastatin at 20 to 40mg per day) were used, at a cost of about $700 per patient per year, it would cost about $41,000 to avoid one stroke. If all 4,800 TIA/stroke people with hypercholesterolemia were to be treated, it would cost about $3.36 million to avoid about 81 strokes.

Antiplatelet Therapy

Antiplatelet therapy is appropriate for about 75% (7875) of people with TIA (2000) or ischemic stroke (8,500) and, if given to all, could reduce the annual incidence of stroke from about 7% (551) to 5.8% (457) (odds reduction: 23% + 6% [SD]),[56] thus avoiding about 94 strokes each year (4.7% of all strokes). Treating 83 TIA/ischemic stroke patients for one year (at least) would avoid one stroke each year.

Besides clopidogrel,[57] no single antiplatelet agent exists that is more effective than aspirin. Aspirin reduces the risk of important vascular events by about 13% (17 ± 4.4% odds reduction),[58] from about 7.0% (551) to 6.0% (472), thus avoiding 79 strokes each year (4.0% of all strokes). Clopidogrel reduces the risk of important vascular events by 8.7% (95%CI: 0.3% to 16.5%) compared to aspirin, indicating that it would further reduce the risk from 6.0% (472) to 5.5% (433), thus avoiding about 39 more strokes each year, and 118 strokes compared with control.[57]

The combination of dipyridamole and aspirin may also be more effective than aspirin alone. The addition of the second European Stroke Prevention Study (ESPS-2) to four previous studies that had compared the combination of aspirin and dipyridamole with aspirin alone reveals that the combination of aspirin and dipyridamole is associated with about a 15% relative risk reduction compared with aspirin alone.[59,60] If these results can be confirmed in ongoing trials (e.g., ESPRIT), and the 7875 people with TIA/stroke take the combination of aspirin and dipyridamole for at least a year, the total number of strokes each year could be reduced from 6.0% (472) to 5.1% (402), thus avoiding about 70 more strokes each year than aspirin alone, and 188 strokes compared with control. One hundred patients need to be treated with aspirin, 66 with clopidogrel, and 53 with aspirin plus dipyridamole for at least one year to avoid one stroke each year.

If the cost of aspirin is about Aus$10 per year, then it is likely to cost about $1,000 to treat 100 TIA/stroke patients for one year to prevent one stroke. If the cost of clopidogrel is about Aus$1000 per patient per year, it is likely to cost about $66,000 to treat 66 TIA/stroke patients for one year to prevent one stroke. If the cost of dipyridamole is about Aus$700 per year, it is likely to cost about Aus$37,100 to treat 53 TIA/stroke patients for one year to prevent one stroke.

Anticoagulant Therapy

Oral anticoagulant therapy (INR 2.0 to 3.0) is indicated for about 20% (2100) of patients with TIA/ischemic stroke who have high-risk sources of embolism from the heart to the brain.[51,52] Treating these 2100 people with oral anticoagulants would reduce the number of strokes each year by about two-thirds, from 12% (252) to 4% (84),[61] thus avoiding 168 strokes each year (8.4% of all strokes). About 12 people with TIA/stroke and a potential cardiac source of embolism need to be treated with oral anticoagulants for one year to prevent one stroke each year.

The annual cost of anticoagulant drugs, excluding regular checks of international normalized ratio (INR), extra visits to doctors and travel, and the costs of major hemorrhage in 0.5 to 0.8% of patients, would be about $100. Anticoagulating 12 TIA/stroke patients with a cardiac source of embolism for one year would likely cost at least $1200 and avoid one stroke.

CE for Symptomatic Carotid Stenosis

CE is indicated for individuals who have had recent symptoms of carotid territory TIA or mild ischemic stroke, severe (>70% in NASCET, >80% in ECST) carotid stenosis, and who are fit and willing for surgery. Only about 8% (816) of TIA/ischemic stroke patients meet these criteria.[51,62] If all 816 appropriate TIA/stroke patients undergo CE, the three-year risk of major stroke or death could be reduced from about 26.5% (8.8% per year) to 14.9% (5.0% per year).[63] This is an average absolute risk reduction of 3.8% per year, which equates to about 31 strokes prevented each year (1.5% of all strokes) by performing CE on 816 patients. At least 26 patients would need to be treated with CE to avoid one stroke per year. The number needed to treat to prevent one stroke is higher if the perioperative risk of major stroke or death is higher than about 7%. Performing CE in 26 patients, at a cost about $7000 per patient for the preoperative investigations, operation, and postoperative management costs about $182,000 to avoid one stroke each year for the next three years.

CE for Asymptomatic Carotid Stenosis

About 10,000 (1%) people in the population (4% of the population aged 50–75 years) have asymptomatic carotid stenosis of 60%–99%.[47] If these 10,000 people are accurately identified and undergo CE, the number of strokes could be reduced from 11% (1100) at five years to 5% (500),[49] thus avoiding up to 600 strokes over five years, or 120 strokes per year (6% of all strokes). This means that 83 patients need to be treated with CE, at a cost of about $580,000, to avoid one stroke per year. This analysis does not include the considerable additional costs of screening for asymptomatic carotid stenosis, particularly in populations with a low prevalence of severe carotid stenosis, which may realize a dangerously high absolute number of false positive and false negative results, and inappropriate angiographic and surgical interventions, with their attendant risks and costs.[64]

Carotid Angioplasty and Stenting

Carotid angioplasty and stenting is a promising but currently experimental procedure that is in trial.[65]

POPULATION EFFECTS OF SECONDARY STROKE PREVENTION AMONG TIA/STROKE PATIENTS

Among individuals presenting with TIA and mild ischemic stroke, the above data suggest that the most effective interventions in preventing stroke (and thus reducing the burden of stroke) among the population are effective antiplatelet therapy with the combination of aspirin and dipyridamole (which could prevent 9.4% of all strokes occurring among TIA/stroke patients), anticoagulation of TIA/stroke patients with an embolic source in the heart (which could prevent 8.4% of strokes), and blood pressure lowering therapy (which could prevent 6.6% of strokes) (Table 17.6). Although the effects of each of these strategies of stroke prevention, relative to one another, are likely to be true, they are unlikely to be mutually exclusive (i.e., they are not additive), and the absolute effects of each are likely to be overestimated. The overestimate is because only about 50% of people with TIA come to medical attention, some experience a stroke before treatment is commenced, many are not appropriate patients for certain treatments (e.g., CE), and for those in whom treatment is appropriate, some do not comply with treatment, some experience adverse effects of treatment, and many do not respond to treatment.[15] Consequently, in reality, the treatment of TIA and stroke patients who seek medical attention before they suffer a recurrent stroke is likely to prevent only a minority of the 800 strokes that are potentially preventable each year by treating these patients.

COST EFFECTIVENESS OF SECONDARY STROKE PREVENTION AMONG TIA/STROKE PATIENTS

The average cost (direct and indirect) of a stroke in Australia is about $40,000 (Table 17.7).[66] More precisely, this is the average amount of money spent by the

TABLE 17.6. Summary of the Potential Impact of the Different Strategies of Secondary Stroke Prevention for TIA and Stroke Patients on Stroke Prevention in the Population

STRATEGY/INTERVENTION	% OF ALL STROKES AVOIDED EACH YEAR IN TARGET POPULATION
Aspirin + dipyridamole	9.4
Anticoagulation	8.4
Blood pressure–lowering therapy	6.6
Clopidogrel	5.9
Smoking cessation	4.1
Aspirin	3.9
Cholesterol-lowering statin therapy	3.4
Carotid endarterectomy	1.5

Australian government on each stroke patient; it may not necessarily reflect the true cost of stroke (i.e., what actually should be spent on stroke patients and their caregivers).

The most cost-effective secondary prevention interventions among TIA/stroke patients, in terms of costing less than the cost of the strokes prevented, are listed in Table 17.8. Clearly, the most cost-effective are antiplatelet therapy with aspirin ($1000 per stroke avoided); anticoagulant therapy for TIA/stroke patients with an embolic source in the heart ($1200 per stroke avoided); blood pressure lowering therapy with diuretics ($1350 per stroke avoided), or beta-blockers ($4500 per stroke avoided) (no data are available as yet as to the effect of angiotensin-converting enzyme (ACE) inhibitors [$18,000 per stroke avoided] on stroke prevention); and smoking cessation. All these interventions cost well

TABLE 17.7. Estimated Direct and Indirect Costs of Stroke in Australia[66]

Direct costs	$ million
Acute care	175
Nursing homes	400
Rehabilitation	75
Other[1]	92
Total	$742 million

Indirect costs	$ million
Lost earnings of patient due to premature death	450
Lost earnings of patient due to premature morbidity	582
Lost earnings of spouses/partner due to morbidity of patient (e.g., taking on caregiver role)	340
Total	$1372 million

[1]Outpatient attendances, GP visits, allied health interventions, hospital transport, home modifications, district nursing, home help, meals on wheels, community health care, respite care.

TABLE 17.8. Summary of the Relative Costs of the Different Strategies of Secondary Stroke Prevention for TIA and Stroke Patients to Prevent One Stroke

Less Than the Estimated Average Cost (Aus$40,000) of One Stroke in Australia

Strategy/Intervention	Cost per Stroke Avoided (Aus$)
Aspirin	$ 1,000
Anticoagulant therapy	$ 1,200
Diuretic therapy	$ 1,350
Beta-blocker	$ 4,500
Smoking cessation	$ 0–19,600
ACE inhibitor	$18,000
Aspirin + dipyridamole	$37,000

More Than the Estimated Average Cost (Aus$40,000) of One Stroke in Australia

Statins	$ 41,000
Clopidogrel	$ 66,000
Carotid endarterectomy	$182,000

below $40,000 (the cost of a stroke), when applied to TIA/stroke patients, to prevent one stroke. On the borderline is the cost of antiplatelet therapy with the combination of aspirin and dipyridamole for TIA and stroke patients, which is about the same as the cost of the strokes it prevents. The widespread use of statins for cholesterol-lowering, clopidogrel as an antiplatelet agent, and CE among TIA and stroke patients is not cost effective, and CE for asymptomatic carotid stenosis is particularly not cost effective. However, that is not to say that these treatments may not have a role and be cost effective in certain subgroups of patients. For example, statistical analysis of the European Carotid Surgery Trial cohort of TIA/ischemic stroke patients with 70%–99% carotid stenosis on the symptomatic side reveals that about 16% of these patients benefit from CE and 84% do not.[67] If this model can be validated externally in other data sets, it would reduce the number needed to treat to prevent one stroke by 84%, from 26 to 4. At a cost of Aus$7,000 per CE, this would mean that only $28,000 would be spent to prevent one stroke, which is less than the $40,000 cost of the stroke prevented. Similarly, if high-risk subgroups in the CAPRIE cohort can be identified for whom clopidogrel is more effective than aspirin, then the cost effectiveness of clopidogrel could be vastly improved.

METHODS OF MONITORING THE INCIDENCE OF STROKE IN THE POPULATION

As the primary goal of a stroke prevention policy is to prevent stroke, it is crucial that the incidence of stroke in the population be accurately monitored to judge the effectiveness of the policy. Furthermore, the incidence of subtypes of stroke, which reflect different causes of stroke, and the prevalence of causal risk factors, such as hypertension, smoking, hypercholesterolemia, and diabetes need to be monitored.

However, these data are not routinely collected nationally. This is because stroke is not a notifiable disease; these data are therefore generally derived only from dedicated, community-based studies in which all people with suspected stroke are ascertained through repeated enquiry of multiple sources (to identify all strokes, and not just the 55%–95% who are admitted to hospital[1]); assessed by a highly trained physician (to make an accurate diagnosis of stroke); referred for brain imaging or autopsy (to diagnose the pathological subtype); and followed-up over at least 1, and preferably 6–12, months and longer (to document the process of care, patient outcome, and costs incurred).[1]

The only routinely collected data for measuring and monitoring the burden of stroke are mortality statistics (hospital discharge rates are unsatisfactory without knowledge of the percentage of strokes admitted to hospital). However, over time, mortality statistics may be confounded by changes in diagnostic criteria (e.g., if brain imaging findings influence the diagnosis of stroke); by the accuracy, completion, and coding of death certificates (which is particularly poor in elderly people); by mortality due to other causes of earlier death (e.g., coronary deaths); by the percentage of strokes due to particular stroke subtypes that have a high mortality (e.g., primary intracerebral hemorrhage and total anterior circulation infarction) or low mortality (e.g., lacunar infarction); and by case fatality rate (which influence mortality rates but not incidence rates). Despite these potential flaws, it has been consistently shown that there has been a substantial decline in mortality rates for stroke (and also coronary heart disease), by about 3%–7% per year, among men and women of all ages, over the past decades in most Western countries and Japan (but not eastern Europe).[9] It is less clear, however, whether this reflects any or all of a decline in incidence (fewer strokes occurring), a decline in case fatality (improved survival), a change in case mix (e.g., a decline in the percentage of lethal intracerebral hemorrhages), or (less likely) is an artefact.

CONCLUSION

Stroke is an enormous public health problem, the magnitude of which can be reduced, mainly by effective stroke prevention. Because the majority of strokes (70%) are first-ever strokes, these can be prevented only by effective primary prevention strategies. The greatest effect is likely to be achieved by a mass approach to prevention, which consists of modification of lifestyle behaviors (e.g., lowering of smoking and intake of salt, alcohol, and fat) among the general population through public education and government legislation. The appropriate identification and treatment of high-risk individuals by neurologists is likely to have a smaller but complementary impact on the population burden of stroke, and a substantial impact on the burden of stroke among individuals. The most cost-effective prevention strategies for TIA and ischemic stroke patients are early secondary prevention with vascular risk factor control (e.g., blood pressure control, smoking cessation) and antithrombotic therapy (aspirin, or oral antico-agulant therapy in the appropriate patient). The cost effectiveness of cholesterol-lowering by means of statin drugs, clopidogrel antiplatelet therapy, and CE for symptomatic carotid stenosis remain to be established through better risk-factor stratification and prognostic modeling to identify the minority who benefit from these expensive treatments. CE for asymptomatic carotid stenosis is highly cost-ineffective at present but also may be improved when further data from ongoing trials (e.g., ACST) become available. Screening for asymptomatic carotid steno-sis is more likely to be harmful than helpful, except perhaps among populations with a very high prevalence (pretest probability) of severe carotid stenosis.

The impact of stroke prevention strategies need to be measured and moni-tored by ongoing studies of the incidence, outcome, and cost of stroke. Currently, this is done simply, but unreliably, by examining changes in statistics that are al-ready being gathered, such as mortality (e.g., among those less than about 70 years old, for greater accuracy). A growing priority in many countries is the de-velopment and implementation of valid, reliable, practical, and inexpensive meth-ods of routinely collecting and evaluating data on stroke incidence, outcome, and cost.

REFERENCES

1. Sudlow CLM, Warlow CP. Comparable studies of the incidence of stroke and its patho-logical subtypes: Results from an international collaboration. *Stroke* 1997;28:491–499.
2. Bamford J, Sandercock P, Dennis M, Warlow C, Jones L, McPherson K, Vessey M, Fowler G, Molyneux A, Hughes T, Burn J, Wade D. A prospective study of acute cerebrovascular disease in the community: The Oxfordshire Community Stroke Pro-ject, 1981–1986. Methodology, demography and incident cases of first-ever stroke. *J Neurol Neurosurg Psychiatry* 1988;51:1373–1380.
3. Murray CJL, Lopez AD. Mortality by cause for eight regions of the world: Global Burden of Disease Study. *Lancet* 1997;349:1269–1276.
4. Bonita R, Solomon N, Broad JB. Prevalence of stroke and stroke-related disability: Estimates from the Auckland Stroke Studies. *Stroke* 1997;28:1898–1902.
5. Murray CJL, Lopez AD. Global mortality, disability and the contribution of risk fac-tors: Global Burden of Disease Study. *Lancet* 1997;349:1436–1442.
6. Isard PA, Forbes JF. The cost of stroke to the National Health Service in Scotland. *Cerebrovasc Dis* 1992;2:47–50.
7. Evers SMAA, Engel GL, Ament AJHA. Cost of stroke in the Netherlands from a so-cietal perspective. *Stroke* 1997;28:1375–1381.
8. Taylor TN, Davis PH, Torner JC, Holmes J, Meyer JW, Jacobsen MF. Lifetime cost of stroke in the United States. *Stroke* 1996;27:1459–1466.

9. Bonita, R, Stewart A, Beaglehole R. International trends in stroke mortality, 1970–1985. *Stroke* 1990;21:989–992.

10. Whisnant JP. Modeling of risk factors for ischaemic stroke. *Stroke* 1997;28:1839–1843.

11. Bucher HC, Griffith LE, Guyatt GH. Effect of HMG CoA reductase inhibitors on stroke: A meta-analysis of randomised, controlled trials. *Ann Intern Med* 1998;128:89–95.

12. Rose G. *The Strategy of Preventive Medicine*. Oxford: Oxford University Press, 1992.

13. Counsell C, Warlow C, Sandercock P, Fraser H, van Gijn J (The Cochrane Collaboration Stroke Review Group Editorial Board). Meeting the need for systematic reviews in stroke care. *Stroke* 1995;26:498–502.

14. Agency for Health Care Policy and Research. Acute pain management: Operative or medical procedures and trauma. AHCPR 92-0023. Rockville, MD: AHCPR, 1993.

15. Ebrahim S, Davey Smith G. A systematic review and meta-analysis of randomised controlled trials of health promotion for prevention of coronary heart disease in adults. *BMJ* 1997;314:1666–1674.

16. Tudor-Smith C, Nutbeam D, Moore L, Catford J. Effects of the Heartbeat Wales programme over five years on behavioural risks for cardiovascular disease: Quasi-experimental comparison of results from Wales and a matched reference area. *BMJ* 1998;316:818–22.

17. Ebrahim S. *Clinical Epidemiology of Stroke*. Oxford: Oxford University Press, 1990.

18. Rose G, Day S. The population mean predicts the number of deviant individuals. *BMJ* 1990;301:1031–1034.

19. Law M, Frost C, Wald N. By how much does dietary salt reduction lower blood pressure. III: Analysis of data from trials of salt reduction. *BMJ* 1991;302:819–824.

20. Cutler JA. Randomised clinical trials of weight reduction in nonhypertensive persons. *Ann Epidemiol* 1991;1:363–370.

21. Arroll B, Beaglehole R. Does physical activity lower blood pressure: A critical review of the clinical trials. *J Clin Epidemiol* 1992;45:439–447.

22. Alderman MH. Non-pharmacological treatment of hypertension. *Lancet* 1994;344:307–311.

23. Whelton PK, Appel LJ, Espeland MA, Applegate WB, Ettinger WH, Kostis JB, Kumanyika S, Lacy CR, Johnson KC, Folmar S, Cutler JA, for the TONE Collaborative Research Group. Sodium reduction and weight loss in the treatment of hypertension in older persons: A randomised controlled trial of nonpharmacologic interventions in the elderly (TONE). *JAMA* 1998;279:839–846.

24. Council on Scientific Affairs. The worldwide smoking epidemic: Tobacco trade, use, and control. *JAMA* 1990;263:3312–3318.

25. Warlow CP, Dennis MS, van Gijn J, Hankey GJ, Sandercock PAG, Bamford J, Wardlaw J. *Practical Management of Stroke*. Oxford: Blackwell Scientific Publications, 1996.

26. Sytkowski PA, Kannel WB, D'Agostino RB. Changes in risk factors and the decline in mortality from cardiovascular disease: The Framingham Heart Study. *N Engl J Med* 1990;322:1635–1641.

27. Sigfusson N, Sigvaldason H, Steingrimsdottir L, Gudmundsdottir II, Stefansdottir I, Thorsteinsson T, Sigurdsson G. Decline in ischaemic heart disease in Iceland and change in risk factor levels. *BMJ* 1991;302:1371–1375.

28. Vartiainen E, Puska P, Pekkanen J, Tuomilehto J, Jousilahti P. Changes in risk factors explain changes in mortality from ischaemic heart disease in Finland. *BMJ* 1994;309:23–27.

29. Barrett-Connor E, Palinkas LA. Low blood pressure and depression in older men: A population based study. *BMJ* 1994;308:446–449.

30. Marmot M, Brunner E. Alcohol and cardiovascular disease: The status of the U shaped curve. *BMJ* 1991;303:565–568.

31. Doll R, Peto R, Hall E, Wheatley K, Gray R. Mortality in relation to consumption of alcohol: 13 years' observations on male British doctors. *BMJ* 1994;309:911–918.

32. Law MR, Thompson SG. Low serum cholesterol and the risk of cancer: An analysis of the published prospective studies. *Cancer Causes and Control* 1991;2:253–259.

33. Law MR, Thompson SG, Wald NJ. Assessing possible hazards of reducing serum cholesterol. *BMJ* 1994;308:373–379.

34. Gallerani M, Manfredini R, Caracciolo S, Scapoli C, Molinari S, Fersini C. Serum cholesterol concentrations in parasuicide. *BMJ* 1995;310:1632–1636.

35. Holmen J, Forsen L, Hjort PF, Midthjell K, Waaler HT, Bjorndal A. Detecting hypertension: Screening versus case finding in Norway. *BMJ* 1991;302:219–222.

36. Family Heart Study Group. Randomised controlled trial evaluating cardiovascular screening and intervention in general practice: principal results of British family heart study. *BMJ* 1994;308:313–320.

37. Rose G, Tunstall-Pedoe HD, Heller RF. UK heart disease prevention project: Incidence and mortality results. *Lancet* 1983;i:1062–1070.

38. Fries JF, Bloch DA, Harrington H, Richardson N, Beck R. Two year results of a randomised controlled trial of a health promotion programe in a retiree population: The Bank of America Study. *Am J Med* 1993;94:455–462.

39. Lindholm LH, Ekbom T, Dash C, Eriksson M, Tibblin G, Scherstein B, on behalf of the CELL Study Group. The impact of health care advice given in primary care on cardiovascular risk. *BMJ* 1995;310:1105–1109.

40. Imperial Cancer Research Fund OXCHECK Study Group. Effectiveness of health checks conducted by nurses in primary care: Final results of the OXCHECK study. *BMJ* 1995;310:1099–1104.

41. Campbell NC, Thain J, Deans G, Ritchie LD, Rawles JM, Squair JL. Secondary prevention clinics for coronary heart disease: Randomised trial of effect on health. *BMJ* 1998;316:1434–1437.

42. McCormick J, Skrabanek P. Coronary heart disease is not preventable by population interventions. *Lancet* 1988;2:839–841.

43. Andrade SE, Walker AM, Gottlieb LK, Hollenberg NK, Testa MA, Saperia GM, Platt R. Discontinuation of antihyperlipidemic drugs—do rates reported in clinical trials reflect rates in primary care settings? *N Engl J Med* 1995;332:1125–1131.

44. Whelton PK. Epidemiology of hypertension. *Lancet* 1994;344:101–106.

45. Collins R, MacMahon S. Blood pressure, antihypertensive drug treatment and the risks of stroke and of coronary heart disease. *Brit Med Bull* 1994;50:272–298.

46. Sandercock PAG, Bamford J, Dennis M, Burn J, Slattery J, Jones L, Boonyakarnkul S, Warlow CP. Atrial fibrillation and stroke: Prevalence in different stroke types and influence on early and long term prognosis (Oxfordshire Community Stroke Project). *BMJ* 1992;305:1460–1465.

47. Hankey GJ. Asymptomatic carotid stenosis: How should it be managed? *Med J Aust* 1995;163:197–200.

48. Blakeley DD, Oddone EZ, Hasselblad V, et al. Noninvasive carotid artery testing. A meta-analytic review. *Ann Intern Med* 1995;122:360–367.

49. Executive Committee for the Asymptomatic Carotid Atherosclerosis Study. Endarterectomy for asymptomatic carotid artery stenosis. *JAMA* 1995;273:1421–1428.

50. Hankey GJ, Jamrozik K, Broadhurst RJ, Forbes S, Burvill PW, Anderson CS, Stew-

art-Wynne EG. Long-term risk of recurrent stroke in the Perth Community Stroke Study. *Stroke* 1998;29:2491–2500.

51. Hankey GJ, Warlow CP. *Transient Ischaemic Attacks of the Brain and Eye*. London: WB Saunders, 1994.

52. Jamrozik K, Broadhurst RJ, Anderson CS, Stewart-Wynne EG. The role of lifestyle factors in the etiology of stroke: A population-based case-control study in Perth, Western Australia. *Stroke* 1994;25:51–59.

53. The INDANA (Individual Data Analysis of Antihypertensive intervention trials) Project Collaborators. Effect of antihypertensive treatment in patients having already suffered from stroke. Gathering the evidence. *Stroke* 1997;28:2557–2562.

54. Commonwealth Department of Health and Family Services. Shedule of pharmaceutical benefits for approved pharmacists and medical practitioners. Canberra: JS McMillan Printing Group, 1997.

55. Hankey GJ. Smoking and risk of stroke. *J Cardiovasc Risk* 1999;6(4):207–211.

56. Antiplatelet Trialists Collaboration: Collaborative overview of randomised trials of antiplatelet therapy-I: Prevention of death, myocardial infarction, and stroke by prolonged antiplatelet therapy in various categories of patients. *BMJ* 1994;308:81–106.

57. CAPRIE Steering Committee. A randomised blinded trial of clopidogrel versus aspirin in patients at risk of ischaemic events (CAPRIE). *Lancet* 1996;348:1333–1338.

58. Algra A, van Gijn J. Aspirin at any dose above 30 mg offers only modest protection after cerebral ischaemia. *J Neurol Neurosurg Psychiatry* 1996;60:197–199.

59. Diener HC, Cunha L, Forbes C, Sivenius J, Smets P, Lowenthal A. European Stroke Prevention Study 2: Dipyridamole and acetylsalicyclic acid in the secondary prevention of stroke. *J Neurol Sci* 1996;143:1–13.

60. Hankey GJ. One year after CAPRIE, IST and ESPS 2: Any changes in concepts? *Cerebrovasc Dis* 1998 (in press).

61. European Atrial Fibrillation Trial Study Group. Secondary prevention in nonrheumatic atrial fibrillation after transient ischaemic attack or minor stroke. *Lancet* 1993;342:1255–1262.

62. Hankey GJ, Slattery JM, Warlow CP: The prognosis of hospital-referred transient ischaemic attacks. *J Neurol Neurosurg Psychiatry* 1991;54:793–802.

63. European Carotid Surgery Trialistsí Collaborative Group. Randomised trial of endarterectomy for recently symptomatic carotid stenosis: Final results of the MRC European Carotid Surgery Trial (ECST). *Lancet* 1998;351:1379–1387.

64. Whitty CJM, Sudlow CLM, Warlow CP. Investigating individual subjects and screening populations for asymptomatic carotid stenosis can be harmful. *J Neurol Neurosurg Psychiatry* 1998;64:619–623.

65. Writing Group. Carotid stenting and angioplasty. *Stroke* 1998;29:336–348.

66. National Health and Medical Research Council Working Party and Contractors. Prevention of stroke: Clinical practice guidelines. Australian Government Publishing Service, Canberra, Commonwealth of Australia, 1997, 67–74.

67. Rothwell PM, Warlow CP. Prediction of effect of carotid endarterectomy for individual patients. The Lancet Conference: The Challenge of Stroke. Montreal, October 15–16, 1998;47 (abstract 57).

EPILOGUE

John W. Norris and Vladimir Hachinski

Despite sporadic attempts at prevention in the past, serious and concerted efforts at disease prevention are largely a phenomenon of the twentieth century. In the last few decades death rates from heart disease have dropped by 51% and from stroke by 60%, mostly because of effective treatment of hypertension.[1] Public health measures have eliminated smallpox, scurvy, and bubonic plague, the scourges of earlier centuries, and polio will disappear by the time this book is published.

Hitherto undreamt of success in treating acute ischemic stroke with expensive technology and hospital services available only in highly developed countries, is now a reality for a tiny fraction of patients worldwide. It will not be available to the underdeveloped world, and so to the majority of the world's population for decades. Even then, the cost will be so prohibitive that few will be able to afford it, and pharmaceutical methods of prevention of stroke such as new antiplatelet drugs will be affordable to only a few in the foreseeable future.

Public health measures to alter lifestyle and behavior in preventing disease, not just stroke, have proven much less expensive and more effective. In an ambitious program in the United States, Healthy People 2000, initiated in 1990, attempts were made to meld local, state and federal health programs into a concerted national strategy of disease prevention.[2] The aim was to increase the healthy life span of Americans, reduce health disparities, and achieve universal access to preventive services. For stroke, the aim was to reduce stroke deaths to 20 per 100,000, from 26.8 in 1991 with risk-reduction strategies using evidence-based data. Some risk factors have been reduced, including hypertension and smoking, but physical inactivity, obesity, and diabetes remain unchanged or have even increased. High cholesterol levels were not understood to be a major risk factor for stroke in 1990, and only in recent years have blood lipids been appreciated as relevant risks in certain subtypes of stroke.[3]

The war on tobacco is a global, not regional or continental problem. The World Health Organisation is working with member states to initiate the first steps in global eradication of tobacco smoking. In the first Framework Convention on Tobacco Control, in October 2000, binding international laws were recommended to regulate the public health threat of smoking and prevent the impending epidemic of tobacco-related disorders for the twenty-first century.[4]

High technology may not be available to the global poor within the foreseeable future, but public health measures aimed at stroke prevention can be more easily implemented, if only at basic levels. Much can be achieved by simple education in healthy living addressed both to the population and health care workers. In 1990, 59% of death and disability among the world's poorest 20% was due to communicable disease. In the world's richest 20%, this figure was only 15%, 85% being due to noncommunicable disease, notably stroke and heart disease.[5]

Lifestyle patterns in the developing world are changing rapidly. As the population becomes more affluent, they can buy cars, afford endless smoking, and stop walking to work. By 1990, noncommunicable diseases had overtaken communicable diseases as a leading cause of world mortality (56%), and it is estimated they will account for 73% by 2020 (Fig. E.1).[5] In addition, as fertility and mortality decrease, the aging population will become even more susceptible to degenerative and circulatory disorders.

Unfortunately, good, well intended advice on healthy living is not always heeded. Evidence-based clinical practice guidelines for preventive health care are not always accepted by patients or their physicians. Recently, the Canadian Task Force on Preventive Health Care recommended that annual physical examinations should be discarded in favour of "selective health protection packages" (such as stroke prevention).[6] Further, it suggested that many accepted screening tests, such as prostate specific antigen levels (PSA) for prostate cancer, and routine chest radiography, be discarded, since they do not influence outcome although they detect the disease earlier. When the responses of physicians and patients to these proposals were sampled, strong resistance was found. Both groups could not be dissuaded that routine annual "check-ups" were not invaluable, particularly laboratory tests, because patients perceive tests as more valuable than clinical examinations. The sampling team concluded that more evidence-based prevention education was needed to overcome this credibility barrier.

Even today, the emphasis in medical education is on recognising and treating disease, rather than preventing it. However, stroke prevention clinics and pro-

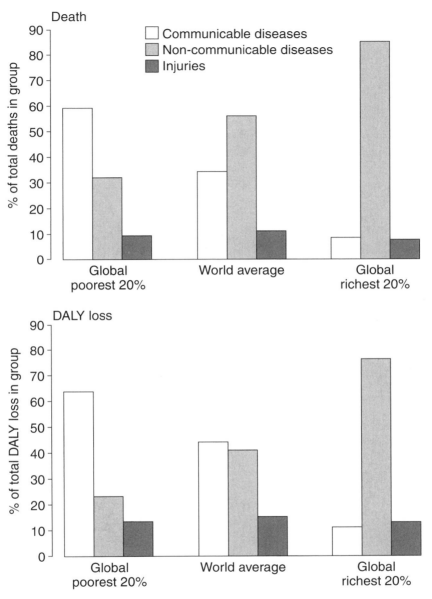

FIGURE E.1. Causes of death and disability, 1990. Reprinted with permission from Ref. 5.

grams are appearing throughout the developed world, mainly for secondary prevention in already symptomatic patients, although asymptomatic patients (such as those with asymptomatic carotid stenosis) also benefit. Still, specialised clinics are the exception, and most individuals with cerebrovascular symptoms rarely obtain advice on lifestyle modifications, diet, smoking, and exercise. If the 10% of the population most at risk of stroke could be identified, it has been estimated that 50% of strokes could be prevented.[7]

The last decade of the twentieth century, the "decade of the brain," witnessed giant strides in the proactive treatment of stroke, mainly because of the growing knowledge of basic mechanisms leading to stroke. Even though thrombolytic therapy is restricted to only a tiny fraction of ischemic stroke patients, and there are substantial risks[8] a seemingly untreatable condition can now be at least, partially reversed. Although many compounds have been tried, no effective neuroprotective drug exists for the acutely ischemic brain.[9]

The potential for replacement of damaged brain using pluripotent human embryonic stem cells can only be surmised at this stage, not just in stroke but also for Alzheimers and Parkinsons diseases. These cells, obtained from aborted fetuses or "spare" early stage human embryos resulting from in-vitro fertilization, raise serious ethical questions, but funding for this research has recently been approved in the United States by governmental agencies. A start has already been made, using human neural cellular transplantation in stroke patients, and although it is premature to announce significant clinical improvement, the technique is clearly feasible.[10]

Parallel with these advances in acute stroke therapy, strategies for stroke prevention are becoming evidence-based. Just as acute stroke units are reducing the morbidity and mortality of stroke as well as costs, so stroke prevention clinics are aimed at reducing complications and recurrent stroke in the survivors. Useful data remain scarce, and, as yet, less than half of stroke patients have obvious risk factors, while the role of some entities, such as plasma homocysteine, remains uncertain.[11] For instance, raised levels of plasma homocysteine associated with atherosclerosis in children have been recognized for years, but this is a rare disorder. The role of this amino acid in adult atherosclerosis has not been established. Another new area for investigation is the emerging role of banal infection from a variety of infectious agents such as Helicobacter and herpes viruses. Chlamydia pneumoniae has been found in the wall of carotid and coronary arteries[12] so that antibiotic treatment to prevent atherosclerosis is an area worth exploring.[13]

Stroke is a global problem that requires a global approach with evidence-based measures. The vast differences in prevalence in different parts of the world demand close study. For example, strategies to overcome sickle-cell disease as a cause of stroke in one location are inappropriate to another, where atherosclerosis is the major cause. With the development of information technology, databases can be linked within countries to produce national, and eventually international, stroke registries. The gap between stroke prevention knowledge and practice and the huge mass of data from epidemiology and clinical trials must be bridged.[14] Using the rapidly expanding database and computerised decision support systems, advances in stroke management and prevention in this new millennium can be made available not to just a privileged few, but to the benefit of the world's population.

REFERENCES

1. Satcher D and Hull FL. The weight of an ounce. *JAMA* 1995;273:1149–1150.
2. McGinnis JM and Lee PR. Healthy People 2000 at mid decade. *JAMA* 1995;273: 1123–1129.
3. Gorelick PB, Schneck M, Berglund LF, et al. Status of lipids as a risk factor for stroke. Neuroepidemiology 1997;16:107–115.
4. Brundtland GH. Achieving world wide tobacco control. *JAMA* 2000;284:750–751.
5. Gwatkin DR, Giuillot M, and Heuveline P. The burden of disease among the global poor. *Lancet* 1999;354:586–589.
6. Beaulieu MD, Hudon E, Roberge D, et al. Practice guidelines for clinical prevention: Do patients, physicians and experts share common ground? *Can Med Ass J* 1999; 161:519–523.
7. Dunbabin DW and Sandercock PAG. Preventing stroke by the modification of risk factors. *Stroke* 1990;21(suppl IV):IV36–IV39.
8. Clark WW, Albers GW, Madden KP and Hamilton S. The rtPA (Alteplase) 0 to 6 hour acute stroke trial. Part A. *Stroke* 2000;31:811–816.
9. Gorelick PB. Neuroprotection in acute ischaemic stroke: a tale of for whom the bell tolls. *Lancet* 2000;355:1925–1926.
10. Kondziolka D, Wechsler L, Goldstein S, et al. Transplantation of cultured human neuronal cells for patients with stroke. *Neurology* 2000;55:565–569.
11. Hankey GJ and Eikelboom JW. Homocysteine and vascular disease. Lancet 1999;354: 407–413.
12. Grayston JT, Kuo CC, Coulson AS, et al. Chlamydia pneumoniae (TWAR) in atherosclerosis of the carotid artery. *Circulation* 1995;92:3397–3400.
13. Gupta S, Leatham EW, Carrington D, et al. Elevated Chlamydia pneumoniae antibodies, cardiovascular events, and azithromycin in male survivors of myocardial infarction. *Circulation* 1997;96:404–407.
14. Goldstein LB. Evidence-based medicine and stroke. *Neuroepidemiology* 1999;18: 120–124.

INDEX